CHOICES

In Health and Fitness for Life

Sally A. Althoff
Portland State University

Milan Svoboda
Portland State University

Daniel A. Girdano
University of Utah

Gorsuch Scarisbrick, Publishers
Scottsdale, Arizona

Dedication

The authors wish to dedicate their efforts to the following people:

Sally,   to my grandmother, to Aunt Sally, and to my parents, all special people who helped me grow

Milan,   to Carol for her faithful love and support, and to my children, Matt, Geoff, and Sarah, for being my children

Dan,   to Joan

Editor: John W. Gorsuch
Consulting Editor: Robert P. Pangrazi
Production Manager: Gay L. Orr
Interior Design: Victoria A. Vandeventer
Cover Design: Ted Wolter
Typesetting: Ash Street Typecrafters, Inc.

Gorsuch Scarisbrick, Publishers
8233 Via Paseo del Norte, Suite F-400
Scottsdale, Arizona 85258

10   9   8   7   6   5   4   3

ISBN 0-89787-608-3

Preface

Being all that you can be is a dynamic, ever-changing process, and this process is directly affected by the personal choices you make every day. Indeed, these choices affect both the quality and quantity of your life. *Choices in Health and Fitness for Life* addresses this dynamic process and is written to serve as a helpful tool in your personal journey.

Your life has many dimensions—physical, emotional, social, intellectual, and spiritual—and research confirms that your choices in the areas of *fitness, nutrition,* and *stress management* can enhance or detract from your ability to function in all of these dimensions. Of course, your choices in these areas can also alter the likelihood of your suffering from the major chronic diseases that affect so many people.

With the extensive and conflicting information available in the marketplace about fitness, nutrition, and stress, it is sometimes difficult to determine what information is correct and what is not. Which guidelines are reliable? Which guidelines are relevant to your life and goals? There are no easy answers to these questions. The best answer is simply to be as informed as you can, so that you can in turn make informed choices and decisions. Our main objective in writing this book is to provide the basic information you need on the topics of fitness, nutrition, and stress management regardless of your age and whether or not you are athletically inclined.

In presenting this information we have assumed that, ideally, you would like to be fit, to eat well, and not be burdened by stress. However, we have tried also to acknowledge that your choices in these areas are personal and practical, affected by many aspects of your life. Thus, a central theme of this book is personal responsibility to explore and expand your potentials via the choices *you* make—choices that are based on your schedule, your goals, your abilities, your budget, and so on.

To help you decide whether changes are in order in your current lifestyle, methods to assess your current fitness status, your nutritional habits, and the level of stress in your life are included as these topics are discussed. Whenever possible, we have attempted to select tests that do not require specialized equipment. To help you develop as fully as you wish, we have described what we think are the best methods and techniques for building and maintaining positive health practices. Again, we have tried to make our recommendations as practical as possible so that, if you prefer, you can do what you choose to do at home without investing large sums of money for special equipment or clothing.

Briefly, Chapter 1 of *Choices in Health and Fitness for Life* introduces the concepts of quality living, health, and wellness and their interdependent nature. Recognizing that it isn't always easy to act in accord with what you know, we have devoted Chapter 2 to examining the pathways and pitfalls involved in self-directed change. This chapter offers step-by-step methods for successfully undertaking such changes. Chapter 3 describes the aging process, the major diseases and the related risk factors that people in our culture most typically encounter, and suggests behaviors that might lessen their impact.

Chapter 4 introduces the components of fitness, the general principles that underlie all forms of training, and common problems encountered in exercise. Chapter 5 provides the rationale for and the methods to develop and maintain cardiorespiratory fitness. Chapter 6 offers procedures for developing and maintaining flexibility, strength, and muscle endurance. The focus of Chapter 7 is on weight control and the role of both diet and regular exercise in this process.

Chapter 8 discusses what is known and what is controversial about nutritional recommendations to maximize health and minimize disease. Chapter 9 provides instructions for analyzing your diet and building a healthy diet for yourself. Chapters 10 and 11 discuss daily stresses you may experience, their impact on your health, and techniques you may use to manage this problem.

Finally, with the worksheets provided in Chapter 12 you will be able to summarize all of your assessments and, if you choose, develop a personal behavior change strategy to follow now or in the future. The information in this book will provide a basis for your choices; the decisions will be yours.

The authors wish to express gratitude to those who served as reviewers of the book as it developed. In particular, we wish to thank Robert C. Barnes of East Carolina University, Robert Slevin of Towson State University, Bob O'Connor of Los Angeles Pierce College, Delores Seemayer of Palm Beach Junior College, Bob Pangrazi of Arizona State University, Dot Dusek of Paradox Professional Seminars and Publishing of Winter Park, Colorado, and Jack Schendel and Margaret Heyden of Portland State University for helpful, critical reviews. As editor, Gay Orr has been extremely helpful and patient throughout the production process. Her contributions have helped to pull our different writing styles together very nicely. Finally, the heroics of Elizabeth Bull in typing countless drafts of the manuscript while still managing the normal chaos at the office is gratefully acknowledged.

Thanks also to Gary R. Brodwicz, Mary Changsut, René Changsut, Steve Curtis, Dori Frame, Gordon Dunkeld, Nancy Gunther, Jennifer Himmelsbach, Eric Ludlow, and Belinda Zeidler for serving as models for the photographs.

Sally Althoff
Milan Svoboda
Dan Girdano

Contents

7   The Weight Control Struggle   173

8

The Daily Dilemma: What's Good to Eat?   201

9

Checking Up on Eating Well   255

12 Your Self: Your Choice 321

Appendices

Index 432

1

Quality Living:
Your Personal Best

What is your definition of quality living?

How important is health to quality living?

Can you experience quality living even when you are seriously ill or when other aspects of your life are less than perfect?

What does *lifestyle* have to do with quality of life?

Introduction

What is "quality living"? According to the dictionary, the combination of these two terms means "excellent or superior existence." This definition presents a problem, however: after all, your concept of "excellent" or "superior" existence may be quite different from that of the person next to you. Think for a moment about the qualities of life that you feel would contribute to "quality living." Would your family or friends come up with the same list? Probably not. With this in mind, "quality living" needs to be defined in such a way that everyone can relate to the concept, and apply it to themselves.

Some common descriptors for quality living have emerged in psychological literature, particularly from the works of Abraham Maslow, Carl Rogers, and Fritz Perls. Maslow refers to quality living as *the process of self-actualization;* Rogers calls it *personal fulfillment;* and Perls refers to a *condition of wholeness and happiness.* Essentially, the living condition each man describes is *being all you can be.* Maslow refers basically to the process of quality living and the others to the feelings and emotions that quality living generates.

The process Maslow called *self-actualization* is that of becoming and being ever more of what you can be, ultimately expressing your full potential (an ideal, of course). In plain terms, this means making your best effort to develop yourself in all aspects of life and then using your talents and capabilities in creative and productive ways. Logically this includes trying to be as healthy as possible, given that the more healthy you become, the more completely you will be able to fulfill your potential.

$$QL = Health \times Effort$$

Quality living, then, is the product of your health and your efforts. In this formula, *health* means how well you are able to function in each aspect of your life, the physical, emotional, social, and so on. *Effort* actually refers to two things: (1) Action—how much you are doing to improve and/or maintain your health; and (2) Emotion—the feelings of fulfillment, wholeness, and happiness that you derive from making the effort to develop yourself and be creative and productive.

Although each of these factors actually influences the other to a certain extent, each also has a direct impact of its own on quality living. How these factors interrelate and what levels of health and effort bring about quality living are the issues addressed in the rest of this chapter.

The Criteria for Quality Living:
The Hierarchy of Needs

From his studies, Maslow found that in order to be your most creative, productive self, certain basic needs—such as the need for food and shelter, for instance—must be satisfied, at least sufficiently well to allow you to focus your attention and energies on your growth and development. This concept, with which you are probably familiar, has become known as *Maslow's Hierarchy of Needs.* As shown in Figure 1.1, it is typically presented in the form of a triangular stepladder to emphasize the dependency

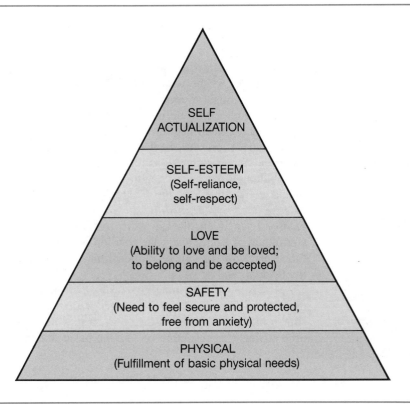

FIGURE 1.1
Maslow's Hierarchy
of Needs.

of the higher, more complex, needs on the fulfillment of the lower level, more basic, needs. In order of the most basic to the most complex, these needs are:

1. Feelings of physical comfort in terms of hunger, sleep, bowel function, sex, and so on, and of energy and well-being in terms of overall health and physiological function.
2. Feelings of safety, security, lack of danger and threat.
3. Feelings of belongingness and acceptance, of being one of a group or having a place; feelings of loving and being loved, of being worthy of love.
4. Feelings of self-reliance, self-respect, and self-esteem.
5. Feelings of self-actualization and fulfillment, of personal growth and development.

Clearly the *foundation* for achieving self-actualization is some basic degree of physical functioning. This is not surprising since life itself depends upon this. In terms of the hierarchy of needs, the more healthy and fit you are physically, the better able you will be to fulfill higher level needs.

Essential as it is, however, physical health by itself is not enough. As the hierarchy of needs indicates, self-actualization requires some degree of satisfactory or healthy functioning in *all* aspects of life—not just the physical. Thus, the emotional, social, intellectual, and spiritual aspects of your life are also important to self-actualization. Indeed, as with physical functioning, the healthier you are in each of these areas, the greater your potential for experiencing quality living.

Health and Quality Living: The Means and the Goal

Health is the term that describes your overall level of functioning at any particular point in time. As the word "time" indicates, health is a dynamic concept, fluctuating even from moment to moment. The range of fluctuation can be illustrated as extending on a continuum from optimal health to death. This *Continuum of Health* is shown in Figure 1.2. Optimal health represents the highest level of function possible. This is an ideal to strive for, but one that is probably never actually achieved. Death, of course, represents the complete loss of function.

Although the word "healthy" is often used to mean only the absence of physical illness or dysfunction, the Continuum of Health clearly shows that the *absence of disease does not mean that you are even average in terms of overall functioning or health*. Even if all disease were eliminated from the world, there would still be a continuum of health and your position on that continuum would be a reflection of how functional you were in *all* dimensions of your life—the physical, emotional, social, intellectual, and spiritual.

To visualize this, imagine that the continuum line representing health is not a two-dimensional line at all, but a cylinder that may be sliced into a series of discs, as shown in Figure 1.3. Each disc may in turn be divided into five pie-shaped segments, each segment representing one of the basic dimensions of life.

$$\text{Health} \ = \ \frac{\text{Effort} \times \text{Other Factors, e.g., Genetics, Disease, etc.}}{\text{Time}}$$

Where you are on the continuum of health, then, is a product of your efforts to develop your level of functioning in each dimension and such factors as genetics, disease, medical expertise, and so on, which can also influence how well you function.

While the formula for health suggests equal weighting of effort and other factors that can affect health, that isn't always the case. It is possible for your level of effort to overcome a factor that usually limits function. For example, you might have lost your legs due to an accident, but you do a marathon anyway, wheelchair division. You're blind, but you learn to ski anyway. It is also possible to exert your best effort and still have your health deteriorate due to uncontrolled disease such as AIDS or advanced-stage cancer.

Time is also an issue in the formula for health. It is possible to have a time lag between effort and its impact on health. For example, beginning to exercise doesn't result in instant fitness, nor does stopping exercise result in instant loss of fitness. In either case, however, you would be one step closer to or farther from your physical best.

Thus far, the examples that have been used to discuss the formula for health have referred mainly to the *physical* dimension of life because most people think of health in primarily physical terms. However, the formula really applies in each dimension of your life, the emotional, social, intellectual, and spiritual as well as the physical.

It is important, then, to know what constitutes healthy functioning in each dimension of life. Knowing this can help you determine what factors may be influencing your health and what efforts you can make to move toward a higher level of overall health and thus, toward a higher quality of living.

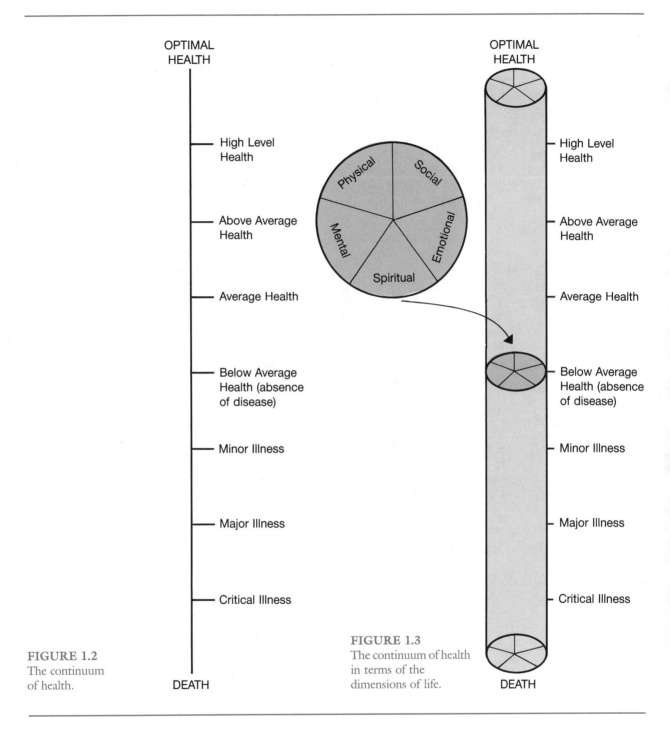

FIGURE 1.2
The continuum
of health.

FIGURE 1.3
The continuum of health
in terms of the
dimensions of life.

Healthy Functioning in Each Dimension of Life

In their recent book, *Health Through Discovery,* Dintiman and Greenberg offer the following definition of healthy function in terms of the five basic dimensions of life:

1. *Physical health:* The ability to carry out daily tasks with energy remaining for unforseen circumstances; biological integrity.
2. *Emotional health:* The ability to control emotions and express them appropriately and comfortably.
3. *Social health:* The ability to interact well with people and the environment; having satisfying interpersonal relationships.
4. *Mental health:* The ability to learn, including intellectual capabilities.
5. *Spiritual health:* The belief in some unifying force such as nature, scientific laws, or a godlike entity.

Factors Affecting Healthy Functioning

As already indicated, how healthy you *really* are in each of these areas depends on many factors. Some of these factors are directly within your control and some aren't. These factors are listed below. Keep in mind while you are reading that although the factors are listed by distinct categories, in reality these categories often overlap and influence one another.

As previously noted, for example, lifestyle choices (your efforts) overlap many, if not most, of the factors to some degree. You can choose to lower your risk of disease by not smoking or by avoiding unsafe sex practices. You may be able to change your physical environment by moving from the city to the country, or improve your medical care by choosing another doctor. While you cannot always prevent disease or accidental injury from occurring, you can choose how you will deal with these or any other factors should they become issues in your life.

1. *Lifestyle Choices:* Many health experts rate lifestyle—the daily choices you make about how you will live your life—as the single most important factor influencing your overall health. Some examples of lifestyle choices that may affect your health:

   a. To exercise or not; how much and how often to exercise
   b. What to eat
   c. How to handle stressors and stress
   d. To seek out or build a supportive environment
   e. To create and/or use opportunities to grow intellectually and spiritually

2. *Genetics:* Genetics determines your ultimate potential in each dimension of life. Manipulating your genetic endowment is not within your direct control, but lifestyle choices help you develop/utilize whatever potential you do have, be it extensive or limited. Some examples of genetic traits that may affect your health positively or negatively:

   a. Hemophilia $(-)$
   b. Extra large lung capacity $(+)$
   c. Above average immune system function $(+)$
   d. Huntington's Disease $(-)$

3. *Accident/Injury:* Accidental injuries may limit your function potential, and their impact is also subject to available medical expertise. Although you cannot always prevent or avoid accidents, the choices you make to protect yourself from these hazards to quality living can reduce the risk of their occurrence in your life. Some examples of injuries that may affect your health:

a. Broken arm

b. Sprained ankle

4. *Disease/Dysfunction:* As with genetics and accidents, you may not be able to avoid these health problems entirely, but your lifestyle choices can actually reduce your chances of disease. By eating well, by exercising, and so on, your risks may be substantially reduced. While a healthy lifestyle cannot assure that you will live free of disease, it can make you better prepared to deal with disease. The "state of the art" of medicine can also be a critical factor in determining the impact of disease on your life. Some examples of diseases/dysfunctions that may affect your health:

a. Physical—Hepatitis, cancer, heart disease, diabetes, AIDS

b. Emotional/Intellectual—Depression, schizophrenia, dyslexia

5. *Medical Expertise:* As mentioned, the state of the art of medicine can be a critical factor in determining the impact of genetic abnormalities, injuries, and diseases. The knowledge level and skill of your personal physician and/or hospital/clinic staff are perhaps the most important of all since these people actually provide the care you receive. While most of the issues in this area are not directly within your control, you can exert some influence by educating yourself and others and by direct action such as voting and working with organized groups on private and government programs for health. Some important examples of how medical issues may affect your health:

a. State of the art medical techniques may/may not be available to you

b. You may/may not be able to afford necessary treatment

c. Government allocations and budget considerations may make certain programs/ treatments accessible or inaccessible

d. Socio-cultural norms can limit access to help via such prejudices as sexism, racism, ageism, and so on

e. Medical solution/cure may simply not be possible/known at this time.

6. *Physical Environment:* The physical environment in which you live and/or work most certainly can affect your health, primarily by increasing your risk of injury and/or disease. Today environmental quality is largely controlled or not controlled by government and politics, business and social policy, not necessarily in that order and not necessarily with human health as the main goal. Economics, politics, and nationalism often take precedence over health concerns. Nonetheless, there are numerous actions you can take every day to lessen your exposure to environmental hazards. Wearing seat belts when driving, avoiding smoke-filled rooms, refusing excessive exposure to X-rays, and not drinking and driving are but a few examples. Some examples of physical environment factors that may affect your health:

a. Overcrowding

b. Air/water pollution

c. Radiation

d. Work hazards

7. *Psycho-Social Environment:* The people in "your world" and the quality of interaction you have with them constitute your psycho-social environment. Most immediately this includes your family and friends, but it also includes workmates and members of your community, state, region, and country. Today everyone is even a member of the world community. The beliefs, values, attitudes, knowledge, and actions of these people can have a significant impact on your opportunities to grow emotionally, intellectually, and spiritually, as well as to be physically safe and well. Of course you don't get to pick the family or the society into which you are born, but you can acknowledge for yourself an "unhealthy" situation and work to establish relationships with people whose values, attitudes and actions encourage you to strive for full function in each dimension of your life. Some examples of psycho-social factors that may affect your health:

a. Exposure to the beliefs, values, and attitudes in your circle of family and friends
b. Peer pressure to smoke, drink, "party" excessively, and so on
c. Being part of a family or group that is physically active and encourages you to be so
d. Social norms and political policies that may support racism, religious biases, and so on

In essence, as shown in Figure 1.4, health is a *means to the goal of self-actualization,* the quality living experience. In plain terms, your health is "what you've got to work with" at any particular point in time. As defined earlier, a healthy level

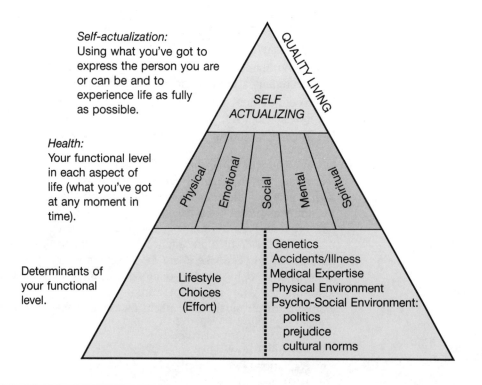

FIGURE 1.4
Health and
self-actualization: The
means and the goal.

of functioning in each aspect of life is basically synonymous with the capabilities Maslow identified in the Hierarchy of Needs as critical to becoming all you can be or moving toward self-actualization.

Of the numerous factors that can influence how healthy you are, your *lifestyle*—that is, your everyday *efforts* to preserve and develop your capacities—is the single most important factor. As indicated earlier, such efforts not only enhance your functioning, but also generate the feelings of a quality living experience: fulfillment, wholeness, and happiness. *Wellness* is the currently popular term for describing a health-promoting lifestyle.

Quality Living: A Wellness Lifestyle

Throughout the previous discussion of quality living and health, *effort* has emerged as a key to quality living. It is critical to all the aspects of quality living—developing healthy functioning in each dimension of life, using your talents and capabilities in creative and productive ways, and experiencing feelings of fulfillment and happiness. Deliberate and consistent efforts to become more and more of what you can be in each dimension of life constitute a wellness lifestyle, the process of self-actualization, a quality living experience. The greater your efforts and the healthier you become, the more "actualized" you will be.

You may be wondering how a physical disability, temporary or permanent, or a decreased level of health affect your capacity to live a wellness lifestyle. It is important to remember that *wellness* refers to the efforts and the choices you make from moment to moment—it does not refer to your *functional status*. In other words, as long as you are striving to develop and expand your potential you can experience a sense of personal fulfillment *regardless of your actual level of health*. Thus, should you find yourself at a low level of health due to inactivity, stress, poor diet, and so on, by beginning to use and develop what capabilities you do have, you can experience increased quality in living as you work to become healthier. In the same way, you can experience quality in living even while struggling against disease/dysfunction. Until the problem condition obliterates the potential for function, it is possible to express and develop the capacity you do have.

In essence, your level of health may not always reflect your level of effort at the moment, but the quality of your living experience will. Full expression of the person you can be may be the ultimate goal in the pursuit of quality living, but becoming what you can be at this moment provides the joy in daily living.

What does it really mean to live a wellness lifestyle? By definition, a wellness lifestyle means striving to develop your abilities in each dimension of life. By doing this, you will be developing the capabilities specified by Maslow's Hierarchy of Needs (Figure 1.1) as being necessary for self-actualization. A wellness lifestyle, then, must include efforts to:

1. Achieve and maintain biological integrity. For example:
   a. becoming physically fit
   b. eating nutritious foods
   c. getting needed rest and relaxation
   d. protecting yourself from physical hazards and injurious agents/substances in the environment

2. Develop self-love and love for others. For example:
   a. acknowledging and expressing feelings and desires constructively
   b. creating a psycho-social environment supportive to your growth and develop-ment
   c. expressing affection and respect for others

3. Interact with other people successfully. For example:
   a. being interested in other people
   b. identifying other people with whom you enjoy talking and doing things
   c. establishing a sense of belonging with other people

4. Develop and apply intellectual capabilities and skills. For example:
   a. expanding your knowledge base
   b. applying your skills to become self-reliant and productive in society

5. Formulate a personal philosophy for living. For example:
   a. examining approaches to life proposed by science, philosophy, and religion
   b. identifying personal beliefs about life
   c. formulating answers for the basic questions "Why am I here?" and "What am I about?"

Adopting a wellness lifestyle doesn't mean suddenly accomplishing all of these goals. It does mean making some effort to grow in each dimension of your life, beginning wherever you need to begin. Your efforts may not be equal in all dimen-sions—it is not unusual for someone to concentrate efforts in one or a few areas. However, a true wellness lifestyle means at least some attention is given to each dimension of your life. The ultimate goal is to balance your efforts, striving to develop as much in one dimension as in another. The more balanced your efforts, the better you will be able to express, experience, and enjoy yourself. The discussion of the *Lifestyle Circle,* below, will help you determine how balanced your efforts are.

The Lifestyle Circle

The *Lifestyle Circle* is designed to allow you to determine whether or not you are living a wellness lifestyle and, if so, how well balanced your efforts are.

By estimating your level of effort in each dimension of life, using the scale of 1-10 provided on the circle, you can create a picture of your lifestyle. For example, if you rate your efforts in all dimensions relatively high—for instance, 7s, 8s, and 9s—your lifestyle circle will be filled out fairly completely and evenly. That is, it will actually look like a large circle, as shown in Figure 1.5a. This "picture" shows a balance of efforts across dimensions.

On the other hand, if you rate your efforts in one dimension as fairly high, but only average in three others and actually low in another, your lifestyle circle will appear lopsided, as shown in Figure 1.5b. This circle reflects effort in each dimension of life, but certainly not a balanced effort.

In essence, the more closely your lifestyle picture approximates a circle and the bigger the circle, the more completely you are becoming the person you can be, given your level of health at the moment. Likewise, the smaller and/or the more lopsided your lifestyle picture, the less you will experience an overall sense of well-being.

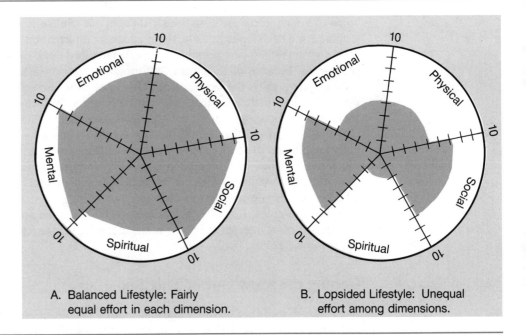

FIGURE 1.5
Wellness lifestyle circles.

A. Balanced Lifestyle: Fairly
   equal effort in each dimension.

B. Lopsided Lifestyle: Unequal
   effort among dimensions.

In Chapter 12 you will have a chance to fill in your own lifestyle circle. For now, consider the different dimensions of your life and take a brief mental inventory of your efforts in each area. How uniform are your efforts to live a wellness lifestyle?

In summary, the concept of quality living presented in this chapter is based on the observations of Maslow, Rogers, and Perls that richness in living is experiencing the thrill of becoming and being all you can be. Becoming as healthy as you can be will provide the knowledge, the skill, the confidence, the fitness and the energy for you to achieve whatever heights are possible for you. In the interim, the process of becoming—the practice and preparation, the hard work and effort it takes to develop your capacities—generates a feeling of quality living all its own. In essence, quality living is not just reaching a goal, it's also *reaching for the goal!*

The Focus and Purpose of This Book

It is probably not within the scope of any book to offer information and guidelines for successfully engaging in efforts in all the dimensions of life. This book provides a starting point for beginning such an effort by focusing on three areas: physical fitness, nutrition, and stress management. These areas make up the *basic building blocks* for health in all aspects of your life.

Choices Influence Quality Living

Making informed choices and taking personal responsibility for your choices in the areas of fitness, nutrition, and stress management are themes that run throughout this book. Almost everything you do involves making choices. If you are like most people, some of your choices are consciously thought out while others may not be. Sometimes a choice or a decision is made without adequate information, and as a result the choice may not be the best one possible. You can probably think of an example in your own past when, because of inadequate information, you made a choice that in hindsight did not prove to be the best choice. This book is written to provide you with basic, up-to-date information so that you will be better able to make informed decisions in the areas of fitness, nutrition, and stress management.

It is recognized that simply having access to this information will not automatically enable you to adopt behavior patterns different from those you have been following for some time, presuming changes seem warranted. Modifying behavior requires more than up-to-date information. Often less tangible factors are at play in determining whether or not you are able to change; your attitudes, goals, fears, and motivations are good examples. Because factors such as these can be so important in determining the success of an attempt at behavior change, suggestions for dealing with these issues are presented in this book.

Getting the Most Out of This Book

Even though there are great similarities among people, individuals are unique biological organisms. This uniqueness demonstrates itself in the ways people are able to integrate fitness, nutrition, and stress management into their lives. For example, one person may have no difficulty maintaining an adequate exercise program while another may find it extremely difficult to find the time or desire to exercise at all. Thus, to get the most out of this book it might be helpful to realize where you are in the behavior change process with respect to any particular issue. This process, shown in Figure 1.6, consists of four basic steps: considering, attempting, achieving, maintaining. Accordingly, as you read the following chapters:

1. If some portion of the information is new to you, consider it with an open mind. Consider what it would mean to act on the information, to incorporate it regularly as a part of your lifestyle. Consider what you would be gaining and what you would be losing.

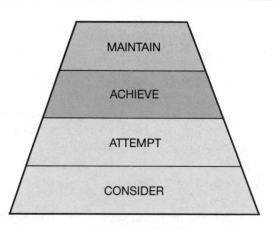

FIGURE 1.6
The process of changing behavior.

2. If you are already familiar with the information but have never attempted to apply it yourself, make an attempt. See what it feels like. Is it something you would find difficult to continue indefinitely? What changes could you make to help it be more to your liking?

3. If the information is something you have attempted to apply in the past but for one reason or another you have been unsuccessful, then spend some time analyzing what it is you need to change to be successful. What was it that caused you to discontinue the new behavior? What type of maintenance schedule would you be comfortable with?

When is the best time to make a change if one is needed? The answer, of course, depends on you and your circumstances. In general, the sooner you make a positive lifestyle change the better because such a change will enable you to operate at a higher quality of living for a greater length of time. Nevertheless, not everyone is willing or able to undertake self-directed change at a specific point in time. Certainly not everyone aspires to the same life goals or to the same health habits. For one person, eating in the most healthful way may be an appropriate goal under all circumstances. For another, it may create too much stress to be preoccupied with good nutrition at all times. Such a person may find it more in keeping with good mental health to be more spontaneous regarding nutrition decisions. All in all, you are the best guide as to whether and when a change is needed in your life. Only you can make that decision; no one can do it for you. Decision making and developing appropriate plans for implementing your goals are also discussed later in this book.

As you read this book you should not try to make every one of the changes you might feel appropriate at the same time. To attempt to do so would be unrealistic, and it is unlikely that any changes you undertook would be maintained. Rather, it is recommended that you take small steps, one at a time. Small steps might be deciding to go for a 15-minute walk twice during the next week, switching to low fat milk from whole milk, or taking 5 minutes during the day to sit quietly and reduce the frenzy in your mind. By taking steps such as these you will slowly and realistically move yourself toward the end of the health continuum (Figure 1.2) described as optimal health.

This book will provide you with the information, the methods and the techniques you need to try one or more small steps toward becoming and being your very best. In fact, just by reading these pages and doing the suggested self assessments, you are taking the first step in the process of behavior change. You are CONSIDERING. If your analysis reveals that *continuing* that behavior change process is what you really need to do, you'll be halfway there: you've started!

References

Ardell, D. 1985. *Fourteen days to a wellness lifestyle*. Mill Valley, CA: Whatever Publisher.

Carlyon, W. 1984. "Disease prevention/health promotion—bridging the gap to wellness. *Health Values: Achieving High Level Wellness* 8 (May/June): 27–30.

Dintiman, G., Greenberg, J. S. 1986. *Health through discovery*, 3rd ed. New York: Random House.

Greenberg, J. 1985. "Health and wellness: a conceptual differentiation." *Health Education* 16 Oct./Nov.: 4–6.

Maslow, A. 1968. *Toward a psychology of being*, 2nd ed. New York: Van Nostrand Reinhold.

Maslow, A. 1970. *Motivation and personality*, 2nd ed. New York: Harper and Row.

Perls, F. 1966. "Gestalt therapy and human potentialities." Chapter 35 in *Explorations in human potentialities*. Herbert Otto, ed. Springfield, IL: Chas. C. Thomas.

Rogers, C. 1968. *On becoming a person*. Boston: Houghton Mifflin.

2

Making Choices About Health

Willpower isn't the key to changing behavior; do you know what is?

Do you know how to motivate yourself to make changes in your life? What steps can you follow to deliberately change your behavior?

What are common pitfalls you may encounter when trying to change behavior, and how can you avoid these pitfalls?

When is the best time to try to make changes in your life?

Introduction

The purpose of this chapter is to describe a process you can use to deliberately change your behavior without relying on willpower and wishes, should you decide that doing so would enhance your quality of living. The basic actions involved in changing yourself in some way are considering, trying, achieving, and maintaining. These actions were shown in order of progression in the staircase drawing in Figure 1.6 in Chapter 1. The smaller size of each successive step represents the number of people who generally reach it. As indicated, many people consider changes in their lives but never quite get to the point of trying them. Of those who do try, many stop before actually achieving their goal, and of those who do reach their goal, many do not maintain their new behavior in the long run.

Why do only some people advance from step to step in the behavior change process? Is it a matter of willpower? If so, what do you do if you just don't have the necessary willpower? Without it, is there some procedure to follow that guarantees success in changing your behavior? Is there some "best time" to try to make changes in your life? To help you take charge of your life and make the changes you wish to make, these questions are addressed in this chapter.

Choosing and Changing Our Behavior

Decide how you want to be
Do what you have to do
Epictetus, Discourses

Making Choices vs. Relying on Willpower

Amazingly, this simple ancient directive provides a succinct summary of what modern researchers have been learning about how people actually do make behavior changes. At this point you may be wondering, "How can something that sounds so easy be so hard?!" Perhaps the reason is that we try to change ourselves without following Epictetus's basic steps: we don't first *decide* how we want to be. Many times we try to change ourselves according to someone else's beliefs and values, without determining if we actually believe in and value that behavior ourselves. Most often we simply *wish* we were like this or that, or hope that someday we will be; but we don't actually *decide* that we will be—that is, we don't take action.

Next, we usually don't analyze ourselves and our behavior sufficiently well, if at all, to *determine* what it is that *we* need to do in order to change. We may try to make total changes overnight when, in fact, we are only ready or able to take one small step toward the change we want to make. Or, we may try to make changes according to someone else's guidelines, which may not be right for us, or indeed may not even be right at all. Witness the plethora of weight loss diets offered to us in magazines and paperbacks, many of which result only in short term loss, malnourishment, and increased body fat!

We may understand Epictetus's directive but this does not mean we know *how* to accomplish the steps he recommends. Many of us who try to change something about ourselves proceed in ways destined to fail, or perhaps manage to succeed without really knowing how we did it. Thus, willpower or the lack of it has become the mystical explanation for success or failure. If you succeed, you are one of the lucky few with enough willpower; if you fail, you just don't have it. If you have ever made a New Year's Resolution or some similar type of self promise to change something about yourself, you probably understand this problem all too well.

The "PRE" Factors vs. Willpower

Fortunately, research has shown that willpower isn't the key to changing behavior after all. Specifically where health is concerned, there appear to be three key categories of factors that determine our behavior: Predisposing factors, Reinforcing factors, and Enabling factors.

Predisposing factors are thought to be the basis for motivation or the predisposition to act one way versus another. These factors include our knowledge, beliefs, attitudes, and values, plus those personal characteristics such as age, sex, race, socioeconomic status and so on, which can influence the extent of our knowledge and what we believe and value. As used here, the term *belief* means a conviction that something is true or real. *Attitude* refers to a relatively constant feeling of positivity or negativity about something or someone. And *value* refers to something that we act to keep or gain. **Reinforcing factors** refer to persons or events who/which support or encourage certain behaviors. **Enabling factors** are our personal skills and resources—that is, what we know how to do and the resources available to help us do what we want to do. Such resources could include money, a swimming pool, a car, a clinic or hospital, a stop-smoking class, and so on.

The PRE factors and how they influence our behavior are illustrated in Figure 2.1. As the arrows in the figure indicate, we tend to choose behaviors that we know about, that we believe to be helpful in some way (or at least not immediately and drastically harmful), and that we enjoy or feel good about (arrow 1). Our choices may, however, be modified and/or limited by the absence or inadequacy of personal skills or "know how," and/or facilities and services necessary to carry out the behavior as we need to (arrow 2). The behaviors we eventually choose impact events and people in our lives in positive, negative, or neutral ways (arrow 3). They, in turn, influence our behavior. Behaviors associated with the desired outcome of events and/or found acceptable by other people, especially other people we care about, will be positively reinforced. We will feel encouraged to repeat such behaviors. On the other hand, behaviors that are not favored by others or that don't produce desired results or good feelings will be negatively reinforced or discouraged (arrows 4 and 5).

This model of how the PRE factors influence behavior provides a way of analyzing why we have succeeded or failed at trying to change ourselves in the past. More importantly, it provides a way to plan successful behavior changes in the future. The prescribed plan involves developing a set of predisposing factors that moves us to behave in the desired way, a set of enabling skills and resources that allows us to perform the desired behavior successfully, and a sufficient number of supporters to reinforce our forward steps and encourage us to keep going forward. In essence, we have to create a new chain of events or PRE factors which leads to the desired behavior.

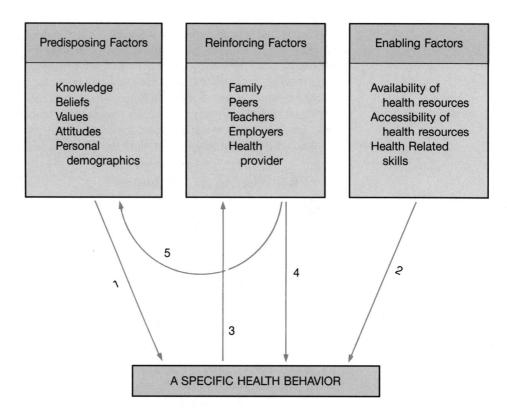

FIGURE 2.1
The "PRE" factors: How they influence health behavior. The numbered lines indicate the direction of influence in usual order of occurrence.

Adapted from Green, L., et al. *Health Education Planning: A Diagnostic Approach* © 1980 by Mayfield Publishing.

A Guide for Planning Successful Behavior Change: The Health Belief Model

Researchers in the area of health-related behavior change have found that we are most likely to succeed in changing our behavior when *we believe* the following to be *true:*

1. That our health is in some way being jeopardized by our current behavior.
2. That we could end up experiencing considerable pain, time lost from work, money problems, family problems, and so on due to our current behavior.
3. That the benefits of a new way of behaving are ultimately achievable and worth the cost in terms of the time, effort, and money we might have to expend to change ourselves.
4. That we can, in fact, do this new behavior and that whatever we need to do it in the way of facilities, equipment, or assistance is within our grasp.
5. That once these beliefs are in place, there is a "cue to action" or precipitating force that makes us feel the need to take action.

Officially known as the *Health Belief Model,* these five conditions provide a basic guideline for constructing the chain of beliefs, attitudes, values, capabilities, and reinforcements that can link us with the way we want to be. Specifically, they suggest that the pathway to change is made up of three segments or steps linked together:

1. Analyzing current and possible alternative behaviors;
2. Deciding that a new way of behaving is desirable and worth working toward; and
3. Identifying and planning for the particular conditions, facilities, equipment, and/ or assistance that seem most likely to promote success, *and* specifying a particular time for getting started.

The Pathways and Pitfalls In Making Behavior Changes

Each of the three sequential segments or steps in *the pathway to change* is presented below. For this discussion, the steps are titled: (1) "Analyze Current Behavior"; (2) "Decide How You Want to Be and Begin an Action Plan"; and (3) "Do What You Have to Do: Individualize Your Action Plan." Suggestions are offered for successfully accomplishing each step. In addition, common "pitfalls" or traps that lead away from successful change are identified for each step. Finally, ways to "get back on track" are discussed.

The first steps in the behavior change process are designed to work on predisposing factors: our knowledge, beliefs, attitudes, and feelings. We need to become aware of our real actions, how we feel about our behavior, and the options open to us. Once we are aware of these factors we can plan how to enable and reinforce ourselves to change.

The Pathway to Change, Step 1: Analyze Current Behavior

The goal of the first step along the pathway to change is to determine the answer to two questions: (1) Is our current behavior jeopardizing our health, and/or our ability to work productively, to support ourselves, and to build rewarding relationships? (2) Is there another way of behaving that would produce results more in line with the quality of living we would like for ourselves? To answer these questions with any degree of accuracy, we will need to gather some information about ourselves—what we actually do and how this affects our lives now and will affect us in the future, should we continue our current behavior. We also need to learn what benefits we might gain if we choose a different way of behaving.

Because we are all busy with so many things each day, the only way to get an accurate picture of any particular behavior we engage in is to keep a written record of it for at least one week and perhaps even two or three, if our lives vary a lot from week to week. We need to record not only when the behavior occurs, but also where, with whom, the positive and negative outcomes, and what thoughts/feelings we experience. A sample behavior record or diary focusing on stress is shown in Figure 2.2.

Not all of this information is necessary just to determine if you are endangering your health and well being. However, if you do decide to change your behavior, the additional information will help to identify the people, places, and times that tend to

FIGURE 2.2
A behavior diary
for stress.

When	What happened	Where	With Whom	Outcomes N = negative P = positive	Thoughts/ Feelings
S L E E P					
5					
6					
7					
8					
9					
10					
11					
Noon	Top priority — Visit with mother Low priority — Stopped to get shoes at repair shop	On the way to Mother's	Alone	N: less Time with mother— She felt bad	I felt bad and sad
1					
2					
3	Late for appointment because left mother's late	At office	With colleague	N: Not enough Time to plan meeting	Embarrassed Annoyed
4					
5					
6					
7					
8					
9					

trigger or reinforce the behavior you are trying to change; the needs that you will have to fulfill in other ways; and the "self talk" (the things you say to yourself about your behavior or your capabilities) that may impede or discourage your attempts to change. Knowledge of these things will allow you to *individualize* the behavior change process to fit your own particular circumstances—or, in the words of Epictetus, to "do what *you* have to do."

Another important aspect of the first step is personal assessment. Is your current behavior providing the degree of health and functional capabilities you want for yourself right now? You will also need to do some "personalized study" to determine the probable long term impact of your behavior. Personalized study means more than just reading; it means actually projecting what you might be like ten, twenty, or thirty years from now, based on your personal assessments and what is currently known about the long term benefits/consequences of various behaviors. This projection should show you whether you are headed up or down the quality living scale. The information and assessment tools/techniques needed to gather this data on a basic level are provided in the remaining chapters of this book.

If more information is needed to firmly substantiate or convince you of the impact of a specific behavior, talking with or reading about people who are enjoying the benefits or suffering the consequences of the behavior may help. The many clubs, self-help groups, and official organizations supporting or fighting almost any form of health behavior or condition will help you locate others who are like you or like you want to be. You can also obtain more in-depth self-assessment data from a thorough physical exam, blood tests, an EKG, blood pressure screening, exercise stress test and so on. These tests generally cost money and require trained personnel as well as additional time. However, if the results of sophisticated tests and consultation with experts will impact your belief system to a greater degree than self-assessments, the money and time will be well spent.

Pitfalls to Change in Step 1:   Minimizing the importance of any or all of the components of this first step may lead to some erroneous conclusions or assumptions about our behavior and ourselves. For example, it's easy to decide not to do the record keeping, the personalized study exercises, and/or the assessments—we assume we already know such information, or that we don't have the necessary time for such things.

In reality, however, we all do much of the information gathering required by Step 1 *automatically,* as we listen to news broadcasts, our friends and families, and read magazines, newspapers, and books. What we usually don't do, however, is make a concerted effort to find out the nitty-gritty facts about recommended behaviors versus what we actually do. Consequently, we are generally aware of behaviors that are supposed to be harmful or helpful to our health, but we don't really know how our own behaviors compare to these and, therefore, what risks or benefits are ours. Rather, we simply assume we are in fairly good shape, or eat a well-balanced diet, or handle stress well enough.

One reason we make these assumptions is that our bodies seem to be working all right, and spending time and effort and perhaps even money to check up on something that works is hard to justify in our busy lives. Ironically, we behave differently when it comes to our cars.* We do take time to watch the gauges and look under the hood even when the car *is* working well. We do spend the money to refuel, change the oil

---

*The authors recognize that not everyone has or cares about a car. However, the points being made in this analogy apply to any machine you use for transportation, be it a motorcycle, bike, balloon, or bus. (You may not own it or care for it, but you want someone to!)

and belts and so on, before the car sputters to a halt. We do these things to assure that the car will get us where we want to go when we want to go. That's the body's job, too, but our cars have some advantages when it comes to eliciting caring behavior from us: they come equipped with gauges and warning lights to tell us how they are running and if something needs our attention. They also come with maintenance schedules and repair manuals to tell us what it is we have to do to keep them operating in top form. If we ignore all of this "enabling" information, the car simply won't run, so we are quickly "reinforced" to take proper care of it.

The body, on the other hand, doesn't have gauges to indicate from moment to moment how much fat is accumulating on our blood vessels, if our fuel mixture is adequate, or how high our blood pressure or muscle tension is. It also doesn't come with a maintenance/repair manual. This manual is still being written, in fact, as we learn bit by bit why the body breaks down and how to prevent it or fix it. So unless we make a special effort to assess the body's functioning level and obtain information about the best way to treat it, we may unknowingly let it deteriorate.

The body may give warning signals when it is starting to "break down," but this is not always the case. Furthermore, because it is more durable and adaptable than our cars, the body can continue to run, although certainly not at full capacity, for a long time even without proper care. Thus, the body actually reinforces lack of attention and sloppy maintenance. Unless we learn from others or through experience what higher quality functioning (living) is like we might ignorantly sputter along through life thinking our bodies are working just fine.

Our cars have one more advantage over our bodies: we know the value of our cars. They cost thousands of dollars. Most of us cannot afford to replace them very often, and we certainly don't want to be without one. So we are "predisposed" or motivated to take good care of them. It's hard to be similarly motivated to take good care of the body, however. We never paid anything for it; it came "free." Furthermore, since we've never been without it, it's hard to realize how valuable the body is even though we know all the money in the world couldn't buy a new one should we need it.

Only when the body breaks down do we get an inkling of its value. In fact, the body is our one vital vehicle in life, providing us with the potential to do what we want and to become what we can. Perhaps this is what Hugh Prather meant when, in his book, *Notes on Love and Courage,* he wrote, "Learning to love [to value] yourself is the definition of change." Taking the time to learn about ourselves, what we are doing and how we can enhance our living experience *is* an act of valuing. One thing is clear—we do spend time, effort, and money on the things we value.

Sometimes it is not the time or money that makes us reluctant to assess our behavior, but rather that we don't really want to confirm our suspicions that we are behaving in harmful or at least unbeneficial ways. If we force ourselves to acknowledge this by recording our behavior, then we might feel guilty or uncomfortable, or feel that we have to give up things we like doing and/or do things we won't like.

If comparing our actual behavior with what we think is right or best for us produces uncomfortable feelings, then something *does* need to be changed—either our behavior or our opinion of it or both. Such emotional discomfort indicates values/attitudes in conflict with each other. It is possible, however, to like or value doing something that we know could shorten our lives or at least reduce our vitality and vigor. Smoking, over-using salt, a regular diet of bacon and eggs or burgers and shakes are just a few examples of this. It is clear now that these behaviors are or can be harmful, but this wasn't always the case. Thus, while we now have new information/options to consider, we may still not be free to choose the healthiest way of behaving.

We may find ourselves trapped in long-term habits or in behavior patterns that we find pleasurable or have always believed to be "okay" or perhaps even value as part of our family or ethnic heritage. In such cases, just knowing that another way of behaving would be more beneficial to our health might not be enough to overcome the influence of these beliefs and attitudes.

If the new information is strong enough, we might be moved to try the new behavior. However, since any new behavior is initially awkward and uncomfortable, we have a tendency to quickly return to old habits. Our habits, whether good or bad, will feel more comfortable and natural than the new behavior. Until we can free ourselves from the reaffirming attitudes, beliefs, and values attached to our current behaviors, trying to change ourselves might be a losing battle. We may even conclude that we lack willpower, or decide we want to remain just as we are.

While deciding we like ourselves as we are is certainly an acceptable possibility, we need to make sure that choice hasn't been made simply because, even though we would like to be different, we don't want to give up the satisfaction or pleasure our current behavior brings. It's important to make this distinction because what many of us fail to realize is that we don't (won't) give up something we like or habitually do unless another way of behaving becomes equally or more attractive. In his book *Toward a Psychology of Being,* renowned psychologist Abraham Maslow made the following observations about how we grow or change:

> *We don't do it because it's good for us . . . or because someone told us to or because it makes us live longer . . . growth [change] takes place when the next step forward is more intrinsically satisfying than the previous gratification with which we have become familiar and even bored . . . .*

To summarize, we don't have to worry about giving up something we like doing, because we probably won't. What we do have to be concerned about is finding a different behavior that provides as much or more satisfaction as the old behavior. Our chances of accomplishing this are best if we gather the information about our current behavior and about alternative ways of behaving, as indicated in Step 1. We will then have personal guidelines for shaping the remaining steps in the behavior change process. These steps deal with learning and coming to value behaviors that are more representative of how we would like to be and of the quality of life we desire.

The Pathway to Change, Step 2: Decide How You Want To Be and Begin an Action Plan

After studying the probable consequences of our current behavior versus other ways of behaving, the next step begins with deciding how we *want* to be. This is not to be confused with a conclusion such as "that's how I am." You may decide not to make changes, of course, but whatever your decision, you must be able to say "I want to be like that." This step requires making a statement of desire: "I want to be a person who exercises regularly and is fit" or "I want to be a smoker" are examples.

Stating such desires doesn't presume that tomorrow or from now on we must be that way, or even that we want to go through the sometimes uncomfortable and awkward process of changing ourselves, if that's required. Such a statement simply identifies what we would like to become and, thus, what we need to start becoming now.

In essence, this is a decision that commits us to action—the action of becoming. Unless we complete this critical step, we probably won't be successful in changing ourselves because we won't do what we have to do.

To ensure that our decision about how we want to be evolves into a commitment to act, we will need to *build an action plan*. Otherwise our decision could easily become just another silent promise to ourselves that gets forgotten in the daily hubbub of our lives, over-ridden by old habits and thoughts. Thus, the first concern in our action plan must be to keep our attention focused on the new way we want to be and the rewards and benefits we hope to gain. We can do this by developing and practicing new ways of thinking about ourselves that affirm and remind us of what we want to become. In his book *Increasing Human Effectiveness*, Bob Moawad calls this positive self-talk "constructive affirmation." He emphasizes that we need to practice this technique two to three times a day for two to three weeks in order to begin displacing the attitudes and beliefs that have supported our old behavior. This might seem rather silly and unnecessary, but just as the body needs some time to "get in shape," the mind needs time to move from such thoughts as "I don't have time to exercise" to "I take time to exercise."

"I take time to exercise" is an example of an affirmative statement that can be used if becoming a regular exerciser is your goal. "I enjoy exercising 15 minutes a day, three to four times a week" is another example. Both of these statements reflect the following guidelines for formulating constructive affirmations:

- Describe what you want to be rather than what you are or don't want to be.
- Use the personal reference, "I."
- Use present tense, not future tense.
- Use "feeling" words such as *enjoy, am proud of,* and so on.
- State specifically what you are doing.
- Use realistic standards such as "regularly" or "consistently" versus "always" or "every day".
- Refer only to your own behavior without making comparisons to other people.

By reviewing the feelings and self-talk you recorded in your behavior diary for Step 1, you can see the attitudes and beliefs—the thinking patterns—that have sustained your old behavior. Using the guidelines just given, you can work on changing these thoughts by substituting constructive affirmations that will encourage you to choose behavior to fit your goals. Thus, to complete Step 2 in a way that keeps you moving forward along the pathway to change, you will need to:

a. Clearly state your goal: how you want to be and why (that is, the rewards and benefits you expect to gain);
b. Make a commitment to that goal by initiating an action plan; and
c. Formulate constructive affirmations and practice them 2–3 times daily as the first component of your action plan.

One way to operationalize this process is to carry with you a 3 × 5 card with your goal and its rewards written on one side and three to four affirmations written on the other side. An example of this action plan reminder card is shown in Figure 2.3. While you are working on affirming how you want to be, you can begin to determine what it is you have to do to change yourself, which is Step 3 in the pathway to behavior change.

GOAL AND REWARD/BENEFITS

```
                    ┌──────────────────────────────────────────┐
                    │                                          │
                    │  GOAL:  Decrease and prioritize the      │
                    │         number of things I do in a day.  │
   3″ × 5″          │                                          │
   CARD             │                                          │
                    │  REWARDS:  Enjoy what I do more.         │
                    │            Feel more relaxed.            │
                    │            Produce higher quality work.  │
                    │            Have more time for people     │
                    │            and relationships.           │
                    │                                          │
                    └──────────────────────────────────────────┘
```

AFFIRMATIVE STATEMENTS

```
                    ┌──────────────────────────────────────────┐
                    │                                          │
                    │  I enjoy planning for people in my day   │
                    │  as well as things.                      │
   FLIP             │                                          │
   SIDE             │  I make time for myself on a regular     │
                    │  basis.                                  │
                    │                                          │
                    │  I budget time to do quality work.       │
                    │                                          │
                    └──────────────────────────────────────────┘
```

FIGURE 2.3
An action plan
reminder card.

Pitfalls to Change in Step 2: Deciding how we want to be but not taking any action usually means we haven't actually decided. Instead, we are *considering* how we might want to be. We are, in fact, still at Step 1. As was indicated in Figure 1.6, many of us remain at this stage, never really committing ourselves to action. Why? And how do we get out of this pit of inaction and back on the pathway to change?

The primary reasons that we seem to get stalled at the considering stage of behavior change are (1) we don't really believe that our health or quality of living are being jeopardized by our current behavior or that we could change ourselves even if we wanted to, and/or (2) we can see that we need to change, but we are simply not motivated. In both of these cases, collecting additional data regarding the consequences of our current behavior and the benefits of changing might be the stimulus we need. Just doing more reading may not be potent enough, however. We may have to deliberately expose ourselves to those who are currently suffering the consequences of potentially damaging behavior or who have changed their behavior and are currently enjoying those benefits. We can find such people through such organizations as Alcoholics

Anonymous, stroke clubs, Overeaters Anonymous, the Cancer Society, the Heart Association, and so on, as well as through teachers, counselors and friends.

We can also do something to get ourselves motivated. According to Art Turock, who specializes in methods for generating motivation to exercise, motivation is "a function of what we choose to focus on." Thus, by focusing our thoughts on how we would like to be and the benefits that would be ours, we may be able to develop the motivation we've been waiting for. Probably the easiest way to do this is to formulate and use the constructive affirmations described earlier—whether or not we feel motivated. What we say to ourselves has a great deal to do with how we behave.

We may have to work on these issues for some time to get ourselves back on the pathway to change. That's okay. No step in the pathway has a time limit. Each step does, however, require action. The key to changing ourselves is to keep acting. We will only succeed if we have tried.

The Pathway to Change, Step 3:
Do What You Have to Do:
Individualize Your Action Plan

To determine what we have to do to successfully change our behavior, we must deal with two key problems. Maslow described these problems in his analysis of how we grow, or make constructive changes, in our lives. He wrote that "the only way we can ever know what is right for us is that it feels better . . . than any alternative." However, he also pointed out that we are "both actuality and potentiality" and that basically we don't (won't) move from safe, secure actuality (how we are now) toward potentiality unless the dangers are minimal and the attractions or rewards clearly evident.

To address these issues we will have to try a new way of behaving for a long enough time to really see if it provides the benefits we want. In addition, we will have to do this in a way that minimizes the stress and discomfort that usually accompany change and maximizes our chances of being successful and feeling positive about what we are doing. The only way we can hope to meet all of these conditions is by carefully preparing and planning for the change we want to make.

There are several ways you can enhance your chances of success when trying a new behavior:

a. *Make sure you know how to work toward your goal step by step, safely and effectively.* Taking a class and reading books and articles written by legitimate experts are ways of doing this. If you injure yourself the first time you try to exercise or find yourself ravenous and depressed after not eating for three days, it is highly unlikely you will want or be able to continue your efforts to change.

b. *Identify a short term goal—some action, no matter how small, that you know you can do to begin working toward your goal.* If becoming a non-smoker is your goal, but quitting completely isn't something you think you can do immediately, then your goal needs to be reduced to something you can do, even if it's only cutting out one cigarette a day. Success breeds success, *and* the confidence that we can change our behavior.

c. *Locate sources of and/or arrange for support and reinforcement.* Designate a support person or group. Any change you try to make, no matter how small, can be stressful. Such discomfort can cause you to abandon your new efforts and return to old habits. Having someone to talk with when you feel distressed or discouraged can make the difference between continuing to try and abandoning the effort.

It is important, however, to select a support person who appreciates the effort you are making and can provide the encouragement and reinforcement you need when you need it. The ideal would be someone who has lived through the experience you are attempting. If no personal acquaintance matches this description, self-help groups and behavior change classes are excellent sources of help.

d. *Stipulate a reward that will be yours for* each day *you achieve your goal.* This must be something you can do or have *only* if you are successful. A sauna or luxurious bath, 30 minutes just to read the paper or an interesting book, watching a television program, a favorite snack, some "play time" with friends are examples of such rewards.

Caution: No matter how tough, determined, or capable you think you are in pursuing your goal, it is important to arrange for reinforcement of your efforts. As noted earlier, reinforcement is one of the major factors in shaping behavior, which is exactly what you are trying to do.

When you have completed these preparations, you can finalize the action plan you began in Step 2 above by accomplishing the tasks discussed below.

▪ *Deciding what you will do and how you will do it is really the key to "doing what you have to do."* Very often the goal we are working toward means eliminating or reducing some behavior, like smoking, drinking, eating cookies, or watching television. The key is to concentrate not on what we must *stop* doing, but on what we will do in its place. Furthermore, if we decide to eat an apple rather than a cookie during our break, how will we manage if no apples are available or if everyone else is having luscious looking brownies? We can, of course, bring an apple with us to solve the availability problem, take a walk instead of going to the snack room at break, interest a friend in eating apples instead of brownies so we have some support, and so on.

There are many possible ways to resolve problems such as these, but not all of them would be right for any one of us. Identify for yourself constructive behaviors that will be consistent with the long term goal you are trying to achieve. It's important to keep in mind that each time we do not engage in our old behavior we will be practicing a new way of being. Replacing one bad habit with another is unlikely to be anyone's goal.

We also have to determine how we will avoid or deal with the social and/or environmental cues or conditions that might trigger our old behavior instead of the new one we are trying to learn. The information you recorded in Step 1 about where and when and with whom your old behavior occurred should provide some guidance in meeting these challenges.

▪ *Deciding when to begin trying a new behavior sounds simple enough.* You simply have to name a date. However, this decision may in actuality be one of the most difficult to make and/or adhere to. "Tomorrow," "soon," or "next week, perhaps" are the dates we prefer. The primary reason for our hesitation is that changing is scary. It is uncertain. It is different. All of this can make us feel uncomfortable enough to decide not to decide when to begin.

We can do several things to minimize our concerns and get ourselves started. First, we can try visualizing our action plan. If we have carefully planned exactly what we will do, we should be able to "see ourselves" doing it. This mental rehearsal can help to alleviate our fears and boost our confidence. If we can't see ourselves behaving as we have planned, then perhaps we need to revise our plan to better reflect what we can do.

Next we need to promise ourselves a review date, at which time we will evaluate how well we've done and how we feel, and alter our plans accordingly. In general, a week or two of trying our new behavior will be long enough for us to determine how we are doing. Knowing that we don't have to suffer interminably if our plan isn't working will let us feel more comfortable about trying it. If we have been able to do what we planned, and we feel confident and comfortable about it, then we can expand our plan. If we have only been partially successful or don't yet feel comfortable with what we are doing, we can work with the same plan or revise it to better reflect what we can do.

Keeping a record of or charting our behavior and our feelings each day is probably the best way to ensure that we have the data we need to evaluate our progress and revise our plan. Since record keeping is also an effective motivation technique, making the effort to do this might just help us succeed.

▪ *Finally, we can help ourselves actually get started on the date we have set by utilizing a motivational device called a "Self Contract."* A sample self contract form is presented in Figure 2.4. Essentially, this is a written promise to ourselves to try the action plan we have developed for a designated period of time. In a way, it is also a public declaration of our intent since our helper or support person must read and sign the contract to confirm his/her participation.

Putting our intentions in writing, telling someone else we're going to do something, and asking someone to do something with us are all good ways to get ourselves going. In fact, asking our support person to help us with what we are trying or to check with us each day to see how we are doing can also be helpful in maintaining our momentum once we do get underway.

Self-contracting is a tool to help you get your plans out of your imagination and into action *now*. It works. You may not need such a device to get you started (or to keep you going), but for many of us such a tool will make the difference between just studying the map and actually taking the trip!

Pitfalls To Change in Step 3:   Preparing and planning for changing ourselves step by step is not something most of us want to nor expect to have to do. We want instant success without too much effort or too much discomfort. We ignore the fact that we may be trying to change behavior we have engaged in for ten to twenty years, which could mean, for example, that we have practiced not exercising between 3,560 and 7,300 times, eating in some particular way between 10,950 and 21,900 times and smoking (one pack per day) between 73,000 and 146,000 times. We may encounter disappointment, then, when we simply expect to eliminate behaviors like these from our lives in one fell swoop.

In essence, we try to do major surgery on our behavior without preparing for the operation by learning the steps involved in the procedure, whether or not we should expect discomfort and for how long, and what kind of help or support we will need to get us over these rough spots. We also don't plan how we are going to live without our old behavior, what we will do in its place, or how we will learn these new

SAMPLE CONTRACT
A CONTRACT WITH MYSELF

I, _____Candy Daley_____, hereby declare that I am ready and willing to commit myself to the following goals and activities. I realize that to achieve my long term goals I must be willing to work for small gains, I must seek support and I must be adequately prepared. Therefore, for the next week I resolve to myself to do the following:

1. Long term goal(s): _____Eat more nutritious foods and less junk_____

2. Specific goal: During the next week, I plan to: _____Have a piece of fruit instead of a candy bar or chips for my afternoon snack when I'm at school on Monday, Tuesday, Wednesday, and Thursday.

3. I will ask my helper to assist me by: _____Meeting me at snack time (before class) and bringing or buying something nutritious to eat with me.

4. I realize I can easily avoid fulfilling my action plan by: _____Forgetting to take a piece of fruit to school. Buying a candy bar instead of some fruit at school "just for today."

5. So I plan to avoid doing this by: _____Putting a reminder note on the refrigerator door and on the notebook I take to school. Meeting my "helper" for snack time someplace away from candy machines and counters.

6. My reward to myself when I fulfill the terms of my action plan each day will be: _____Put 50¢ in kitty each day to use for a snack or movie on the weekend.

TODAY'S DATE: __2/22/87__   SIGNATURE: _____

REVIEW DATE: __3/1/87__   HELPER: _____

7. Action Plan Evaluation/Revision

   a. After working on my action plan for one week, I found that: _____Every day that my helper and I met as planned, I was successful and I saved money and felt pretty good about myself! However, on the day my helper was sick, I bought my usual candy bar. After I ate it, I was sorry I'd done that.

FIGURE 2.4
"Contracting" can help you stick to goals.

(continued)

b. To continue working toward my goal in small steps during the next week, I plan to:

_____✔_____   Follow the same action plan because: _Even though I wasn't totally successful my first try, I do think I can do this. I want to try it one more week. If I don't succeed completely this week, I'll cut my goal back to three days per week instead of four so that I can feel fully successful._

_____   Expand my action plan to include: _____

_____

_____

_____

_____   Cut back on my original plan for now because: _____

_____

_____

_____

behaviors. Consequently, many of our behavioral surgeries just get cancelled or ultimately have to be repeated again and again because the procedure we followed produced only temporary improvement, and our old behavior gradually grew back into place. So once again we fall off the pathway to change and into the pit of inaction, concluding that we lack willpower or are simply not motivated, or that we are what we are and can't change.

The truth is that the pathway to lasting change can only be traveled step by step because it requires learning and practicing, not just eliminating. What we must learn are the thoughts and feelings, skills and support systems that predispose, enable, and reinforce us to change—to become who we want to be. Thus, the way out of the "inaction pit" is to *learn* what *you* have to do to change yourself and to *start* doing those things as best you can. Building an action plan and using self-contracts can help you to succeed in accomplishing these goals.

The best time to change is always *now. Now* gives us the longest time to enjoy the quality of life being the person we want to be. If our current behavior is actually damaging to life itself, *now* may also give us a longer time to live.

If, for some reason, *now* just isn't right for you, the next best time is always *as soon as you possibly can.*

Summary

Now is the time to take possession of my life, to start the impossible journey to the limits of my aspirations, for the first time to step toward my loveliest dream "If I had only known then what I know now"—but now I know enough to begin.
Hugh Prather, Notes on Love & Courage

The primary focus of this chapter has been a process for changing behavior based on personal analysis of current behavior patterns and taking into account the possible alternatives that might better reflect the person you would like to be. Factors known to influence behavior are discussed in terms of how they predispose, reinforce, and enable you to act one way versus another. Important among these factors are your attitudes, beliefs, values; the people around you, especially those you care about; your personal skills; and access to needed resources.

The Health Belief Model offers a guideline for developing the beliefs, attitudes, values, reinforcements, and capabilities that can lead to positive change in your life. This model suggests that the pathway to change consists of three basic steps. These steps and the specific actions involved in each are listed in the following outline; suggestions for accomplishing these steps as well as the potential pitfalls that can lead away from successful change are discussed in the chapter itself.

The Pathway to Change

1. Analyze Current Behavior:
   a. Keep a behavior diary for at least a week.
   b. Assess current physical and/or psycho-social status.
   c. Project probable long term impact of current behavior.
   d. Obtain additional information if needed by reading, talking with others, and in-depth assessments.
2. Decide How You Want to Be and Begin an Action Plan:
   a. Write a first person statement of your goal or how you would like to be.
   b. Begin an action plan by formulating and practicing constructive affirmations.
3. Do What You Have to Do: Individualize Your Action Plan:
   a. Learn how to progress toward your goal step by step and safely.
   b. Identify a short term goal you know you can accomplish.
   c. Locate sources of support—person or group.
   d. Stipulate a reward for each day you achieve your goal.
   e. Finalize your action plan:
      - Decide exactly what you will do and when you will start doing it;
      - Visualize the situation, what you will do, and how you will handle obstacles;
      - Use the self contract to get started; and
      - Evaluate your progress and revise your plan accordingly within one to two weeks.

References

Becker, M. 1974. "The health belief model and personal health behavior." *Health Education Monographs* 2 (4):409-19.

Branden, N. 1983. *Honoring the self.* Los Angeles, CA: Jeremy P. Tarcher, Inc.

Each Day a New Beginning 1982. Center City, MN: The Hazelden Foundation.

Farquhar, J. 1978. *The American way of life need not be hazardous to your health.* New York: W. W. Norton.

Frankel, H. 1983. "Reducing cardiovascular risk by changing your lifestyle." Kaiser-Permanente Health Services Research Center, Portland, OR. Mimeo.

Green, L. et al. 1980. *Health Education Planning: A Diagnostic Approach.* Palo Alto, CA: Mayfield Publishing.

James, J. 1983. *Life is a game of choice.* Seattle, WA: Jennifer James, Inc.

James, J. 1984. *Windows.* Seattle, WA: Jennifer James, Inc.

Maslow, A. 1968. *Toward a Psychology of Being.* New York: Van Nostrand Reinhold.

Melby, C. 1986. "The personal laboratory for health behavior change." *Health Education* 16(January):29-31.

Moawad, B. 1980. *Increasing human effectiveness.* Tempe, AZ: Edge Learning Institute.

Prather, H. 1977. *Notes on love and courage.* New York: Doubleday.

Schuller, R. 1983. *Tough times never last, but tough people do.* New York: Bantam Books.

Schutz, S. 1978. *Yours if you ask.* Boulder, CO: Blue Mountain Press.

Turock, A. 1984. *Getting physical: motivate yourself to stay fit.* Seattle, WA: Excel Fitness Publishing.

3

The Major Hazards to Quality Living: Aging and Chronic Disease

Did you know that almost seven out of ten deaths are due to only two diseases?

Do you know how susceptible you are to these diseases and what factors minimize your risk?

How you age is largely up to you—do you know how to maintain vitality and vigor as you get older?

Why do so many people develop disabling conditions such as diabetes, high blood pressure, arthritis, and so on, as they grow older?

How can you tell if you are developing these problems and what can you do about it?

Introduction

Many things in life can keep you from feeling and doing your best: genetic problems, accidents, the weather, a cold, failing a test, an argument, drugs, and a myriad of other things can all have this effect. But if you ask people to list the things that might decrease quality of life over a span of years, most of the things they identify, over which they have any direct control, will fall into the categories of aging changes or chronic diseases. This is probably not surprising news, but you might be wondering why, in a book about health and fitness, it is important to devote a whole chapter to the things that diminish well-being. If you have ever won or succeeded at anything that required more than a momentary effort, be it winning a game or graduating from college, then you will understand why this chapter is so important. If you are going to win the race or the game or get the job or sell more than your competition, then you need to know what you are up against; that is, you need to know the strengths and weaknesses of your competition. In this case, the competition is disease and aging. You also have to know yourself: in what ways you are strong or vulnerable, and how you can make your strengths formidable and your weaknesses minimal.

This chapter focuses on two of the major opponents to quality living—aging and chronic disease—and how to best defeat them. In the following pages you will find a summary of what is known about aging changes, why they occur and, importantly, what is known about preventing or minimizing them. The diseases that are primarily responsible for ending life prematurely and/or limiting the quality of life are identified and described and ways of reducing your risk of death and disability are discussed. The choices open to you in your quest for health and life will become clear as the chapter unfolds.

The Aging Process

Coming to Terms with Aging

Aging is not a popular word in this society, probably because most people equate the concept of "aging" with the state of being "old." *Old* is not a popular word either since we tend to equate it with inevitable losses. In our culture inevitable losses are doubly offensive: we dislike losing and we dislike not having control over what happens to us! In truth, however, all of these interpretations of the word *aging* are misconceptions. Being "old" is only one part of the aging process, and although ultimately deterioration of function and death do appear to be inevitable, many of the losses associated with aging are not.

Actually, the term *aging* and the phrase *the aging process* means *changes that happen due to the passage of time.* In reality, then, aging occurs from the moment of conception until the moment of death. Since this span of time just happens to be the same time period generally referred to as "living," aging is really synonymous with living. For research purposes, however, the definition of aging has been restricted to post-maturation changes or changes that occur during adulthood. The National Institute on Aging uses age 21 as that demarcation—to the shock of many who didn't know they were among the "geriatric set"! This reference alerts us to two other terms to be defined: *geriatrics* is a medical speciality that focuses on the diseases and physical problems that occur in old age. *Gerontology* is the study of the aging process that spans all adulthood. Compared to such disciplines as chemistry and physics, gerontology is a very young science, and much remains to be learned about how and why people age. The discussion that follows is based on the current literature in this area.

If asked if they want to grow old, most people say no. But the alternative—dying young—is equally unacceptable to most. The confusion here stems from the fact that in actuality most people don't care about age itself. Instead, they care about what happens to them as the years pass by, and basically they don't like what they see. The result is negative feelings about the process of aging. People often say that although they don't want to die young, they don't want to live to be "decrepit and helpless" either. Death, it seems, is basically accepted, although not desirable; but aging is neither acceptable nor desirable. Perhaps this is the way it should be because thus far gerontological research seems to support such feelings: death appears to be inevitable, but many of the losses generally attributed to aging are not.

Research in aging seems to confirm that the human life span is fixed. *Life span* refers to the age at which the average person would die if there were no such thing as disease or accidents. At this time that age is calculated to be about 85 years. However, people have lived to almost 120 years, so estimated *maximum life potential* is somewhere around that figure. The *average life expectancy* you hear so much about is the expected age of death for the average person given current mortality rates from diseases and accidents. Average life expectancy has increased during the 20th century from about 48 years in 1900 to almost 74 years in the 1980s. This figure reflects an average life expectancy for men of about 71 years and for women, about 81 years. Human life span and maximum life potential have not changed during this century, nor, it is thought, for the last 100,000 years. To illustrate this point, human survival curves for this century are shown in Figure 3.1. Consequently, current research efforts are devoted primarily to determining how and why aging occurs so that interventions can be developed that will minimize functional losses and maximize capabilities for as long as possible. Today, the concept of finding the "fountain of youth" refers to achieving high quality living during the time you are alive, and much is being learned about how to do just that.

How We Age

Before discussing how the body's ability to function changes with age, it is important for you to be aware of the limitations of the information that follows. First, as previously noted, gerontological research is a relatively young science; thus, what is known to date should not be considered as the permanent handwriting on the wall of your future, but rather as a possible indicator. Genetic inheritance is known to be a major factor in how you will age, but it is not known how to determine the strength of this for any given individual or body system, or its potency in relation to beneficial or harmful behavior.

In addition, information about aging changes has come primarily from three types of studies: animal studies, human cross-sectional studies, and human longitudinal studies. All of these present limitations when used to draw inferences for individuals. For example, it is not possible to say for sure that what happens to animals with age will happen to humans. Also, variations in life experiences, health care, diets, exercise

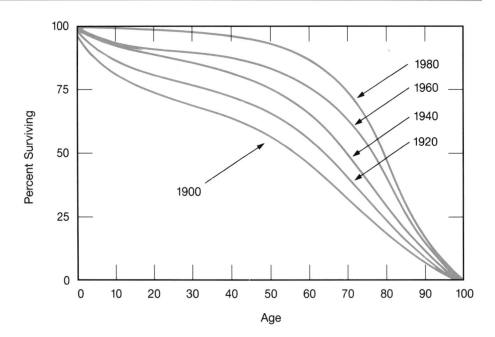

FIGURE 3.1
Human survival curves
for the twentieth century.

From *Vitality and Aging,* by
James F. Fries and Lawrence
M. Crapo. © 1981 by W. H.
Freeman and Company.
Reprinted with permission.

habits, and so on may account for some of the differences that have been found between older and younger people in cross-sectional studies. Last, data available from longitudinal studies (the best research model) spans only some 25 years and largely reflects the aging process in males. Until about 10 years ago, almost all subjects in longitudinal studies were men.

Thus far, research has shown that the basic trend in body functioning is one of decline with the passage of time, with some systems "going" faster than others (see Figure 3.2). A general estimate for the rate of decline in the organs and systems that allow us to do physical work is .75–1% per year after the age of 30. On the other hand, the decline in speed of nerve impulse transmission is only about 10% by age 75. These graphs also emphasize an earlier point that the aging of many functions is already underway by early adulthood.

Probably the most important loss that occurs with age is the loss of cells in muscle, organ, and nerve tissue. Because of this *and* disease, muscle strength and muscle mass tend to decline 25–30% by age 75. Maximum cardiac output (the amount of blood the heart can pump per minute) decreases about 1% per year and respiratory function as indicated by vital capacity (the amount of air you can expel with one "big blow"), declines 40–50% by age 75. The kidney loses about 50% of its nephrons (functional units) between the ages of 30 and 75, and brain weight may decline as much as 1/4 pound.

Again due to the loss of cells, there is a decline in basal metabolic rate (BMR) averaging about 3½% per decade. Basal metabolic rate refers to the number of calories being used just to keep basic body organs functioning, such as the heart, kidneys, and lungs. This small drop in the number of calories needed per day for these functions has been estimated to be no more than 5 calories per day over a 50 year span. This seemingly negligible amount can actually amount to almost a 30 pound weight gain

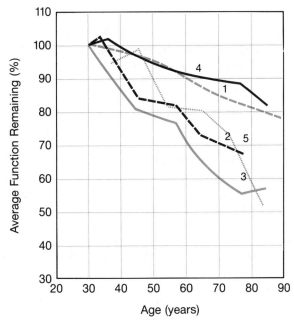

Percentage changes with age for five different physiological functions are shown in this
diagram. The average value for each function
at age 30 is taken as 100 percent. Small drop
in basal metabolism (1) is probably due simply to loss of cells.

1 Basal Metabolic Rate
2 Cardiac Output
   (At Rest)
3 Vital Capacity of Lungs
4 Nerve Conduction
   Velocity
5 Filtration Rate
   of Kidney

FIGURE 3.2
Percentage changes with
age for various body
functions.

From *The Physiology of Aging,*
by Nathan W. Shack. © 1962
by Scientific American, Inc.
All rights reserved.

if calorie intake isn't decreased by the same amount. This is one reason why body
fatness or the percent of body weight that is fat increases with age. Average percent
body fat for males at age 25 is about 15% and for females, 25%. By age 50, this has
increased to almost 28% for males and 44% for females. Even if there were no weight
gain, however, the loss of muscle or fat free tissue, would still create a higher percentage of body fat.

By age 75, bone mass has declined about 10% in males and about 30% in females.
This process begins in the early 30s in women and mid to late 40s in men. When
severe enough, this loss is classified as the disease *osteoporosis*. By age 50, almost
all people show joint wear in the form of osteoarthritis, especially in the weight-bearing
joints, hips, knees, and ankles. Digestion and absorption of some nutrients becomes
less efficient with age, proteins and calcium being examples. The calcium absorption
problem undoubtedly aggravates the bone mass loss, but doesn't fully account for it
by any means. Glucose tolerance declines after the age of 45 and in some people
becomes severe enough to be classified as diabetes. Glucose is the digestive end
product of sugars and starches and the cells' preferred fuel source. Glucose tolerance
refers to the body's ability to move glucose out of the blood into cells at an adequate
rate for efficient functioning.

Hearing begins to decline in the second decade of life, but loss is usually not noticeable until thirty or more years later, if at all. For some reason men experience this loss more prominently than women. Vision changes are generally evident by the early 40s, with loss of near point vision being the most obvious change. The lens of the eye gradually becomes somewhat cloudy, requiring 2/3 more light by age 65 for clear sight. The universality of visual changes is reflected by the fact that almost 95% of people over 65 wear glasses.

With the passage of years, susceptibility to disease increases. Osteoporosis, osteoarthritis, and diabetes have already been mentioned. Heart disease, cancer, stroke, and high blood pressure also increase in incidence with time. These are all *chronic* conditions, which means they tend to take a long time to develop. It is possible that all of these have some relationship to the aging process itself, as indicated with osteoporosis, for example, or diabetes. Abnormalities in functioning of the immune system, the body's basic defense mechanism, also occur with age. Some of these problems are called *autoimmune responses,* which means that antibodies (the cells that normally fight outside invaders like viruses and bacteria) for some reason begin to attack and damage our own tissue—blood vessels, for example. The antibodies may also fail to attack and destroy cells that become abnormal (like cancer cells), as if the system were being suppressed in some way.

These are some of the major ways that body functional capacities change with age. Many more could be listed if space permitted, but perhaps the more important questions at this point are "why do these things happen?" and "what can be done about it?" Numerous theories have been proposed to explain why cells gradually dysfunction and die, but there is no clear answer at this time. There is, however, a growing body of knowledge about how to minimize, and in some cases even prevent, some of the aging changes and disease processes that accompany aging.

Aging: Do We Have Any Choices?

Although death does seem to be the final reality, the quality of life between now and then does appear to be more a matter of choice than many people realize.

As early as ten years ago, experts in the field of aging and exercise began to report that perhaps as much as 50% of the decline in function attributed to aging is actually due to disuse. In fact, current research suggests that by following a program of regular exercise for the heart, other muscle groups, and joints (flexibility), a person 60–70 years of age can have the functional capacities or biological age of someone 20–30 years younger.

As you will read later in this chapter, lack of exercise is a risk factor for cardiovascular disease as well as for several other chronic disabling diseases that can downgrade quality of life. In Figure 3.3, the impact of regular vigorous exercise is compared to the changes that occur with age in critical functional capacities. There can be no question about the difference. In all cases, exercise combats the downward trend in function and the increased susceptibility to disease, especially cardiovascular disease. Chapters 4 and 5 will describe what types of exercise you can do to gain these benefits.

What and how much you eat also seems to have a potent impact on many of the changes attributed to age. The increase in percent body fat and loss of bone mass are but two of these. Perhaps most important is the fact that no cell can function without adequate oxygen and nutrient. If cell death is the major underlying reason for aging, then quality nutrition is certainly critical in thwarting the premature demise of cells.

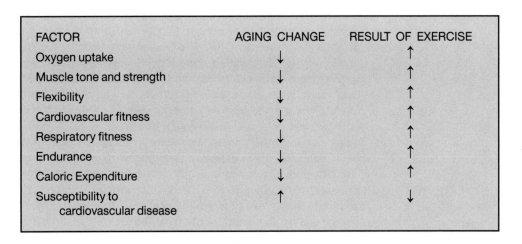

FACTOR	AGING CHANGE	RESULT OF EXERCISE
Oxygen uptake	↓	↑
Muscle tone and strength	↓	↑
Flexibility	↓	↑
Cardiovascular fitness	↓	↑
Respiratory fitness	↓	↑
Endurance	↓	↑
Caloric Expenditure	↓	↑
Susceptibility to cardiovascular disease	↑	↓

FIGURE 3.3
Changes due to aging vs. the benefits of exercise.

Dietary practices also greatly impact the capability of the cardiovascular system to deliver oxygen and nutrients to cells. In fact, a high fat level in the blood, especially cholesterol, is one of the most potent risk factors for cardiovascular disease. The nutritional choices that can minimize aging changes and susceptibility to disease will be discussed in Chapters 8 and 9.

Lastly, although not so clearly as with exercise and nutrition, the amount of stress you experience seems to influence age-related changes. In animal studies, high stress produces acceleration of aging changes, perhaps by causing disturbances in the immune system. The importance of dysfunction in the immune system is sufficient to have been proposed as a major theory for why aging occurs. Susceptibility to disease also increases during periods of high stress and/or prolonged stress. Especially prominent and serious is the association of chronic stress with cardiovascular disease. Thus, stress management is another tool available for use in minimizing aging changes. Information about stress and stress management techniques is presented in Chapters 10 and 11.

It does seem possible, at least to a point, to avoid one of humankind's oldest laments—having the wisdom and maturity that comes with age, but not the health and vigor to enjoy it. Making the right choices day by day seems to be the best way of achieving this.

Chronic Diseases

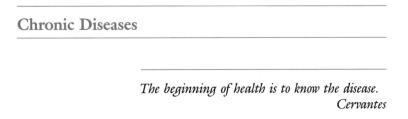

The beginning of health is to know the disease.
Cervantes

If the human life span is as high as 85 to 120 years, as gerontological studies seem to indicate, then why with all the advancements in modern medicine is average life expectancy less than this? What is killing people prematurely, and is there anything that can be done about it? Since the discovery of antibiotics in the early 1940s, infectious diseases have almost disappeared from the list of major causes of death and disability in America. Chronic diseases have become the major hazards to our health and longevity. They can't be cured by pills and injections like most infectious deseases; in fact, there are no cures for them at present. Chronic diseases develop slowly, often over many years; once their symptoms appear, they generally become life-long problems. Currently the best way to eliminate or minimize their impact on life and health is to prevent or curtail their development. How to do this is not fully clear yet, but many so-called risk factors that seem to increase susceptibility to these diseases have been identified. Eliminating or avoiding as many of these risk factors as possible and strengthening functional capacity is the best prescription available today for chronic diseases. No medicine does all of this; instead, the prescription relies on individual action. In the following pages the behaviors that seem critical to protecting and preserving the quality and length of life from the ravages of chronic disease will be identified.

Leading Causes of Death: Cardiovascular Disease and Cancer

A quick glance at Table 3.A, listing the top 10 causes of death in 1985, reveals that heart disease and cancer are by far the major killers, accounting for almost 60% of all deaths in the United States. Of these two, heart disease stands out as our number one killer, exceeding cancer by more than 1½ times. Two other entries among the 10 leading causes of death are blood vessel diseases: stroke, and atherosclerosis, the most common form of hardening of the arteries. These two diseases accounted for 8.4% of all deaths. Thus, heart and blood vessel disease, commonly referred to as cardiovascular disease, together caused 45.6% of all deaths in 1985. That's almost one-half of all deaths and in numerical terms, that's almost one million. A little-known but important fact about these one million deaths from cardiovascular disease (CVD) is that almost one-fifth, or about 200,000 deaths, occurred at ages under 65! In comparison, cancer causes approximately 22% of all deaths, or about 472,000. This number is certainly significant, and far exceeds other individual causes of death, but it stands a distant

Table 3.A   Leading causes of death in the United States, 1985.

ORDER		% OF ALL DEATHS
1	Heart Diseases	37.2
2	Cancers	22.0
3	Stroke	7.3
4	All Accidents	4.4
5	Chronic Obstructive Pulmonary Diseases	3.6
6	Pneumonia and Influenza	3.2
7	Diabetes Mellitus	1.9
8	Suicide	1.4
9	Chronic Liver Diseases and Cirrhosis	1.3
10	Atherosclerosis	1.1

Data from National Center for Health Statistics, *Monthly Vital Statistics Report,* Sept. 19, 1986.

second to CVD in prematurely shortening life. It is important to note here, however, that between the ages of 1 and 44—that is, during the first half of life—cancer exceeds heart disease on the list of the leading five causes of death. The *five* leading causes of death for various age groups are given in Table 3.B. Clearly, both CVD and cancer present major hazards to our quality of life and longevity.

The potency of different forms of CVD in causing death is identified in Figure 3.4. In the category of heart disease, meaning disorders of the heart and its blood vessels, heart attack is by far the biggest enemy causing 55.3% of all the deaths due to CVD. In second place, but far behind heart attack statistically, is stroke or cerebrovascular disease. This is a blood vessel disorder that results in insufficient blood being available to the brain and subsequent dysfunction of those body parts controlled by the affected area of the brain. Stroke accounts for about 16% of all deaths due to cardiovascular disease.

Although heart attack and stroke are most noteworthy as causes of death and are considered in that context in this discussion, they also fit into the category of major disablers. About 1½ million people have heart attacks each year and about 953,000 survive. The approximate number of heart attack victims still living to date is more than 4½ million. Likewise, of the approximately 500,000 people who have strokes every year, 344,000 survive. There are nearly 2 million survivors of stroke living today. Although some of these survivors do regain their former quality of life, many are left disabled and faced with the task of redefining the term "quality."

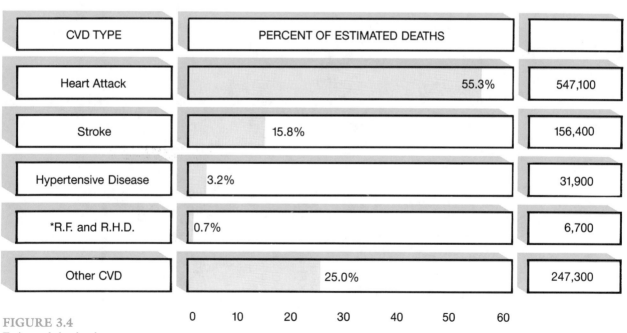

FIGURE 3.4
Estimated deaths due to
cardiovascular diseases
by major type of disorder
(United States, 1983).

*Rheumatic Fever and Rheumatic Heart Disease

From *Heart Facts and Figures, 1986*. American Heart Association, Dallas, TX. Reproduced with permission.

Table 3.B Leading causes of death in the United States by age group, 1985.

AGE GROUP (YRS)	1–14	15–24	25–34	35–44	45–54	55–64	65–74	75–84	85+
Rank Order Cause of Death									
1	Accidents (15.1)	Accidents (48.1)	Accidents (35.2)	Cancer (46.0)	Cancer (165.4)	Cancer (448.2)	Heart Disease (1087.4)	Heart Disease (2727.0)	Heart Disease (7333.6)
2	Cancer (3.8)	Suicide (12.0)	Suicide (15.9)	Heart Disease (40.2)	Heart Disease (155.5)	Heart Disease (437.4)	Cancer (837.8)	Cancer (1272.7)	Cancer (1569.4)
3	Congenital Anomalies (2.6)	Homicide (11.5)	Homicide (14.3)	Accidents (32.0)	Accidents (31.2)	Stroke (55.3)	Stroke (171.7)	Stroke (592.4)	Stroke (1849.8)
4	Homicide (1.5)	Cancer (4.8)	Cancer (12.7)	Suicide (13.6)	Stroke (21.8)	Accidents (36.5)	Chronic Obstructive Lung Disease (142.5)	Chronic Obstructive Lung Disease (292.0)	Flu & Pneumonia (1018.1)
5	Heart Disease (1.3)	Heart Disease (2.5)	Heart Disease (8.0)	Homicide (11.0)	Chronic Liver Disease & Cirrhosis (21.7)	Chronic Obstructive Lung Disease (48.3)	Diabetes (63.7)	Flu & Pneumonia (235.9)	Atherosclerosis (460.1)

Note: Numbers in parenthesis indicate the Age-Specific Death Rate per 100,000 population based on 10% sample of deaths.

Monthly Vital Statistics Report, Vol. 34, #13. DHHS Pub #86-1120, PHS, Sept. 19, 1986

Hypertensive disease, better known as high blood pressure, is responsible for 3.2% of deaths due to cardiovascular disease. This is far fewer deaths than caused by heart disease and stroke, but high blood pressure far exceeds heart disease and stroke combined when you consider the number of people who are living with this problem. Almost 55 million adults have high blood pressure; the combined number of living victims of stroke and heart disease is just over 6½ million. For this reason, high blood pressure is considered more of a disabler than major cause of death. Nonetheless, high blood pressure is one of the leading causes of heart disease and stroke and thus should certainly command attention as a threat to life and to quality living. Because of the tremendous impact cardiovascular disease has on the length and quality of life today, a more detailed discussion of the forms and development of these diseases is provided later in this chapter.

Like cardiovascular disease, cancer is not just one disease. It is a large number of diseases characterized by the development, uncontrolled growth, and spread (often referred to as *metastasis*) of abnormal cells. If this growth is not checked, eventually these abnormal cells literally "hog" so much of the nutrient and oxygen supply that normal cells can no longer survive and death ultimately occurs.

The percent of cancer deaths in 1985 from each of its various forms is shown in Figure 3.5. By far the most prominent killer is lung cancer, taking an estimated 130,000 lives per year. Almost 70% of these victims are men, although the number of women dying from lung cancer has been increasing steadily over the years. In 1985, for the first time ever, lung cancer became the number one cancer killer of women, just as it is for men. The large number of male smokers and the increasing number of

FIGURE 3.5
Cancer deaths by site and sex, 1985 estimates.

Cancer Facts and Figures, 1986. American Cancer Society.

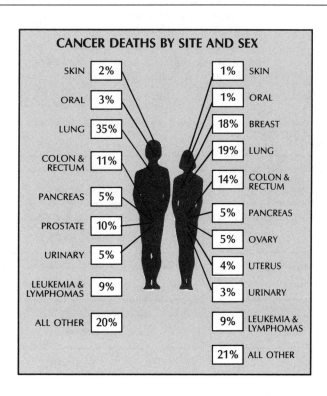

CANCER DEATHS BY SITE AND SEX

	Men		Women	
SKIN	2%		1%	SKIN
ORAL	3%		1%	ORAL
			18%	BREAST
LUNG	35%		19%	LUNG
COLON & RECTUM	11%		14%	COLON & RECTUM
PANCREAS	5%		5%	PANCREAS
PROSTATE	10%		5%	OVARY
URINARY	5%		4%	UTERUS
			3%	URINARY
LEUKEMIA & LYMPHOMAS	9%		9%	LEUKEMIA & LYMPHOMAS
ALL OTHER	20%		21%	ALL OTHER

women smokers explain the prominence of this killer and the death rates by sex. Cancer of the colon and/or rectum, called colorectal cancer, is the second biggest killer overall, causing almost 60,000 deaths per year. Colon cancer is responsible for the large majority of these deaths. For women, however, annual deaths due to colorectal cancer (almost 31,000) are the *third* largest killer; breast cancer holds second place for women, taking about 40,000 lives each year. For men colorectal cancer is the second biggest killer, causing about 29,000 deaths per year. Cancer of the prostate gland ranks third for men, causing some 26,000 deaths per year.

Although cancer is most noted as a cause of death, it also disables. Not all who develop cancer die. Today about 4 out of 10 people who get cancer will be alive five years after diagnosis. Fifty years ago this rate was only 1 out of 5. Currently, there are over 5 million Americans living who have a history of cancer; 3 million of these were diagnosed 5 or more years ago and are considered "cured." The remainder still have some evidence of cancer. Thus, it is appropriate that cancer has also earned the label of *major disabling disease*.

Why is it that so many people develop and die from heart attack, stroke, and cancer? How do some manage to escape these fates? The answers to these questions are not yet clear, but we do know that there are certain diseases, personal habits, and characteristics that singly or in combination increase the risk of developing and/or dying from these diseases. Fortunately, some of these risk factors, as they are called, can be reduced or eliminated by individual decision; unfortunately, others cannot.

The risk factors for cardiovascular disease are shown in Figure 3.6. Of the eleven risk factors, only four—heredity, sex, race, and age—cannot be modified. Those that can be eliminated or at least modified are smoking, high blood pressure, blood fat levels (cholesterol in particular), diabetes, obesity, lack of exercise, and stress. These risk factors will be discussed in greater detail in the special section on cardiovascular disease later in this chapter.

The major risk factors for cancer are given in Table 3.C; not all apply to every form of cancer. The non-modifiable risk factors are heredity, sex, race, and age.

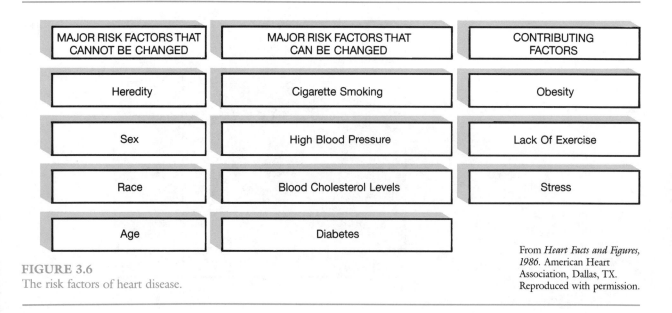

MAJOR RISK FACTORS THAT CANNOT BE CHANGED	MAJOR RISK FACTORS THAT CAN BE CHANGED	CONTRIBUTING FACTORS
Heredity	Cigarette Smoking	Obesity
Sex	High Blood Pressure	Lack Of Exercise
Race	Blood Cholesterol Levels	Stress
Age	Diabetes	

FIGURE 3.6
The risk factors of heart disease.

From *Heart Facts and Figures, 1986.* American Heart Association, Dallas, TX. Reproduced with permission.

Table 3.C   The major risk factors for various types of cancer.

NON-MODIFIABLE	MODIFIABLE	
Heredity Age Sex Race	Occupation	— Exposure to industrial agents such as nickel, chromate, asbestos, vinyl chloride, pesticides, and so on.
	Diet	— High intake of alcohol, fat, and foods cured with salt, smoke, or nitrate; low intake of fiber and foods rich in Vitamin A & C.
	Smoking	
	Radiation	— High exposure
	Sunlight	— High exposure
	Obesity	
	Stress	

From *Cancer Facts and Figures, 1986*. American Cancer Society, New York, NY.

Modifiable risk factors include occupational exposure to various industrial agents, diet, smoking, radiation, sunlight. There is growing evidence that high levels of stress may also increase the risk of developing cancer via depression of the immune system; however, some experts feel more data is needed to firmly establish this relationship. Notably, several of the risk factors for cancer are the same as those for heart disease. Thus, doing what you can to minimize your risk of heart disease may also help to reduce your risk of cancer, or vice versa.

Major Causes of Disability

Chronic diseases not only end life prematurely, they also interfere with the quality of life, causing millions to suffer pain and disability. Most prominent as causes of disability in America are high blood pressure, diabetes, osteoporosis, arthritis, and low back pain. A brief explanation of each of these conditions is provided in this section, and those factors known to influence susceptibility in each case are discussed.

High Blood Pressure

Blood pressure is simply the force exerted by the blood against blood vessel walls. On each beat, blood is ejected from the heart and the pressure rises. The level to which it rises is called *systolic pressure*. Between beats the pressure drops slightly and is called *diastolic pressure*. An air pressure cuff called a *sphygmomanometer* is generally used to measure these pressures. The units of measure are millimeters of mercury (mmHg).

Systolic pressure normally ranges between 110–140 mmHg and diastolic between 70–90, with the standard norm usually given as 120/80. Blood pressure readings below these ranges are generally not harmful unless dizziness or fainting occurs, which would indicate that the blood pressure is so low that blood cannot be pushed upward to the brain in adequate amounts. In such a case, medical treatment would be needed.

However, if you have lower than normal blood pressure but do not experience these problems, you shouldn't be worried. It simply means your heart doesn't have to work so hard to circulate an adequate supply of blood for you.

When the arteries that carry the blood from the heart to the cells become narrowed by fatty deposits on the vessel walls or lose their ability to expand to accommodate the blood being pumped by the heart, blood cannot easily flow through them. The heart must then pump more forcefully to push the blood through the arteries and this creates higher pressure against the blood vessel walls and within the heart itself. If this situation elevates your blood pressure above 140/90 and is the norm for you rather than an occasional occurrence, you have high blood pressure. One elevated blood pressure reading is insufficient to make this judgment; two or more elevated readings over a period of at least three days are needed before a diagnosis of high blood pressure is made.

The danger high blood pressure creates for the heart and blood vessels can be quickly visualized by recalling the effect of water rushing against stone, such as at a waterfall. Over time, the water actually wears grooves in the stone; if the flow is fast enough and hard enough it may even cut through the rock, breaking it apart. Huge sections of such broken-off rock lie at the bottom of Niagara Falls, for example. Constant high blood pressure likewise wears away at the walls of blood vessels and of the heart. Such tissue injury may become the site of fatty deposits and/or become a weak spot that balloons out and eventually bursts, causing a hemorrhage. *Aneurysm* is the term used to describe a section of blood vessel that has bulged or ballooned outward. This extremely dangerous condition is illustrated on p. 56, along with several other vascular conditions described later in this discussion.

In addition to the wearing or eroding effect, high blood pressure causes the heart, which is a muscle, to become enlarged just as any muscle does when it's subjected to higher than normal work loads. A slightly enlarged heart may be able to do its work quite well, but one that grows very much enlarged becomes over-extended and has difficulty meeting the demands of pumping blood against high pressure.

Why does high blood pressure occur? The answer isn't clear yet. In fact, 90% of the cases of high blood pressure are called "essential hypertension," meaning cause unknown. The other 10% of cases can be attributed to some other underlying disease such as a kidney abnormality. Whatever the cause(s), it is clear that many Americans are exposed to them; about one in five Americans has high blood pressure. For black people, the frequency is even greater: one in every three. Thus, race is one of the risk factors for high blood pressure. Increasing age, overweight, lack of regular exercise, stress, and heredity are also risk factors. Eating too much salt may also increase blood pressure, but this does not seem to be the case for all people. Most recently, inadequate intake of calcium has become the focus of attention as a possible precipitator of high blood pressure.

It is estimated that about one-half of the people who have high blood pressure don't know it. The disease is often symptomless, although it can produce frequent headaches and feelings of fatigue. Unfortunately, high blood pressure will do its damage whether or not you have symptoms. Fortunately, having your blood pressure checked is a quick and painless process, frequently offered free of charge at health fairs, shopping centers, public health clinics, and so on. Once discovered, almost all cases of high blood pressure can be controlled; that is, normal blood pressure levels can be attained through diet, exercise, and weight loss measures, or via medications. These measures must generally be continued for the remainder of one's life if normal pressure is to be maintained.

Diabetes

Like cardiovascular disease and cancer, diabetes has several forms. Type I or insulin dependent diabetes generally affects children and young adults. These people are unable to produce needed amounts of a hormone called insulin. Type II or non-insulin dependent diabetes usually occurs in adults older than 40. Type II diabetics can generally produce insulin, but the body cannot use it effectively. The most predominant form of diabetes is Type II or adult-onset diabetes; it accounts for approximately 90% of the diabetic population.

Type I diabetes appears suddenly and acutely, but Type II develops gradually and may go undetected for a long time. Thus, while an estimated 6 million people are known to have diabetes, it is thought than an additional 5 million have it and do not know it. Combined, these estimates indicate that diabetes affects about 1 out of 20 Americans.

Diabetes is called a *metabolic* disease because it affects the way the body uses or metabolizes glucose, the digestive end product of foods containing sugars and starches (pasta, potatoes, rice, cereals, etc.). If not enough insulin is available to help move the glucose into cells, it accumulates in the blood. Then despite the best efforts of the kidney, whose job it is to make sure that only waste, not nutrients, passes out of the body in urine, the high blood sugar levels may overwhelm it and sugar will end up in the urine. Elevated blood sugar and sugar in the urine are prominent indicators of diabetes. At this point, a second means by which cells can obtain energy begins to operate at an accelerated rate: the body begins to utilize large amounts of fat, a process that produces acids called *ketones*. These acids also begin to accumulate in the blood and urine. If this process continues long enough without intervention, the diabetic will lose consciousness and die because the blood has become acidic beyond the body's tolerance.

Diabetes is a serious disease in and of itself, causing 38,000 deaths annually. You may recall that it ranked seventh in leading causes of death in Table 3.A. But when the classification used is "diabetes and its complications," it becomes the third leading cause of death, accounting for some 300,000 lost lives. However, diabetes is considered as a major disabler in this text rather than as a major killer because these complications are most frequently cardiovascular in nature. In fact, diabetics are twice as likely to have heart attacks and stroke and 50 to 100 times as likely to have problems with peripheral vascular disease (disease of blood vessels other than in the heart and brain), which sometimes causes gangrene. Because of this, diabetes accounts for one-half of all the foot and leg amputations performed annually. The high blood fat levels that occur because of the faulty glucose metabolism are one of the primary reasons for the severe cardiovascular complications. In addition to all of this, diabetes is the leading cause of new cases of blindness between the ages of 20 and 74. It also markedly increases the risk of kidney disease and the frequency of birth defects.

Diabetes is obviously a disease worth avoiding when possible, or detecting and controlling otherwise. Avoiding Type I diabetes is difficult because the cause(s) is/are not known. Detection is not difficult because the symptoms are rather severe; they include frequent urination, excessive thirst, extreme hunger, dramatic weight loss, weakness, and nausea. Controlling Type I diabetes requires daily insulin and careful attention to diet and exercise.

Avoiding Type II diabetes may be possible by controlling weight. An estimated 80-90% of people diagnosed with Type II diabetes are overweight at the time of diagnosis and the risk of developing the disease doubles with every 20% of excess weight. Excess fat seems to prevent insulin from working properly. Weight control becomes even more important as an avoidance mechanism since none of the other risk factors for Type II diabetes are modifiable. These factors include having diabetic relatives (heredity), being female, being Black or Hispanic or Native American, and being over 40 years of age.

Symptoms of Type II diabetes can include any of those listed for Type I plus recurrent or hard to heal skin sores; gum or bladder infections; drowsiness; blurred vision; itching; and tingling or numbness in hands or feet. However, these symptoms tend to occur gradually and may be ignored or not recognized as potentially serious. Controlling Type II diabetes may require insulin, but very frequently weight loss and control combined with a careful diet and regular exercise is sufficient. Simple as they sound, these measures generally require numerous changes in long term habits, which may be difficult.

The symptoms or warning signs of Type I and Type II diabetes are listed in Table 3.D. You may want to assess yourself now and keep them in mind in the future. Undetected diabetes can change the quality and quantity of the life you live.

Osteoporosis

In 1965, the estimated incidence of osteoporosis was between 12 and 14 million people, about the same as for diabetes. And yet few people were familiar with the term *osteoporosis,* much less the disease process, though they may have known that old people had brittle bones that were easily broken or bent, sometimes resulting in a "dowager's hump back." Even most doctors accepted this process as an inevitable part of aging.

Today the situation is quite different. The estimated incidence of the disease has increased to about 20 million as the older population has grown in number. As a result, osteoporosis is in the news, on TV, and on people's minds, especially women's minds. Four times as many women suffer from osteoporosis as men, so this fear is a well-founded one. However, men should certainly be aware that osteoporosis is not just a women's disease.

Table 3.D Warning signs for Type I and Type II diabetes.

The following symptoms are typical. However, some people with Type II diabetes have symptoms so mild that they go unnoticed.

TYPE I (usually occur suddenly)	TYPE II (usually occur less suddenly)
frequent urination	any of the Type I symptoms
excessive thirst	recurring or hard-to-heal skin, gum, or bladder infections
extreme hunger	
dramatic weight loss	drowsiness
irritability	blurred vision
weakness and fatigue	tingling or numbness in hands or feet
nausea and vomiting	itching

From *Diabetes Facts and Figures, 1986.* American Diabetes Association, Alexandria, VA.

The term *osteoporosis* describes the outcome of the disease—porous empty-looking bone—rather precisely. These results seem to be caused by an imbalance between the rate of bone resorption and bone building. Most people are not aware that bone is a dynamic tissue; it is constantly being *restructured*—that is, being broken down and reformed. At some time around the age of 35 for women and in the mid to late 40s for men, the bone rebuilding process begins to fall behind the rate of bone resorption; as a result, bone density and mass start declining. Not only do women begin to experience this loss at an earlier age than men, their rate of loss is also greater. The consequence of this is compounded by the fact that the peak bone mass for women is also much less than for men.

The form of osteoporosis just described is called *senile* (meaning "old age") *osteoporosis* or Type I osteoporosis. It affects both men and women and typically results in hip fractures. As you might expect from the above description of the disease, women experience twice the rate of hip fractures than do men. Broken bones are not the only problem osteoporosis presents however. In older persons, hip fractures are often the precipitating event to an overall decline in health that may even result in death.

Type II osteoporosis or *post-menopausal osteoporosis* affects women only and is due to the loss of estrogen following menopause. Besides being a sex hormone, estrogen also supports bone growth. Type II osteoporosis affects primarily the spine, causing disintegration of the vertebrae and the classic stooped posture called the "dowager's hump." The rate of bone loss following menopause becomes quite accelerated for 10–15 years and is then thought to slow considerably. Nevertheless, by then the resulting posture collapse may already be evident in highly susceptible and untreated women. The treatment referred to here is known as *ERT,* estrogen replacement therapy, and it *can* prevent this process. Although ERT has been endorsed by the osteoporosis panel created by the National Institutes of Health in 1985, its use is not without risk: when ERT is stopped, the bone loss immediately resumes, some evidence suggests at an accelerated rate. This means a woman would need to take estrogen from menopause on, possibly a period of 25–35 years, and no one knows the effect of such long term estrogen intake. It is known, however, that some women on ERT have developed endometrial cancer. This risk is probably reduced by using lower levels of estrogen and by combining its use with progesterone, another sex hormone. However, progesterone is suspected of causing increases in a form of blood cholesterol known to be a high risk factor for cardiovascular disease. Taking all of this into account, it appears that a potent remedy may also be a potent risk. Each woman will have to decide for herself, in consultation with her doctor, what risk to take.

Fortunately, estrogen is not the only weapon available to fight osteoporosis. Some experts believe that diet and weight-bearing exercise are the best approach and the least risky. Increased calcium intake seems to help in building a bigger bone mass to start with and also in retarding bone loss. Minimizing intake of substances such as alcohol and caffeine that interfere with calcium absorption is another helpful dietary measure.

The negative effect of weightlessness on bone density has been known for some time. Astronauts have been found to lose 3–4% of heel bone density within a mere 2–3 weeks in space. Persons confined to bed can lose 1% of heel bone and spinal density per week! In favor of weight-bearing exercise, researchers at the University of Wisconsin found that tennis players may have 20% greater density in the lumbar spine area (low back) than swimmers. In another four year study, women 35–65 years of age who exercised three times per week, 50 minutes per session experienced a 75%

decrease in the loss of arm bone compared to non-exercising women. Their work-out consisted of a 10 minute warm-up, 30 minutes of aerobics, and a 10 minute cool down period using *arm weights*. However, over-exercising to the point of menstrual cessation, which can happen in severely strenuous training programs, means loss of estrogen and thus, bone loss. In one study of young female long distance runners who had ceased menstruating, bone content of the runners was comparable to that of 52 year old women. In sum, weight-bearing exercise, but not to excess, does seem to be a wise choice in minimizing bone loss.

Detecting osteoporosis before its victims have experienced bone fractures is not a well-developed science. X-rays can detect losses only when they have reached 25%. Some of the newer scanning techniques, the CAT Scan and the single and dual photon absorptiometry techniques (SPA and DPA respectively) are very expensive and not readily available to everyone.

Knowing the risk factors for osteoporosis and doing what you can to minimize or eliminate those that are modifiable is a course of action you can take without great expense—to the pocketbook anyway. These risk factors are listed in Table 3.E. Being female, having a fair complexion and slight build (low weight), and having a family history of osteoporosis can't be changed. However, you can do something about low calcium intake, high alcohol consumption, smoking, and scoliosis. As with the other diseases discussed so far, there are many choices to make in minimizing this hazard to quality of life.

Arthritis

Arthritis is the number one crippling disease in America and over 37 million people suffer from one or more of its forms. There are more than 100 forms of arthritis, but only three of these occur with notable frequency; they are osteoarthritis, rheumatoid arthritis, and gout. Of these, osteoarthritis is by far the most common, causing painful problems for an estimated 16 million Americans. Rheumatoid arthritis, generally a very severe form of arthritis, affects nearly 2½ million people, and slightly less than 2 million people, mostly men, suffer from gout. Because of its predominance, osteo-arthritis will be the main focus of this discussion.

The term *arthritis* literally means inflammation of the joint, although not all forms of arthritis, osteoarthritis being a prime example, cause inflammation as a primary symptom. As shown in Figure 3.7, the ends of the bones in a joint are covered with cartilage to provide a smooth gliding surface between the bones and to protect the bone ends from damage. Ligaments and tendons hold the bones together and allow movement in the right directions. All of these tissues are enclosed in a capsule lined with a special lubricating tissue called the *synovial membrane*. All forms of arthritis damage this structure, each in its own way. The outcome is a joint that is stiff and

Table 3.E Risk factors for osteoporosis.

NON-MODIFIABLE	MODIFIABLE
Female	Low calcium intake
Fair complexion	High alcohol consumption
Slight build	Smoking
Family history of osteoporosis	Scoliosis

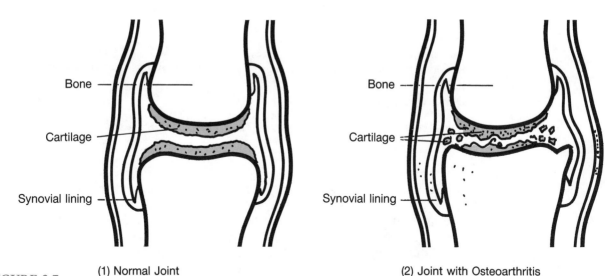

Bone

Cartilage

Synovial lining

(1) Normal Joint

Bone

Cartilage

Synovial lining

(2) Joint with Osteoarthritis

FIGURE 3.7
Joint structure:
Normal and with
osteoarthritic damage.

From *Osteoarthritis—Medical
Information Series.* Arthritis
Foundation, 1985.

painful to move and even touch, sometimes swollen and inflamed and, ultimately, permanently damaged.

Osteoarthritis is called a "wear and tear" disease and everyone develops it to some degree if they live long enough, although not everyone will experience serious symptoms. Women are affected about twice as often as men. Those who are over-weight, who have some imperfections in joint structure, and who have subjected their joints to more than the usual wear are the most likely to develop symptoms of osteo-arthritis. Generally symptoms begin slowly and don't appear before the age of 40, but severe injury or overuse can hasten the onset.

Basically, osteoarthritis involves a wearing away of the cartilage pads covering the ends of the bones in the joint, leaving them unprotected to be ground away with movement. Due to the irritation, the bone ends may thicken, developing bony growths called "spurs," which cause additional irritation. As it would seem, all of this can cause considerable pain, especially upon movement. At this point the tendency is to not move the joint. This in turn causes the muscles around the joint to weaken, leaving the joint stiff and hard to move. The weight-bearing joints, the hips, knees, feet, neck, and low back areas of the spine are the most frequent problem sites, although fingers, thumbs, and big toes sometimes show wear too.

Diagnosing arthritis is often based solely on your medical history, symptoms, and general physical condition, although sometimes X-rays and tests of joint fluid may be done to determine the extent of damage and joint involvement. The symptoms that might tell you to take action to save your joints from severe damage are listed in Table 3.F. The most common of these include joint swelling and morning stiffness, recurrent pain and tenderness in any joint, and inability to move a joint normally. Should any of these symptoms persist for more than two weeks, you could be in trouble with arthritis.

Table 3.F The warning signs for arthritis.

Swelling in one or more joints	Unexplained weight loss, fever, or weakness combined with joint pain
Early morning stiffness	Symptoms such as these that last for more than two weeks.
Recurring pain or tenderness in any joint	
Inability to move a joint normally	
Obvious redness and warmth in a joint	

From *Arthritis: Basic Facts (1986)*. Arthritis Foundation, Atlanta, GA.

Because so many people experience arthritic pain, arthritis "cures" probably constitute one of the biggest quack industries. From copper bracelets to special foods, vitamins and minerals, a myriad of "cures" exists. *But,* the fact is that there *is no known cure for arthritis;* instead, there is a treatment regime that can be relatively successful if followed carefully. Treatment generally includes a combination of medication, rest, exercise, and methods of joint protection.

The most widely used treatment drug is aspirin, which in addition to being a pain reliever, is also a very effective anti-inflammatory agent. Other anti-inflammatory drugs may be prescribed, but often they are no more effective than aspirin and cost more. Corticosteroid drugs (substances similar to cortisone, a natural body hormone) can offer marked relief from inflammation, but their long term use can produce serious side effects, so physicians try to use them sparingly.

Regular exercise is extremely important in controlling osteoarthritis. Without it, joints become increasingly stiff and hard to move, and muscles become weak, making the joint even more susceptible to injury. The type of exercises referred to here are called *gentle exercises,* and do not include marathon jogs or strenuous bouts of weight lifting. Gentle exercises increase and maintain joint flexibility and muscle strength without overstressing the joint. Examples of these exercises will be presented in Chapter 6. Exercise that causes a lot of pain is too much, too hard, and potentially damaging for arthritics and anyone else. For that matter, carrying too much body weight can be just as stressful to a joint as over-exercising it. Weight control, then, is another way to minimize and/or control arthritis problems. Exercise is most helpful in that effort, too.

In sum, it does not appear possible to avoid arthritis, especially if you live a long time. However, there are ways to curtail its impact on your life.

Low Back Pain

This is the last condition to be discussed in this section on major disabling diseases, but in fact, it is the most common cause of occupational and domestic disability. Eighty percent of Americans, about 192 million, will have trouble with low back pain at some time and approximately 74 million are chronic sufferers.

With so many people affected by low back pain, you may wonder why you don't hear more about it. Chances are that you have heard about it, only in different terms. Many people use the term *lumbago,* which simply means "pain," to describe a back problem. Others may say their "back is out"; they have a "slipped disc"; or they have "sciatica." Of these, *sciatica* is the only correct term. It refers to pain in the sciatic nerve, which runs through a large part of the spinal column and into the leg. If pressed upon or squeezed by the spine in some way, severe pain can result. Regarding the other references used to describe back pain, the fact is backs don't "go out" and discs don't "slip." In the former case, an actual injury has occurred. More often than not, a muscle has been strained or torn as a result of a sudden movement or forceful exertion while the spine is out of alignment. Because so many people have poor posture, this is not a rare occurrence. The latter condition is not a slipped disc, but rather a disc (the cushion or pad between vertebrae) that is being squeezed out of shape by abnormal pressure from the spine or one that has actually ruptured under this pressure.

Pain in the back, most often the low back area, is the main symptom. However, muscle weakness in the extremities (arms and legs), numbness and tingling in the feet or hands, and morning stiffness may be experienced. It should be noted, however, that low back pain can also be symptomatic of diseases of the kidney, pancreas, abdomen, or bowel, and of osteoporosis.

The two conditions that seem to cause most low back problems are: (1) spinal misalignment or poor posture that causes the pelvis to tilt out of position, and (2) weak postural muscles, essentially back, hamstring, and abdominal muscles. Thus, a position such as bending forward to pick something up can be very harmful for discs, ligaments, and muscles in the back. In such a position the spine is out of alignment with the body, and weak or overstretched muscles won't be able to support it, especially if any sort of sudden or extra force is exerted.

Faulty posture, then, is the major problem underlying low back pain. Although poor posture is most often the result of habit and improper weight distribution, it can be inherited. Scoliosis, for example, is a sideways curvature of the spine and is thought to be inherited in most cases. Primary indications of scoliosis are a tilting pelvis and leg length differences, but unless these are sufficiently noticeable only X-ray can detect the problem. For many this condition may not be severe enough to cause great pain, but for others discomfort may be great.

Two other common abnormal curvatures of the spine are primarily related to improper weight distribution and to habit. A weight imbalance might be due to overweight, such as with a "pot belly," but it can also be created by wearing high heels. The abnormal curvature associated with these conditions is called *lordosis* or swayback. A woman who is nine months pregnant is one of the best illustrations of this condition. The other abnormal curvature, called *kyphosis,* is usually associated with rounded shoulders and a sunken chest. Tall girls often adopt this posture in an attempt to minimize their height.

Diagnosing the immediate source of back pain is not always an easy task. Often the primary clue is what you were doing when pain became severe, if it was sudden in onset or related to the kinds of work, postures, and so on, that you've generally engaged in for years. X-rays may be of some help in detecting degenerative problems in the spine. A special form of X-ray called the myelogram is particularly useful in searching for disc problems. Also, the normality of nerve conduction can be tested by means of an electromyograph. The best immediate treatment for acute low back pain is spinal manipulation. Osteopaths and chiropractors have training in this technique. However, the relief is likely to be short-term. Hot baths or heat may help by relieving muscle tension. Cold is also useful as a pain reliever.

The best long term treatment for low back pain is exercise aimed at strength deficiencies in postural and lifting muscles, the quadriceps, glutei, abdominals, hamstrings, and back muscles. Such exercises are also one of the best ways to *prevent* low back pain. Controlling stress and tension as well as body weight are additional measures to help prevent back problems. Finally, *practicing* good posture when standing, sitting, lifting, and so on, is probably the only way to take full advantage of the benefits offered by the other preventive measures.

Cardiovascular Disease: An In-Depth Look

As reported earlier in this chapter, over 55 million Americans, almost one out of every five, are afflicted with some form of heart or blood vessel disease. Of all deaths each year, almost one-half are caused by cardiovascular disease. Because it is so lethal, so prevalent, and so hazardous to the length and quality of our lives, this special section on CVD is offered to clarify exactly what these diseases are, how they develop, and what can be done about them.

The CVD Process

From the previous section, it would appear that the most common cardiovascular problems are heart attack, stroke, and high blood pressure. While it's certainly true that these are the primary manifestations of CVD, the most common problem is *arteriosclerosis* or the hardening and narrowing of the arteries that occurs gradually with the passage of time. It happens to a greater or lesser degree to everyone. The most common form of arteriosclerosis is called *atherosclerosis,* the gradual accumulation of fat on blood vessel walls. This is the major condition underlying cardiovascular disease. It seems to begin very early in life, developing quietly until mid-life or later when it shocks its victims to attention with a heart attack or stroke. However, atherosclerosis can become severe earlier than mid-life, as autopsies of young American soldiers in the Korean War revealed. These young men, only 18–22 years of age, already had developed extensive fatty deposits on their blood vessels. It is now known that men are especially prone to early development of this problem.

In atherosclerosis the walls of arteries become thickened and rough, and the passageway narrowed, all due to fatty deposits, especially cholesterol, calcium, and other cellular debris. When sufficiently hardened into place, this is called *fatty plaque*. This process can continue to the point of completely occluding an artery or, at least, so narrowing the blood vessel channel that the movement of blood is difficult, possibly depriving tissues in that area of adequate oxygen. This is called *ischemia,* meaning inadequate blood flow in a certain body area. It is usually accompanied by a great deal of pain. When ischemia exists in the heart, the pain experienced is called *angina pectoris,* meaning pain in the chest. This is a major warning sign for heart disease.

Fibrofatty plaque most frequently develops at points where the arteries branch and blood flow is turbulent. The rough surface of the plaque can cause the blood to clot, further obstructing the artery. An obstruction of this sort is called a *thrombus.* It can form very quickly, causing a sudden total blockage of an artery. When this happens, the tissue supplied by the artery can't get any oxygen and will become nonfunctional and die if the oxygen supply is not quickly restored. A clot forming in and blocking an artery in the heart is called a *coronary thrombosis*—a heart attack. Should the clot occlude the coronary artery long enough to cause tissue death, the heart attack would be called a *myocardial infarction,* which means death of heart muscle tissue.

The heart does have a back-up network of small collateral blood vessels that may open up as major arteries become gradually or suddenly blocked. If adequately developed, this collateral system can prevent heart damage even if the major coronary arteries do become occluded. However, this system does not always develop adequately. It appears that the primary stimulus for developing collateral circulation is inadequate tissue oxygenation or ischemia. Since exercise increases the energy demands of the heart and therefore, the blood flow requirements, it has been suggested that regular vigorous exercise might induce collateral circulation. However, researchers have failed to confirm that this is a consistent benefit of exercise. Vigorous exercise may enhance development of collateral circulation in some people, but there is no guarantee of this result.

Coronary thrombosis is the most common form of heart attack. This same process can occur in the brain, where it would be called a *cerebral thrombosis*—one form of stroke. Actually, a thrombosis can occur anywhere in the body, but these particular sites, as statistics show, are the most lethal. It is also possible for a clot to form at one spot, be dislodged by the constant flow of blood, and float through the vascular system until it becomes lodged in a vessel too small for it, thereby occluding the vessel. Such a floating clot is called an *embolism* and can cause the same damage as a thrombus. See Figure 3.8 for illustrations of a thrombus, an embolism, and the previously described aneurysm.

Why does all of this happen? What causes atherosclerosis? The answer to these questions isn't complete at this time, but some pieces of the puzzle have been identified. Most clearly connected with atherosclerosis is a high level of fat in the blood, particularly the form of fat called cholesterol. It is carried in the blood in combination with several other types of fat and protein. These fat and protein packages are called *lipoproteins*.

Recently several different lipoprotein carriers of cholesterol have been identified. These are shown in Figure 3.9. One form is called *low density lipoproteins* or *LDLs*. This form of lipoproteins is made in the liver for distribution to body cells and contains a large amount of cholesterol. Elevated levels of LDLs are associated with increased atherosclerotic risk of cardiovascular disease. The lower the level of LDLs in the blood, the better. The best way to minimize LDLs in the blood seems to be to eat as little fat as possible, especially saturated fat and cholesterol. How to do this is discussed in Chapters 8 and 9.

Very low density lipoproteins, VLDLs, are another form of lipoprotein produced in the liver. These contain even more fat than LDLs, but very little of that fat is cholesterol. Consequently, LDLs are of greater concern. However, high levels of VLDLs are also undesirable since about half of these are eventually reformulated into LDLs.

A third form of lipoprotein is high density lipoprotein, or HDL. This form of lipoprotein actually seems to minimize atherosclerosis, possibly because it carries less than half the cholesterol carried in LDLs. Unlike LDLs and VLDLs, HDLs are thought to be formed by cells to carry unused cholesterol back to the liver for reuse or disposal. The more HDLs in the blood compared to LDLs and VLDLs, the less the risk of life-threatening atherosclerosis. The best way to raise HDL concentrations in the blood is by frequent, vigorous exercise. The best way to have naturally higher levels of HDLs is to be a woman: the average level of HDLs for females is 55 mgs.; the average for males is 45 mgs. Smokers tend to have lower than average HDLs.

Some people have very high levels of LDLs and VLDLs in their blood due to an inherited tendency to overproduce these substances. Others who suffer from diabetes,

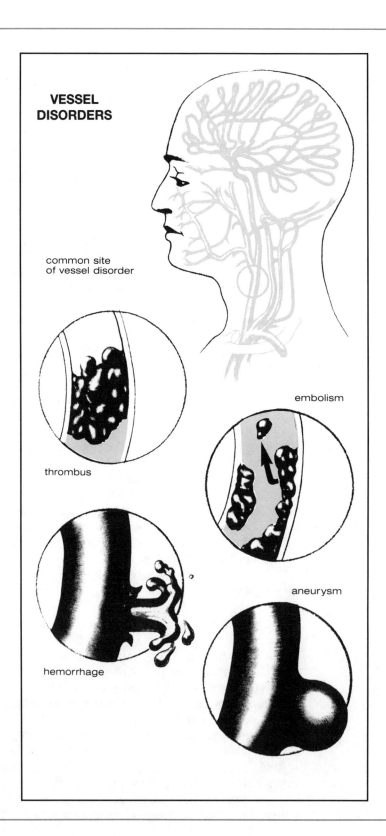

FIGURE 3.8
Vessel disorders.

From *Heart Facts and Figures, 1986*. American Heart Association, Dallas, TX. Reproduced with permission.

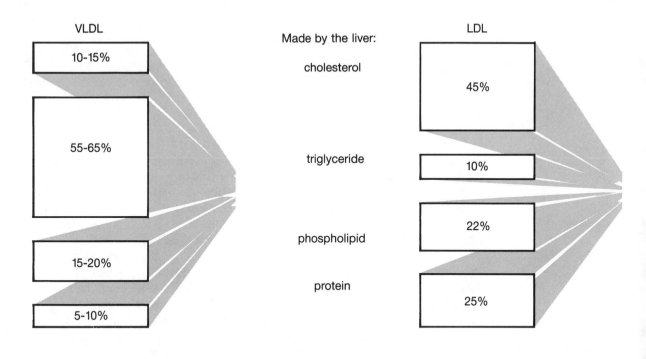

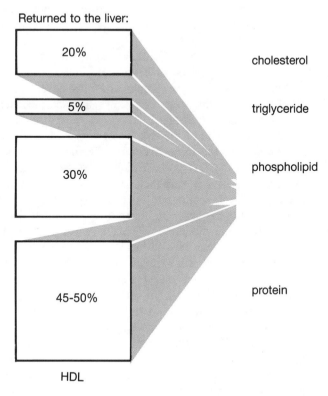

FIGURE 3.9
Types of lipoprotein.

hypothyroidism, and kidney disease also have high LDLs and VLDLs. All of these people are especially prone to atheroscelerosis. Regardless of the reasons for it—diet, genetics, or secondary diseases—high levels of fat in the blood mean increased risk of atherosclerosis and CVD.

The Risk Factors for CVD: Modifiable and Non-Modifiable

Atherosclerosis and high blood pressure seem to work hand-in-hand to some degree, each helping the other to progress. Atherosclerosis can enhance the development of high blood pressure, and high blood pressure can worsen the development of atherosclerosis. It shouldn't be surprising, then, to learn that the three major predictors of risk for CVD disease are high blood cholesterol, high blood pressure, and smoking. High blood cholesterol, as just discussed, is the most prominent factor in the development of atherosclerosis. High blood pressure, in addition to enhancing atherosclerotic development, can directly damage the heart muscle and blood vessels to the point of insufficiency and hemorrhage. Last but not least, smoking facilitates both atherosclerosis and high blood pressure, probably by lowering the level of HDLs, causing arteries to constrict, and by decreasing the amount of oxygen available to cells from the blood. (The carbon monoxide in smoke is about 210 times more able to combine with the hemaglobin in red blood cells than is oxygen and thus reduces the oxygen in the smoker's blood.) The fortunate aspect of these three risk factors is that they are modifiable; their potential damage can be increased or decreased, depending on the choices you make.

Although high cholesterol levels, high blood pressure, and smoking have emerged as the major risk factors for heart disease and stroke, there are others. These were all mentioned earlier in this chapter and now deserve some clarification, for they, too, can play a potent role in determining risk of cardiovascular disease. Fortunately many of these are also modifiable.

Diabetes is one of the risk factors for cardiovascular disease listed as modifiable. It ranks next to the three major risk factors in its ability to promote cardiovascular disease. In fact, CVD is the major complication diabetics face. You may recall from the earlier discussion of diabetes that diabetics are twice as likely to experience heart attacks and strokes and 50–100 times as likely to have peripheral vascular disease. Uncontrolled diabetics have high fat levels in the blood and 80–90% of diabetics are overweight when diagnosed. The relationships of high levels of fat in the blood to CVD should be clear by now, but how overweight affects CVD has not been addressed other than to note that it is a risk factor for heart disease and especially for high blood pressure. It is thought that blood pressure becomes easily elevated in overweight people because of the higher pumping pressure required from the heart to circulate blood through the extra blood vessels added by each pound of fat. As previously noted, high blood pressure can often be controlled without medication, simply by the loss and/or control of weight. The recommended procedure for accomplishing this is generally a combination of careful dieting and exercise.

Losing and/or controlling weight is also recommended for avoiding diabetes, and careful dieting and exercise are also included in the usual treatment plan for controlling diabetes. Thus, the threat of three risk factors—high blood pressure, diabetes, and obesity/overweight—can be reduced through one effort: weight control.

The link between lack of exercise and cardiovascular disease is not so clear as the link between diabetes or hypertension and cardiovascular disease. However, for over thirty years epidemiological data have shown lower rates of CVD among more physically active people. Recently, evidence has been accumulating to suggest why that might be. Some of the effects of exercise that may help reduce the risk of CVD include elevation of HDLs, maintained or decreased body fat and weight, possible stimulation of collateral circulation, increased pumping capacity of the heart, and decreased potential for clots to develop. As these benefits are basically the opposite of those conditions that seem to promote or characterize the CVD process, it would appear that including regular physical exercise in your life can definitely help in reducing the risk of cardiovascular disease. A more thorough discussion of the benefits of exercise is offered in Chapter 4.

The ways in which people respond to the stress in their lives have also been associated with CVD. This association has been most highly linked to a personality type called "Type A." Type A people are described as competitive, having a sense of time urgency, striving for achievement, inclined toward aggressiveness and/or hostility, and suppressive of feelings of fatigue. In modern vernacular, they are "up tight" as compared to their "easy-going" counterpart, the "Type B" person. Some studies, not all, have found Type As to have higher rates of heart attack, high blood pressure, and higher levels of fat in their blood. While there is some controversy about these personality types at this point in time, there is substantial agreement that the kinds of feelings and responses to life attributed to the Type A person are stressful, and that the body's response to stress creates many of the very conditions associated with cardiovascular disease. A few of these are elevated blood fats, increased blood pressure, and constriction of blood vessels. Fortunately, stress management has become a rather well-developed discipline today, and you can learn to reduce your feelings of stress and/or deal with them more effectively. Some of these techniques are described in Chapters 10 and 11.

In addition to modifiable risk factors for cardiovascular disease, there are unfortunately non-modifiable ones—things you can't change. These include heredity, sex, race, and age. Since everyone will find one or more of these risk factors applicable to him/herself, this situation may seem at best alarming. It's important to remember, however, that while you can't change who you are or how old you are, you can reduce or eliminate those risk factors that *are* modifiable and thus minimize your overall risk of CVD.

If your parents or other relatives have developed and/or died from CVD, then it is likely you may have inherited some tendency to develop those conditions, too. High blood cholesterol levels and high blood pressure are examples of cardiovascular problems that can be related to family history.

The death rate for men from heart attacks is almost 2.5 times that for women between the ages of 15 to 45 years of age. Even after menopause, when their death rate from heart attack increases, women don't catch up with men until age 75. Today it is thought that the female's higher level of HDLs may account for at least some of this disparity.

Black Americans develop high blood pressure at a rate 1½ times higher than the average American. The reason for this is unknown, but obviously it is especially important for Black people to monitor blood pressure levels.

And finally, the longer you live the more likely you are to die from cardiovascular disease. This is easy to understand, given the atherosclerotic process described earlier. Nonetheless, 45% of all heart attack victims are under the age of 65; 5% are under

40 years of age. One out of every five deaths from heart attacks also occurs *before* age 65. Thus, *young* does not mean *safe* where this risk factor is concerned.

At the beginning of this section on chronic disease, it was stated that there are no cures for these diseases at present. Nonetheless, it is clear that you can curtail the risk of developing these conditions. How you can do this will be the focus of the remaining chapters. That such endeavors might be worth your time and effort is suggested by the recent decline in deaths from heart disease or stroke, the first downward trend ever recorded. This decline is partly attributable to advanced medical techniques, but researchers have also noted that Americans are smoking less, controlling blood pressure better, exercising more, and reducing blood cholesterol levels.

One risk factor not discussed in detail in the remaining chapters is *smoking,* a behavior that is clearly hazardous to the length and quality of life. Two recommendations to be made regarding smoking are: (1) Don't start, or stop as quickly as you can; and (2) avoid smoke-filled environments as much as possible. There are a myriad of books, programs, classes, and individual therapies available to help anyone who wishes to stop smoking. One thing the stop-smoking classes have demonstrated is that the people most likely to "make it" are the ones who have tried before and failed. Once or a hundred times doesn't matter, but having tried does. The really good news about stopping smoking is that lung tissue that has not been permanently damaged will actually return to normal, just as if you've never smoked. Your risk of cardiovascular disease then becomes the same as someone who has never smoked.

Normalcy Checks For Your Cardiovascular System

How can you determine your status in relation to cardiovascular disease? Are you heading for a heart attack or are you fairly well protected from that potential fate? It's possible to calculate your risk by completing the risk assessment exercise at the end of this chapter. You can do this just by rating your own behavior and personal characteristics. However, actually measuring some of the physiological functions known to indicate the cardiovascular risk might give you more precise information. Some of these "normalcy checks" you can monitor by yourself; others require medical assistance.

The rate and rhythm of your heart beat is one indicator of heart function. A doctor or nurse practitioner can best evaluate these, but you can at least monitor your pulse rate regularly. Several ways to take your pulse rate are explained in Chapter 5. The average heart beats about 70 times per minute, the normal range being 60–80 beats per minute. Thus, the heart beats about 100,000 times per day pumping more than 4,300 gallons of blood throughout the body.

If your average heart rate is below 60 beats per minute, you have *bradycardia,* which simply means a slowed heart rate. Anyone who engages in regular vigorous exercise is likely to have bradycardia because his or her heart is stronger than average and can pump more blood with each beat. Thus, the trained heart doesn't have to work so hard to do the job. If you don't exercise regularly and vigorously, and your average heart rate is lower than 60 beats per minute, you may have inherited such a tendency or you may be in trouble with cardiovascular disease. One sign of the latter would be failure of the heart rate to increase appropriately with exercise or emotion. Low heart rate combined with extreme fatigue and/or faintness brought on by even mild exercise should signal a visit to the doctor.

If your average heart rate is 100 or more you have *tachycardia*. It is possible that this is an inherited trait, but the three most frequent causes of tachycardia are fever, nerve reflexes that stimulate the heart, and toxic conditions in the heart such as lack of adequate oxygen, overuse of stimulants like caffeine and nicotine, lack of sleep, anxiety, or some other debilitating condition. Besides increasing the heart rate, these toxic conditions may also cause some irregularity in the heart rhythm. This is called *dysrhythmia.*

Usually the heart maintains a steady rhythm, although deep breathing can cause some fluctuation in this. There are numerous people who experience dysrhythmia but appear to have no detectable cardiovascular problem. So prudence, and not panic, is in order should you detect this in your own pulse rate. Nonetheless, tachycardia and dysrhythmia certainly can be indicators of cardiovascular disease and should be checked by a physician.

Your physician generally uses a stethoscope to listen to your heartbeat, but he or she could also record your heartbeat and its rhythm pattern on graph paper. This is called an *electrocardiogram* or *ECG*. This graph can actually pinpoint specific areas of the heart that might not be receiving adequate oxygen or that might be damaged. Each person's ECG recording will have its own unique but normal features, some of which might actually be considered abnormal for most people. Thus, it is best to have a baseline ECG performed *before* you experience some sort of cardiovascular symptoms. It is possible that electrocardiograms taken while you are resting may be quite normal while your exercising ECG could be abnormal. Exercise ECGs are not routinely done, however, and they are expensive. Nonetheless, you should discuss the need for such a test with your physician if you have had any shortness of breath, chest pain, or abnormal heart rhythms while exercising.

Having your *blood pressure* checked regularly is another normalcy check you can make. You will need some trained assistance to do this, but it can be obtained very easily. Free blood pressure screenings are offered frequently in most communities. Media announcements of these screenings are usually made in newspapers or on television or radio. You can also call your health department, Red Cross, Heart Association, local hospital, or senior center to learn where and when these screenings might be offered. There are self-testing machines in some stores, usually pharmacies, and you can even purchase blood pressure testing devices to use at home. These are generally very easy to use and even give digital readings or printouts for you, but unless these devices are properly calibrated their results may not be accurate. If you buy a home unit, take the time to make sure it's accurate. For example, take it with you when you have your blood pressure checked by a trained person at one of the free screenings or at your doctor's office.

The normal standard and ranges for blood pressure and those indicating you are at risk are given in Table 3.G. Systolic readings of 140 or more and diastolic readings of 90 or more suggest high blood pressure and warrant medical follow-up. You may want to reread the explanation of these pressure readings given earlier in the discussion of high blood pressure as a major disabling disease.

Finally, monitoring the *level of fat in your blood,* especially the total amount of *cholesterol* you have *and* how much of that is in the form of *VLDLs, LDLs or HDLs,* is a *very* important normalcy check. You can't do this without trained help, and *only you* can seek that assistance. There will be a fee for this test because it entails a chemical analysis of a sample of your blood. Some hospitals and other health care organizations are now beginning to offer such tests at health fairs for a reduced price. Again, by calling your local health department, heart association or hospital (health

Table 3.G Normal and elevated blood pressure readings.

BLOOD PRESSURE MEASUREMENT	NORMAL	ELEVATED	LEVELS OF RISK FOR CARDIOVASCULAR DISEASE
Systolic	120 (Range 110–140)	140 +	At risk
Diastolic	80 (Range 70–90)	90–105 105–120 120 +	Mild risk Moderate risk Severe risk

Data from American Heart Association.

education unit), you can find out if such opportunities are available to you. If not or not soon enough for you, you can ask your physician to have your blood tested. Regardless of who does it, be sure you find out the results. A simple "it was normal" isn't sufficient information if you are really interested in your degree of risk for cardiovascular disease based on your blood cholesterol level. Normal blood cholesterol levels for Americans range from 140 to 250 mgs., but for every 20 mgs. over 200, the risk of cardiovascular disease increases markedly. In fact, most heart attacks occur in people with cholesterol levels between 210–265 mgs. Table 3.H lists the level of risk associated with different levels of blood cholesterol in terms of the following ratios: Total cholesterol/HDLs and LDLs/HDLs.

Table 3.H Atherosclerosis risk ratios.

	TOTAL CHOL./HDL	LDL/HDL	RISK FACTOR
Men	3.43	1.00	½ × Average
	4.97	3.55	Average
	9.55	6.25	2 × Average
	23.39	7.99	3 × Average
Women	3.27	1.47	½ × Average
	4.44	3.22	Average
	7.05	5.03	2 × Average
	11.04	6.14	3 × Average

Note: Average Risk implies a 20-25% chance of developing CHD by age 60. Lipoprotein concentrations in patients past age 60 are variable and should be interpreted with care.

Castelli, W. P. 1977. High Blood Lipid Levels. JAMA 11:1065.

Do You Have A Choice?

"Man does not die; he kills himself." A Roman philosopher named Seneca is credited with having made this observation centuries ago. If this is so, today's men and women haven't changed very much. It seems that almost daily researchers are finding yet another way that the development, or at least the *extent* of development, of the major chronic diseases can be influenced by what you do. A summary of the risk factors for these diseases is presented in Table 3.I. The daily choices you make about what to eat, whether or not to exercise, and how to handle the stress in your life are the behaviors that seem most critical. Indeed, there is something you can do in one or more of these areas to minimize the development and/or severity of each of the diseases discussed in this chapter.

A special note about cancer is needed here regarding the potential influence of nutritional practices, exercise, and stress management. Even though the evidence is not yet definitive, the possibility that your behavior choices in these areas may have an impact on cancer is suggested here for the following reasons. By 1985 the Cancer Society felt that research findings relating dietary practices to at least some cancers were sufficiently strong to warrant publishing *Simply Nutritious,* an educational cookbook that identifies certain *dietary* practices that have the potential to provide some protection from cancer, the book suggests recipes that emphasize these practices. Thus, it seems prudent to pay attention to these recommendations even though such practices are not yet known to *guarantee* protection from cancer.

Whether or not stress management can provide some protection against cancer is even less firmly established. However, doctors have for years recognized the detrimental impact of stress on any disease process even though the reason for this was not clear. Recently researchers have actually demonstrated that among the numerous effects of chronic, uncontrolled stress is depression of the immune system. This immediately suggests that managing the stress in your life could be important in preventing cancer given the role of the immune system in destroying viruses and other foreign bodies that appear in the body, such as carcinogens and even your own cells should they become abnormal. Since exercise is recommended as one way to manage stress, a connection between regular exercise and cancer may eventually be documented.

Table 3.I   Modifiable and non-modifiable risk factors for major chronic diseases.

RISK FACTOR	CVD	CA	HBP	DIABETES	ARTHRITIS	LBP	OSTEO
Non-Modifiable							
Heredity	●	●	●	●	●		●
Race	●		●	●			●
Age	●	●	●	●	●		●
Sex	●	●	●	●	●		●
			(Oral Contraceptive)				
Modifiable							
Smoking	●	●	●				●
HBP	●						
High Blood Fats	●		●				
Diabetes	●		●				
Obesity	●	●	●	●	●	●	
Lack of Exercise	●		●			●	●
Stress	●	●?	●		●	●	
Diet	●	●	●	●	●		●
					(gout only)		

Key: CVD = Cardiovascular disease;   CA = Cancer;   HBP = High Blood Pressure;   LBP = Low Back Pain;   Osteo = Osteoporosis.

Table 3.J summarizes the potential impact of your daily choices—what to eat, whether or not to exercise, how much stress to expose yourself to, how to handle stress—on the diseases that kill and/or disable us prematurely. The information in this table should be encouraging to those who wish to have at least some control over the quality of their lives. Nonetheless, numerous other factors are involved in the development of these diseases about which little is known, and thus it is not yet possible to determine comprehensive protective actions. Choosing to follow current health guidelines can minimize your risk and reduce the severity of these hazards, but it will not *guarantee* freedom from the major chronic diseases.

As a first choice in your favor, you might want to take the self assessment tests that follow to check your current level of risk for cardiovascular disease and cancer.

Table 3.J   The impact of behavior choices on aging and disease.

CHOICES	EFFECT ON BODY FUNCTIONS	IMPACT ON DISEASE	
Reduce and manage stress	↑ Effectiveness of immune response ↑ CV efficiency ↓ Muscle tension/anxiety ↓ Blood fat/stress related hormones ↑ Cellular functioning ↓ Intracellular destruction	↓ CVD ↓ Cancer ↓ Diabetes ↓ Aging	↓ HBP ↓ Arthritis ↓ LBP

Recommended exercise:
  Aerobic and strength
    flexibility
	↑ CV efficiency/effectiveness
	↑ Bone strength
	↑ Metabolism/weight control
	↑ Strength and flexibility
	↓ Blood fat
	↑ Respiratory efficiency
	↑ Cellular functioning
		↓ CVD
		↓ Cancer
		↓ Diabetes
		
		↓ Aging
			↓ HBP
			↓ Arthritis
			↓ LBP
			↓ Osteo

Recommended dietary practices	↑ Weight/fat control ↑ CV efficiency/effectiveness ↑ Bone strength ↑ GI function ↕ Cellular functioning ↓ Blood fat ↑ Effectiveness of immune response	↓ CVD ↓ Cancer ↓ Diabetes ↓ Aging	↓ HBP ↓ Arthritis ↓ LBP ↓ Osteo
The specific choices in each category are explained in Chapters 4–11.	↑ = improve/increase ↓ = decrease	↓ = prevent, delay, minimize	

Summary

In this chapter, aging and chronic diseases are discussed in terms of the limitations they present to both the quality and length of life. Factors known or suspected to promote the aging process and/or the development of chronic disease are identified. Ways to reduce or eliminate many of these factors via daily lifestyle choices are suggested.

Aging is defined as *changes that occur during adulthood due to the passage of time.* The basic trend of these changes in terms of body functioning is one of gradual decline, with some functions "aging" more rapidly than others. Loss of cells and declines in basal metabolic rate, immune system function, strength, cardiac output, and respiratory efficiency typify these changes. Susceptibility to disease tends to increase with age, and it appears that death is ultimately inevitable.

Nonetheless, as much as 50% of the decline in function generally attributed to aging may actually be due to *disuse.* Current research suggest that by following a program of regular vigorous exercise and consuming a quality diet, a person 60–70 years of age could actually have the functional capacities or biological age of someone 20–30 years younger. Exercise and diet are also significant factors in combatting susceptibility to disease. In addition, constructively managing stress appears to minimize immune system dysfunction and susceptibility to disease. In sum, the degree to which you experience loss of function with age is determined, at least in part, by the daily choices you make in the areas of exercise, diet, and stress management.

Chronic diseases have become the major threat to the health and longevity of Americans. Cardiovascular disease and cancer together account for almost 70% of all deaths in the United States. Cardiovascular disease is by far the most prominent of these, being responsible for 46% of all deaths. High blood pressure and diabetes are also noteworthy as causes of death, but they affect the greatest number of people as risk factors for heart disease and as disabling diseases. Additional major causes of disability for Americans are osteoporosis, arthritis, and low back pain.

As the number one killer/disabler of Americans, cardiovascular disease warrants special attention. The gradual accumulation of fat on blood vessel walls, called atherosclerosis, is most commonly the underlying cause of cardiovascular problems. When this condition becomes severe enough, ischemia and thrombus development can occur, both of which can result in heart attack and stroke. High cholesterol levels in the blood, especially in the form of the low density lipoproteins (LDLs) are most prominently associated with the development of atherosclerosis. Smoking and high blood pressure are also at the top of the list of risk factors for cardiovascular disease. As fatty deposits on blood vessels can only be detected with complicated, expensive, and potentially dangerous procedures, monitoring basic indicators of cardiovascular functioning can be critical to health and life itself. These basic indicators include heart rate and rhythm, EKG, blood pressure, and blood fat levels, especially cholesterol and its various forms.

Chronic diseases develop slowly, often over many years; but once their symptoms appear, they generally become lifelong problems. Currently the best way to minimize their impact on the quality and length of life is to avoid or limit exposure to those factors known to increase susceptibility to these diseases. Although some risk factors such as sex, age, race, and heredity are not modifiable, others can be directly influenced by lifestyle choices. These modifiable risk factors include smoking, high blood pressure, high levels of fat in the blood, diabetes, obesity, lack of exercise, diet, and stress.

In terms of aging and chronic diseases, how you choose to live today can make a difference in how you will live in the future.

Self Survey: Heart Attack and Stroke Risk

RISK HABIT OR FACTOR		INCREASING RISK				
I. Smoking Cigarettes		None	Up to 9 per day	10 to 24 per day	25 to 34 per day	35 or more per day
	Score	0	1	2	3	4
II. Body Weight		Ideal weight	Up to 9 lbs. excess	10 to 19 lbs. excess	20 to 29 lbs. excess	30 lbs. or more excess
	Score	0	1	2	3	4
III. Salt Intake *or*		⅕ average hard to achieve; no added salt, no convenience foods	⅓ average no use of salt at table, spare use of high-salt foods	U.S. average salt in cooking, some salt at table	Above average frequent salt at table	Far above average frequent use of salty foods
Blood Pressure Upper Reading (if known)		Less than 110	110 to 129	130 to 139	140 to 149	150 or over
	Score	0	1	2	3	4
IV. Saturated Fat and Cholesterol Intake *or*		⅕ average almost total vegetarian; rare egg yolk, butterfat & lean meat	⅓ average 2 meatless days/week, no whole milk products, lean meat only	½ average meat (mostly lean), eggs, cheese 12 times/week nonfat milk only	U.S. average meat, cheese, eggs, whole milk 24 times/week	Above average meat, cheese, eggs, whole milk over 24 times/week
Blood Cholesterol Level (if known)		Less than 150	150 to 169	170 to 199	200 to 219	200 or over
	Score	0	1	2	3	4
V. Self-Rating of Physical Activity *or*		Vigorous exercise 4 or more times/week 20 min. each	Vigorous exercise 3 times/week 20 min. each	Vigorous exercise 1 to 2 times/ week	U.S. average occasional exercise	Below average exercises rarely
Walking Rating		Brisk walking 5 times/ week 45 min. each	Brisk walking 3 times/ week 30 min. each	Brisk walking 2 times/ week 30 min. each *or* Normal walking 4½ to 6 miles daily	Normal walking 2½ to 4½ miles daily	Normal walking less than 2½ miles daily
	Score	0	1	2	3	4

RISK HABIT OR FACTOR	INCREASING RISK				
VI. Self-Rating of Stress and Tension	Rarely tense or anxious *or*	Calmer than average	U.S. average Feel tense or anxious 2 to 3 times/day	Quite tense Usually rushed	Extremely tense
	Yoga, meditation, or equivalent 20 min. 2 times/day	Feel tense about 3 times/ week	Frequent anger or hurried feelings	Occasionally take tranquilizer	Take tranquilizer 5 times/ week or more
Score	0	1	2	3	4

Enter your total score here _____.

Notes:

(1) Subtract 1 point if dietary fiber intake is high (almost all cereals whole grain, almost no sugar, and considerable fruit and vegetable intake).
(2) Add 1 point if all exercise is competitive.
(3) If you are a female taking estrogen or birth control pills, add 1 point if score is 12 or below, 2 points if risk score is 13 or above (especially if you smoke, are overweight, have high blood pressure or high blood cholesterol).

INTERPRETATION

Maximum points = 24

ZONE	SCORE	
F	21–24	The probability of having a premature heart attack or stroke is about four to five times the U.S. average. Action is urgent. Try to drop four points within a month and three more points within six months.
E	17–20	Incidence of heart attack or stroke is about twice the U.S. average. Action is urgent. Try to drop four points within six months and continue reduction.
D	13–16	The U.S. average is 14. This is an uncomfortable and readily avoidable zone. Careful planning can result in a five- to six-point reduction within a year.
C	9–12	The likelihood of having a heart attack or stroke is about one-half the U.S. average. This is a zone rather easily achieved by most people within a year if they are now in Zone D or E. Careful planning can result in a four- or six-point reduction within a year.

James Farquhar, *The American Way of Life Need Not Be Hazardous to Your Health.* © 1987 by Stanford Alumni Association. Reprinted with permission of Addison-Wesley Publishing Co., Inc.

Cancer: Assessing Your Risks

A Personalized Test

A Service of the American Cancer Society, 1981.

INTRODUCTION

Some people may have more than the average risk of developing certain cancers. These people will be identified by certain risk factors.

This simple self-testing method is designed by the American Cancer Society to help you assess your risk factors for certain common types of cancer. These are the major risk factors and by no means represent the only ones that might be involved.

TEST SCORE CARD DIRECTIONS

Read each question concerning each site and its specific risk factors. Be honest in your responses. Place the number in parentheses in the correct space on your score panel to the right.

For example, Question #2 on lung cancer, above right: if you are 53 years old (age 50–59) then enter 5 as your score.

FOR WOMEN

In addition to completing the score panels for lung, colon-rectum, and skin cancer, complete the panels for breast, cervical, and endometrial cancer.

ABOUT YOUR ANSWERS

You may check your own risks with the answers contained on pages 71–73.

IMPORTANT: REACT TO EACH STATEMENT

Individual numbers for specific questions are not to be interpreted as a precise measure of relative risk, but the totals for a given site should give a general indication of your risk.

Developed by the American Cancer Society

LUNG CANCER

1. SEX
     a. Male (2)   b. Female (1)
2. AGE
     a. 39 or less (1)   b. 40–49 (2)
     c. 50–59 (5)   d. 60 + (7)
3. a. Smoker (8)   b. Nonsmoker (1)
4. TYPE OF SMOKING
     a. Current cigarettes or little   b. Pipe and/or cigar, but not
        cigars (10)   cigarettes (3)
     c. Ex-cigarette smoker (2)   d. Nonsmoker (1)
5. AMOUNT OF CIGARETTES SMOKED PER DAY
     a. 0 (1)   b. Less than ½ pack per day (5)
     c. ½–1 pack (9)   d. 1–2 packs (15)
     e. 2 + packs (20)
6. TYPE OF CIGARETTE
     a. High tar/nicotine (10)*   b. Medium T/N (9)
     c. Low T/N (7)   d. Nonsmoker (1)

*High T/N	20 mg. Tar/1.3 mg. nicotine
Medium T/N	16–19 mg. Tar/1.1–1.2 mg. nicotine
Low T/N	15 mg. or less Tar/1.0 mg. or less nicotine

7. DURATION OF SMOKING
   a. Never smoked (1)
   c. Up to 15 years (5)
   e. 25 + years (20)
   b. Ex-smoker (3)
   d. 15–25 years (10)

8. TYPE OF INDUSTRIAL WORK
   a. Mining (3)
   c. Uranium & radioactive products (5)
   b. Asbestos (7)

TOTAL _____

COLON RECTUM CANCER

1. AGE
   a. 39 or less (10)
   c. 60 and over (50)
   b. 40–59 (20)

2. HAS ANYONE IN YOUR IMMEDIATE FAMILY EVER HAD:
   a. colon cancer (20)
   c. neither (1)
   b. one or more polyps of the colon (10)

3. HAVE YOU EVER HAD:
   a. colon cancer (100)
   b. ulcerative colitis (20)
   e. none (1)
   b. one or more polyps of the colon (40)
   d. cancer of the breast or uterus (10)

4. BLEEDING FROM THE RECTUM (other than obvious hemorrhoids or piles)
   a. Yes (75)
   b. No (1)

*TOTAL*_____

SKIN CANCER

1. Frequent work or play in the sun.   Yes (10) No (1)
2. Work in mines, around coal tars or around radioactivity.   Yes (10) No (1)
3. Complexion - fair skin and/or light skin.   Yes (10) No (1)

*TOTAL*_____

BREAST

1. AGE GROUP
   a. 20–34 (10)
   b. 50 and over (90)
   b. 35–49 (40)

2. RACE GROUP
   a. Oriental (5)
   c. White (25)
   b. Black (20)
   d. Mexican American (10)

3. FAMILY HISTORY
   a. Mother, sister, aunt or grandmother with breast cancer (30)
   b. None (10)

4. YOUR HISTORY
   a. Previous lumps or cysts (25)
   c. No breast disease (10)
   b. Previous breast cancer (100)

5. MATERNITY
   a. 1st pregnancy before 25 (10)
   c. No pregnancies (20)
   b. 1st pregnancy after 25 (15)

*TOTAL*_____

CERVICAL CANCER* Lower Portion of Uterus
*Doesn't apply to women with total hysterectomy

1. AGE GROUP
   a. Less than 25 (10)   b. 25–39 (20)
   c. 40–54 (30)   d. 55 & over (30)

2. RACE
   a. Oriental (10)   b. Puerto Rican (20)
   c. Black (20)   d. White (10)
   e. Mexican American (20)

3. NUMBER OF PREGNANCIES
   a. 0 (10)   b. 1 to 3 (20)
   c. 4 and over (30)

4. VIRAL INFECTIONS
   a. Herpes and other viral infections   b. Never (1)
      or ulcer formations on the
      vagina (10)

5. AGE AT FIRST INTERCOURSE
   a. Before 15 (40)   b. 15–19 (30)
   c. 20–24 (20)   d. 25 and over (10)
   e. Never (5)

6. BLEEDING BETWEEN PERIODS OR AFTER INTERCOURSE
   a. Yes (40)   b. No (1)

                                     *TOTAL*_____

ENDOMETRIAL CANCER* Body of Uterus
*Doesn't apply to women with total hysterectomy

1. AGE GROUP
   a. 39 or less (5)   b. 40–49 (20)
   c. 50 and over (60)

2. RACE
   a. Oriental (10)   b. Black (10)
   c. White (20)   d. Mexican American (10)

3. BIRTHS
   a. None (15)   b. 1 to 4 (7)
   c. 5 or more (5)

4. WEIGHT
   a. 50 or more pounds overweight (50)
   b. 20–49 pounds overweight (15)
   c. Underweight for height (10)   d. Normal (10)

5. DIABETES (elevated blood sugar)
   a. Yes (3)   b. No (1)

6. ESTROGEN HORMONE INTAKE
   a. Yes, regularly (15)   b. Yes, occasionally (12)
   c. None (10)

7. ABNORMAL UTERINE BLEEDING
   a. Yes (40)   b. No (1)

8. HYPERTENSION (high blood pressure)
   a. Yes (3)   b. No (1)

                                     *TOTAL*_____

LUNG

1. Men have a higher risk of lung cancer than women equating them for type, amount and duration of smoking. Since more women are smoking cigarettes for a longer duration than previously, their incidence of lung and *upper respiratory tract (mouth, tongue and larynx)* cancer is increasing.
2. The occurrence of lung and *upper respiratory tract* cancer increases with age.
3. Cigarette smokers have up to 20 times or even greater risk than nonsmokers. However, the rates of ex-smokers who have not smoked for ten years approach those of nonsmokers.
4. Pipe and cigar smokers are at a higher risk for lung cancer than nonsmokers. Cigarette smokers are at a much higher risk than nonsmokers or pipe and cigar smokers. *All forms of tobacco, including chewing, markedly increase the user's risk of developing cancer of the mouth.*
5. Male smokers of less than ½ pack per day have five times higher lung cancer rate than nonsmokers. Male smokers of 1–2 packs per day have 15 times higher lung cancer rates than nonsmokers. Smokers of more than 2 packs per day are 20 times more likely to develop lung cancer than nonsmokers.
6. Smokers of low tar/nicotine cigarettes have slightly lower lung cancer rates.
7. The frequency of lung and *upper respiratory tract* cancer increases with the duration of smoking.
8. Exposures to materials used in these industries have been demonstrated to be associated with lung cancer. Smokers who work in these industries may have greatly increased risks. Exposures to materials in other industries may also carry a higher risk.

   If your total is:

   24 or less . .   You have a low risk for lung cancer.
   25–49 . . . .   You may be a light smoker and would have a good chance of kicking the habit.
   50–74 . . . .   As a moderate smoker, your risks of lung and *upper respiratory tract* cancer are increased. If you stop smoking now, these risks will decrease.
   75–over . . .   As a heavy cigarette smoker, your chances of getting lung and *upper respiratory tract* cancer are greatly increased. Your best bet is to stop smoking now — for the health of it. See your doctor if you have a nagging cough, hoarseness, *persistent pain or sore in the mouth or throat.*

COLON RECTUM

1. Colon cancer occurs more frequently after the age of 50.
2. Colon cancer is more common in families with a previous history of this disease.
3. Polyps and bowel diseases are associated with colon cancer.
4. Rectal bleeding may be a sign of colorectal cancer.

   If your total is:

   29 or less . .   You are at a low risk for colon-rectum cancer.
   30–69 . . . .   This is a moderate risk category. Testing by your physician may be indicated.
   70–over . . .   This is a high risk category. You should see your physician for the following tests: digital rectal exam, guaiac slide test and protoscopic exam.

SKIN

1. Excessive ultraviolet causes cancer of the skin. Protect yourself with a sun screen medication.
2. These materials can cause cancer of the skin.
3. Light complexions need more protection than others.

   If your total is:

   Numerical risks for skin cancer are difficult to state. For instance, a person with dark complexion can work longer in the sun and be less likely to develop cancer than a light complected person. Furthermore, a person wearing a long sleeve shirt and wide brimmed hat may work in the sun and be less at risk than a person who wears a bathing suit for only a short period. The risk goes up greatly with age.

The key here is if you answered "yes" to any question, you need to protect your skin from the sun or any other toxic material. Changes in moles, warts or skin sores are very important and need to be seen by your doctor.

BREAST

If your total is:

Under 100 . . . .   Low risk women should practice monthly breast self-examination and have their breasts examined by a doctor as part of a cancer-related checkup.

100–199 . . . . .   Moderate risk women should practice monthly BSE and have their breasts examined by a doctor as part of a cancer-related checkup. Periodic breast x-rays should be included as your doctor may advise.

200 or higher . .   High risk women should practice monthly BSE and have the above examinations more often. See your doctor for the recommended (frequency of breast physical examinations and x-ray) examinations related to you.

1._____
2._____
3._____
4._____
5._____
_____

CERVICAL

1. The highest occurrence is in the 40 and over age group. The numbers represent the relative rates of cancer for different age groups. A 45 year old woman has a risk three times higher than a 20 year old.
2. Puerto Ricans, Blacks, and Mexican Americans have higher rates of cervical cancer.
3. Women who have delivered more children have a higher occurrence.
4. Viral infections of the cervix and vagina are associated with cervical cancer.
5. Women with earlier intercourse and with more sexual partners are at a higher risk.
6. Irregular bleeding may be a sign of uterine cancer.

    If your total is:

    40–69 . . . .   This is a low risk group. Ask your doctor for a pap test. You will be advised how often you should be tested after your first test.

    70–99 . . .   In this moderate risk group, more frequent pap tests may be required.

    100 or more   You are in a high risk group and should have a pap test (and pelvic exam) as advised by your doctor.

1._____
2._____
3._____
4._____
5._____
6._____

ENDOMETRIAL

1. Endometrial cancer is seen in older age groups. The numbers by the age groups represent relative rates of endometrial cancer at different ages. A 50 year old woman has a risk twelve times higher than a 35 year old woman.
2. Caucasians have a higher occurrence.
3. The fewer children one has delivered the greater the risk of endometrial cancer.
4. Women who are overweight are at greater risk.
5. Cancer of the endometrium is associated with diabetes.
6. Cancer of the endometrium may be associated with prolonged continuous estrogen hormone intake. This occurs in only a small number of women. You should consult your physician before starting or stopping any estrogen medication.
7. Women who do not have cyclic regular menstrual periods are at greater risk.
8. Cancer of the endometrium is associated with high blood pressure.

*1.*_____
*2.*_____
*3.*_____
*4.*_____
*5.*_____
*6.*_____
*7.*_____
*8.*_____

If your total is:

45–59 . . . .   You are at very low risk for developing endometrial cancer.

60–99 . . . .   Your risks are slightly higher. Report any abnormal bleeding immediately to your doctor. Tissue sampling at menopause is recommended.

100 and over   Your risks are much greater. See your doctor for tests as appropriate.

_____

YOUR TEST SCORES

Check your own risks with the answers contained on pages 71–73. Individual numbers for specific questions are not to be interpreted as a precise measure of relative risk, but the totals for a given site should give you a general indication of your risk.

Additional educational information is available from your American Cancer Society.

You are advised to discuss this assessment with your physician if you are at high risk.

References

Arthritis: Basic Facts. 1986. Atlanta, GA: Arthritis Foundation.

Cancer Facts and Figures. 1986. New York: American Cancer Society.

Diabetes Facts and Figures. 1986. Alexandria, VA: American Diabetes Association.

Finch, C. and Hayflick, L., eds. 1977. *Handbook of the biology of aging*. New York: Van Nostrand Reinhold.

Friedman, M. and Ulmer, D. 1984. *Treating type behavior—and your heart*. New York: Alfred A. Knopf.

Fries, J. and Crapo,L. 1981. *Vitality and aging*. San Francisco: W.H. Freeman.

Garfield, C. 1979. *Stress and survival*. St. Louis: Mosby.

Havlik, R. and Feinleib, M., eds. 1979. *Proceedings of the conference on the decline in coronary heart disease mortality*. USDHEW, PHS, NIH #79-1610.

Heart Facts. 1986. Dallas, TX: American Heart Association.

Keim, H. 1981. *How to care for your back*. Englewood Cliffs, NJ: Prentice-Hall.

Osteoarthritis. 1986. Atlanta, GA: Arthritis Foundation.

Pelletier, K. 1977. *Mind as healer, mind as slayer*. New York: Delta.

Piscopo, J. 1985. *Fitness and aging*. New York: John Wiley and Sons.

Pollner, F. 1985. *Osteoporosis: looking at the whole picture*. Medical World News, January 14.

Sheehan, G. 1985. *The causes and treatment of low-back pain*. The Runner 7: 16-18.

Simply nutritious. 1985. Portland, OR: Oregon Division; American Cancer Society.

White, P. and Mondeika, T. 1982. *Diet and exercise: synergism in health maintenance*. Chicago: American Medical Association.

Whitney, E. and Hamilton, E. 1984. *Understanding nutrition*. New York: West Publishing.

Zacharkow, D. 1984. *The healthy lower back*. Springfield, IL: Charles C. Thomas.

4

General Guidelines
For Fitness

What is *fitness* and what aspects of fitness relate to health? To performance?

Why should you know something about overload, progression, and specificity in training?

How should you organize a typical exercise session to achieve maximum benefit?

What should you do if you experience sore muscles, tendinitis, or other problems that commonly result from training?

How should you alter your workout when exercising in the heat? In the cold? Or if the humidity is high or the air is polluted?

Introduction

Physical fitness is a term that is often used rather loosely to mean a variety of things. To the runner fitness may mean the ability to run ten kilometers in a particular span of time; to the non-athletic, working person it may refer to a trim appearance; to the student it may refer to both of the above or possibly to the strength or speed needed in a favorite sport. Is the term *fitness* used correctly in all of these contexts? What precisely does fitness mean? This chapter will address these questions and will provide general guidelines for exercising correctly. In addition we discuss common fitness injuries and environmental problems that you may encounter while training. The chapter concludes with suggestions to help you personalize a fitness program to fit your individual needs.

Fitness Defined

In the broadest sense, physical fitness is *the capacity to meet the demands of modern day life with relatively little strain*. A physically fit individual is able to work and play with ease because of regular and continuing preparation for activity. Should an emergency arise, or even an unusual event such as a day of skiing or hiking, this individual has the capacity to stretch farther than usual and rise to the occasion as needed. To be prepared for any eventuality may sound like an idealistic goal that is really not attainable for the average person. But do such people exist only in the movies? Can you be prepared to meet all untoward circumstances? Before attempting to answer these and other questions we will describe the components of fitness and discuss several important generalizations about methods to improve fitness.

The Components of Fitness

Fitness encompasses such a wide variety of elements that it is useful to break it into components (Table 4.A). *Health related fitness* refers to those components that are related to health and well-being. These include: (1) cardiorespiratory fitness, (2) body

Table 4.A The components of fitness.

HEALTH-RELATED FITNESS	PERFORMANCE RELATED FITNESS
Cardiorespiratory (aerobic) fitness	Flexibility of other parts of the body
Body composition	Power
Strength and muscle endurance	Speed
(Particularly in the abdominal muscles)	Agility
Flexibility of the lower back and hip region	

composition, (3) strength and muscular endurance in the major muscle groups and particularly in the abdominal region, and (4) flexibility of the low back and hip region. The remaining components, including power, speed, agility, and flexibility in other regions of the body, are labeled as components of *performance related fitness*. Note that all of the health related components contribute to both health and physical performance. Since the focus of this book is on those aspects of fitness that have significance for all individuals and not just the athletically inclined, we will devote more time to the health related fitness components than to the performance related fitness components.

Health Related Fitness

Cardiorespiratory Fitness

This refers to the combined abilities of the respiratory and circulatory systems to provide adequate oxygen to muscles during continuous, rhythmic exercise for extended periods of time. Sports events that depend heavily on this component include running, cycling, cross-country skiing, and swimming long distances. Cardiorespiratory fitness is also important for hiking, jogging, and walking, except that in these activities the individual is usually not taxing himself/herself to a maximum degree. Cardiorespiratory fitness is said to be the most important component of fitness because evidence suggests that activities that promote this form of fitness are associated with a lowered incidence of death from all causes (particularly atherosclerosis), with favorable changes in lipid profile, and with enhanced collateral circulation in the heart as well as other positive changes. The term *aerobic fitness* is often used to mean the same thing as cardiorespiratory fitness. In Chapter 5 the importance of cardiorespiratory fitness and how it can be measured, improved, and maintained will be discussed in detail.

Body Composition

This refers to the relative amount of fat in the body compared to other tissues. More precisely, *fat weight* refers to the weight of all deposits of fat in the body, and *fat-free weight* refers to the weight of all the other tissues combined together including muscle, bone, and the various organs. Excess fatness or obesity puts an individual at greater risk for many cardiovascular diseases, for diabetes, and for numerous other health problems. The topics of weight control and weight loss as well as methods of measuring body composition are more fully discussed in Chapter 7.

Strength and Muscle Endurance

Strength refers to the capacity of a muscle group to exert force under maximum conditions. The greater this capacity, the greater strength is said to be. *Muscle endurance* refers to the ability of a muscle to engage in repetitive exercise for long periods of time with little fatigue. Having sufficient strength and muscle endurance in the major muscles of the body plays an important role in many aspects of health. It can make the difference when it comes to survival in emergencies. Recreational pursuits often require the use of many body parts and particularly the upper body. In daily activities, an individual is often required to lift, to hold, or to carry objects of different sizes, shapes, and weights. Being able to do such activities without undue stress and

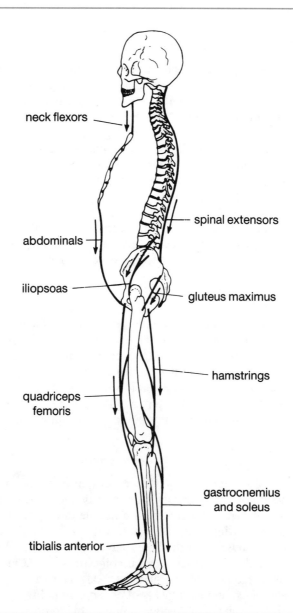

strain and without injury can make a big difference in your health and in your freedom to do what is asked of you and/or what you choose.

It should be noted that women typically have lower levels of strength in their upper body than they do in their lower body. This suggests that women in particular should engage in a program of regular upper body exercise with a special focus on strength.

Evidence suggests that the lower back problems discussed in Chapter 3 are strongly related to low levels of strength and muscle endurance in the abdominal muscles. The abdominals are one of several antigravity muscles that are responsible for maintaining the upright posture. (Figure 4.1). When the abdominals become weak

neck flexors

spinal extensors

abdominals

iliopsoas

gluteus maximus

hamstrings

quadriceps femoris

gastrocnemius and soleus

tibialis anterior

FIGURE 4.1
A lateral view of the human skeleton, indicating the location of the major antigravity muscles, which are responsible for helping the body maintain an erect posture.

Reprinted with permission of Macmillan Publishing Company from *Structural Kinesiology* by Barham, J. N. and Wooten, E. P. Copyright © 1973 by Macmillan Publishing Company

they permit the pelvic girdle to tilt forward, which puts pressure on the spinal nerves in the lower back region. The "protruding belly" syndrome is evidence of poor alignment in this region and places the lower back at considerable risk for injury when doing even simple tasks such as bending over (Figure 4.2).

FIGURE 4.2
The "protruding belly syndrome" arises from weakened abdominal muscles and/or excessive abdominal fat and allows the pelvic girdle to tilt forward, placing the lower back region at greater risk for pain and injury.

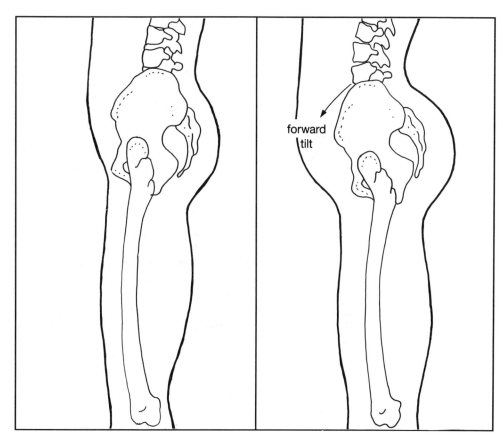

Flexibility of the Lower Back and Hip Region

Flexibility refers to the ability of body segments to move through a range of motion. Poor flexibility of the spine, particularly in the lower back region combined with a poor range of motion in the hips, including the tendons and ligaments supporting such muscles as the hamstrings (see Figure 4.1), is also strongly implicated in problems of the lower back region. As we mentioned in Chapter 3, low back pain represents one of the most significant ways that individuals become temporarily or chronically disabled. Chapter 6 discusses methods of evaluating your flexibility, strength, and muscle endurance and suggests ways to improve each of these fitness components.

Performance Related Fitness

Flexibility in Other Regions of the Body

Having sufficient flexibility throughout the body is an important aspect of fitness even though this additional flexibility has no direct relationship to health in a strict sense. Having a wide range of motion, especially when coupled with sufficient strength and endurance, can permit you to move freely and easily and to perform more fully whatever activity you choose.

Power

Power is the ability to exert force explosively. For example, when a softball player throws the ball as fast as he/she can, the effect on the ball is a combined function of force and speed. The greater the force applied, and also the faster the force applied (i.e., the less the time required to generate the force), the greater the power. While in many athletic events power is a primary requirement if one is to attain a high level of achievement, the non-athletic individual has little need for this fitness component. Training to improve power is discussed more fully in Chapter 6.

Speed and Agility

Speed and agility are fitness components that involve moving the whole body as rapidly as possible. While speed usually refers to rapid movements in a straight line (such as in sprinting), agility refers to the ability to change directions of movement rapidly (such as when a volleyball player moves in a fraction of a second from spiking the ball over the net to driving to retrieve the ball if it is suddenly blocked). The non-athletic person has very little need for a high level of speed and/or agility. However, should you be interested, training procedures for each are briefly discussed in Chapter 6.

General Principles of Fitness

Regular training is required if you wish to improve your fitness. *Training* is used here to mean a process of regular activity that is directed toward building up and/or maintaining any of the components of fitness. It does not imply a spartan-like, regimented commitment of several hours of sweat and toil each day. Nor does it require you to "live half your life in a smelly gym." For some, particularly those who are athletically inclined, training does involve a large investment of time and effort because the goal of reaching one's limits or of achieving a given level of performance is often unattainable without such a commitment. However, for most individuals, training takes the form of a regular period of time several days each week devoted to moderate, submaximal exercise that is enjoyable. It is not a "grit your teeth and bear it" type of experience.

The type of training that will elicit optimum benefits is different for each fitness component. However, for each of the training methods several general principles must be applied if you wish to realize some gain for your efforts. These principles include the *overload principle,* the *principle of progressive exercise,* and the *specificity principle*.

Overload Principle

In the most simple terms, the overload principle states that if you regularly tax a body part or system within certain limits, that system will adapt positively and become more able to withstand stress. The term *overload* refers to the process of using a stressor or some stimulus that taxes the body part in question. The term *body part* can apply to a single muscle or a group of muscles or to entire systems such as the oxygen transport system, in which the coordinated efforts of the circulatory and respiratory systems deliver oxygen to exercising muscles to enable the production of energy. The overload stimulus can take very different forms depending on what body part or system is being overloaded—from lifting weights for improved strength, to slow jogging for an increased ability to mobilize and use fat as a fuel. Often many systems are improved by a given type of overload exercise. For example, if you were to go to a swimming pool and steadily swim several laps of the front crawl, your arm-pulling muscles would be overloaded by the repetitive pulling action against the water. After weeks and months of this type of exercise, the strength and muscle endurance of these muscles would improve. Beyond that, however, your heart and lungs and the blood vessels leading to all the muscles that are engaged in swimming the crawl would become more able to perform their specific functions. Within the active muscles changes would be occurring that improve the capacity to produce energy during exercise. The net effect of all of these latter changes would be an improvement in cardiorespiratory fitness.

Details as to the length of time required before a given overload will result in noticeable changes, and other related questions, will be discussed in Chapters 5, 6, and 7. However, another general principle, that of progressive exercise, works hand-in-hand with the overload principle. How these two principles work together will be the next topic.

Principle of Progressive Exercise

Again in most simple terms, training to improve your fitness must involve progressively increasing the overload stimulus as adaptations occur. With progressive increments of the overload stimulus, the relative degree of stress to the system is maintained at an appropriate level to continue its overload effect, regardless of the fitness status. If no such increments are employed, the improvements will be small and performance will soon level off.

A weight-lifting example will be used to illustrate why this is true (see Figure 4.3). Suppose Suzanne Weakarms decides to begin working on her upper body strength by going into the local weight room. After several days of learning about the weight room and getting some instruction on which exercises she may choose from, she finds that she can do seven repetitions of the benchpress exercise using 60 pounds of weight before she is unable to continue due to fatigue. So she sets herself up on a routine of doing seven repetitions, three days per week and leaves it at that. If she were to continue in such a manner over the course of several weeks and months, she would find that the strength and muscle endurance of the muscles she uses in benchpressing would increase. However, eventually she would stop improving and her strength and muscle endurance would plateau at the new levels they had attained.

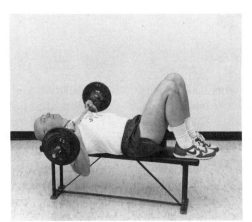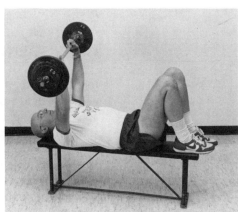

FIGURE 4.3
The "bench press" exercise.

Should Suzanne desire greater improvements in either strength or endurance, she would have to raise the overload stimulus. She might do this in one of several ways. She could do more repetitions as her capacity improves by continuing onward to eight, nine, ten or more repetitions before reaching failure instead of stopping at seven. She could do another set of seven repetitions after a rest period and later build that up to three sets per day. Alternatively, at some point she could raise the resistance to 70 pounds and later to 80 pounds. And of course, she could do any combination of the above.

The point is that after training at a given level for a period of time the stimulus becomes less of an overload because the system has adapted. For the system to continue to be overloaded at a similar level, the stimulus must be increased. This periodic raising of the overload stimulus should continue until the individual attains the desired goal or until what is needed becomes unrealistic.

The process of making progressive steps in overload during an aerobic training program is described in Figure 4.4. The progression depicted in this figure can be used as a model for developing a similar progression for any other form of training. At the beginning of a training program, we advocate a starter fitness program that involves smaller increments in overload to allow the body parts of the system being trained adequate time to adjust to being overloaded. This may last several weeks and certainly long enough for the muscles, joints, and other body parts to not feel overworked. Once this initial period has passed, progressive increments can be made in slightly larger jumps. A good rule of thumb to follow in making any increment, however, is that if the increase is noticeably more difficult than what you had been doing previously, you are probably working too hard and should ease off. Eventually, a maintenance period is reached where progressive increases in overload no longer are necessary. In fact, in some cases evidence suggests that the amount of exercise required to maintain a given level of fitness is less than that required to increase fitness. More will be discussed on this topic in Chapters 5–7.

If you are athletically inclined, or wish to attain a certain level of performance by a given date, you should know that *the harder you work, the faster your improvement will be*. In fact, this is true for any type of training and at any level, so long as you do not exceed your fitness status so much that you are unable to recover between training days. If this happens, performance will begin to fall off. Such "overtraining"

FIGURE 4.4
Progression in aerobic training has been found to be most successful if a 4–5 week, gentle, starter fitness program is undertaken first. Thereafter, increases in exercise should occur every 2–3 weeks until a level is reached that can be maintained indefinitely. For each decade after 30, increase time by 40% to allow for adaptation.

Adapted with permission of Macmillan Publishing Company from *Health and Fitness Through Physical Activity* by Pollock, M. L., Wilmore, J. H., and Fox, S. M., originally published by John Wiley & Sons, Inc. (New York: Macmillan, 1978).

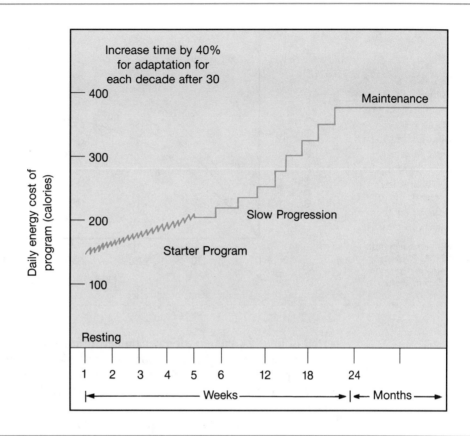

is not uncommon in athletics and can lead to injury or illness. Other signs of overtraining include sleep disturbances, excessive fatigue, and frequent incidence of illness such as colds or flu. The solution is the one that common sense would suggest: ease off in the training.

It should be noted that there is a point of diminishing return in applying what might be called the "harder you work" rule. For example, suppose John Urgentski was a devoted cross-country skier who decided to double his training from 30 minutes per day to 60 minutes per day as an overload increment. While his cardiorespiratory fitness would likely increase to a greater degree as a result, the gain would likely be less than twice that which he had been achieving previously (Figure 4.5). The same would be true if he decided to ski at a faster pace than before to overload his cardiorespiratory system, although admittedly it would be difficult for him to double his initial speed. The point is that potential gains operate on a changing "effort-scale": the greatest gains occur initially, with the least amount of effort; as the effort increases the gains also increase, but to a lesser and lesser degree.

A related phenomenon, depicted in Figure 4.5, is that improvements are inversely related to initial fitness. Those individuals with the lowest level of initial fitness will be able to increase their capacity to the greatest degree, all else being the same. Further, as you train and experience improvements from your efforts, additional improvements become more and more difficult to achieve. Again, there appears to be a point of diminishing return whereby training-induced gains approach zero after a long

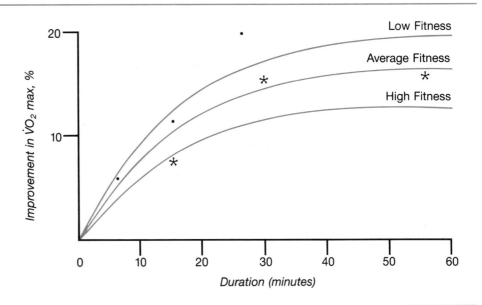

Used with permission from deVries, H. A. *Physiology of Exercise,* 4th Ed. Dubuque: Wm. C. Brown, 1986.

FIGURE 4.5
Improvements from training reflect a law of diminishing return whereby doubling the work done does not double the training effect. Note also that improvements are greater the lower the initial state of fitness.

period of time. Although each person has different limits which appear to be largely determined by genetic predispositions, little has been explored on this question. These limits appear to differ for different components of fitness; for example, strength has been known to improve training to a much greater degree than has cardiorespiratory fitness.

This brings us to the third principle of fitness, that of specificity.

Principle of Specificity

This principle states that training outcomes are specific to the type of training that is done. It applies to all types of training. Let us say, for example, you decide to develop your upper body strength by doing certain weight lifting exercises. Over time your strength will improve but only in those specific muscle groups and only when they are used in the specific ways that you train them. Thus if you had been using the vertical press exercise in which you lift a barbell over your head, you would find it easier to put heavy objects up on the top shelf or to handle anything heavy above your head. However, if you were asked to carry something heavy, such as a big box, in front of you, your greater strength will not be of much assistance since it involves different muscles and/or some of the same muscles used in different ways.

Consider the specificity principle as it applies to training the cardiorespiratory system. While there are many forms of aerobic exercise to choose from, and although each places similar demands on the heart and lungs, each different exercise involves different muscle groups than the others. Thus if you are a trained runner, you may be able to swim a long distance more easily than if you were not trained as a runner, but your ability to engage in aerobic exercise in the water will not have been enhanced as much as your capacity to do endurance exercise while running.

It is most important for the athlete to pay close attention to the specificity principle because athletic training programs should be designed to elicit the greatest gains to performance for time spent training. In such a case, training procedures must overload the body parts or body systems in ways that are very similar to how they will be used while performing. To the extent that such procedures are followed, training is likely to result in the greatest possible improvement, all else being the same.

For the average individual with specific goals, the specificity principle can also be used to devise a training program that will be cost effective. To illustrate, suppose you were interested in being able to pull yourself up over a ledge. Strength-training the specific pulling and pushing muscles of the arms and chest as they mimic such a move would be more appropriate than a general weight training program that emphasized muscle strength in a variety of muscle groups.

If your goals are not limited to certain types of performance, then in light of the specificity principle you might elect to engage in a variety of activities for training. In this manner you would be overloading many body parts and many systems in different ways. Such a comprehensive program could also involve training different fitness components. If you look around you at individuals who are fit, it is not uncommon to find those who are relatively fit in one area and relatively unfit in another. By contrast, a comprehensive training program involves training the whole body for use in a variety of ways.

The Exercise Session

When beginning an exercise session it is important always to begin by warming up and to finish by cooling down. Within the actual workout period, the arrangement of various parts of the training session can be varied. You may wonder whether the order in which you do various parts of your exercise program matters. For example, if you plan to lift weights and run, should you begin with the weights and then go running, or should it be the other way around? These and other questions will be discussed in this section on the specifics of the exercise session.

Warm-Up

Warming up your body is a process of gradually preparing it for more vigorous activity. Just as you should never start your car when it is cold and immediately "floor it" for fear that you might damage parts that need adequate lubrication and/or heat to work properly, so also with exercising your body. *You should never begin vigorous activity without a warm-up.* Your muscles, joints, and organs are designed in marvelous ways to enable you to do many things, but they require proper care and treatment and this includes proper warm-up.

A proper warm-up is important for a number of reasons. First, evidence has demonstrated that presumably healthy hearts can develop unusual patterns of electrical activity called *disrhythmias* if vigorous activity is not preceded by a warm-up. With prior warm-up, the same vigorous activity is much less likely to cause an electrical disturbance. Certain disrhythmias are particularly dangerous to the heart, so this is one of the most important reasons warm-up is recommended as a preventative measure.

A second reason for warming up gradually has to do with the muscles and joints. During vigorous activity such as in jogging/running, the muscles and joints of the lower extremities are subjected to very large forces which can lead to injury. Warming up reduces muscle *viscosity,* which is the resistance to movement. It also causes the cartilage and other tissues within the joints to absorb fluid. Both the above changes reduce the likelihood of injury occurring to these tissues.

Another positive effect of warming up is an increase in performance. This is particularly helpful for explosive tasks such as jumping, throwing, or sprinting. In fact, prior to beginning any explosive, all-out activity, warm-up is an absolute necessity not only as an aid to increased performance but also to reduce the possibility of injury.

Warm-up procedures should begin with a general warm-up of the whole body using gentle exercise such as walking, followed by a specific warm-up of the particular muscles and joints in question using light activity. A basic rule is to gradually build upward with the intensity of exercise. The length of warm-up time may vary, but 5–10 minutes is usually more than adequate.

Prior to engaging in aerobic activity, warm-up is often accomplished by beginning with the same activity except at a very slow pace. Thus if you plan to begin swimming (or jogging), start by swimming (or jogging) very easily for 5–10 minutes. Walking is always a good activity with which to precede jogging/running.

Cool-Down

Following vigorous activity you should cool down by continuing to remain active at a slow pace until your body has recovered substantially. One guideline for determining how long to cool down is a check of your heart rate, which should drop below 110–120 beats per minute. Under most circumstances, this is accomplished with 5–10 minutes of gentle activity that gradually trails off.

Reasons for cooling down before heading to the shower room include factors that relate to health and factors that relate to comfort. It has long been known that the hormones *epinephrine* and *norepinephrine* (also called adrenalin and noradrenalin) rise in concentration in the blood during exercise. Recently it has been shown that levels of these hormones continue to rise for a few minutes following exercise. Such high hormone levels stimulate the heart beat, and researchers believe that this is part of the reason why the period immediately after exercise is one of the most dangerous to people with heart disease. With the continued but light activity of a cool down period, these hormone levels can be brought down gradually rather than allowing the heart to be subjected to great stress at the same time as the skeletal muscles are recovering.

Another reason for cooling down is to avoid blood pooling in the lower extremities. This is a problem particularly when doing upright activity such as running or cycling, in which the large leg muscles have been active. Following such exercise, blood continues to be pumped to these tissues, and without continued muscular activity which pumps this blood back toward the heart, a substantial amount of blood can pool in these regions, leaving little blood in the upper extremities. The effect is a light-headed feeling which in extreme cases can even lead to fainting.

Finally, cooling down hastens recovery. Odd as it may seem, evidence shows that recovery from vigorous activity is more rapid if active cool-down is used.

The Workout

What type of exercise should you incorporate into the workout? How hard should you work, for how long, and how often? The answers to questions such as these depend on your personal goals and your starting point. However, a workout that focuses on developing the components of health-related fitness can serve as a basis for a discussion on this topic. An adequate and relatively comprehensive workout with a health-related focus can be accomplished in 45 minutes using the following guidelines:

- Warm-up: 5–10 minutes
- Workout:
     Strengthening/Flexibility Exercises   10 minutes
     Aerobic Exercise   20 minutes
- Cool Down: 5 minutes

The details of a workout such as the one outlined above may vary depending on your particular goals and needs. For example, a 45-minute workout period would certainly be too long for a beginner, and adjustments would need to be made. This outline simply provides a framework to consider when formulating your own workout. Specific recommendations for improving the various fitness components are provided in Chapters 5, 6, and 7. These chapters will provide the information necessary for you to develop a fitness program that addresses your personal circumstances and preferences.

When integrating several types of training into one workout, you may wonder which parts of your exercise routine to do first. For example, let's suppose you are interested in developing your upper body strength by working out with weights, but you do not want to let your already well-established, 30-minute aerobic exercise period slip. Should you lift weights and then do your aerobic workout, or the other way around? Is it harmful to combine two different types of training together in the same workout?

Unfortunately, there is little concrete evidence on which to base recommendations regarding these questions. Some evidence suggests that though strength training does not interfere with the benefits of cardiorespiratory exercise, you may not gain as much strength as if you trained for strength only. Experienced coaches and athletes who face this problem often use an approach that is dictated by what works best. In other words, complete the workout in whatever order feels best. If you are better able to lift weights after your aerobic workout then do the activities in that order, or vice versa. Certainly your decision should take into account which part of the total workout you deem most essential. By placing the most essential part of your workout into a place of prominence where you are less likely to be plagued by residual fatigue or other carryover that detracts from the quality of training, you are maximizing your potential for positive changes.

The Commercialization of Fitness

As a consumer, you are undoubtedly a little overwhelmed by the endless number of products generated by the fitness industry and by the choices you must make between competing products. Books written by celebrities who are marketing primarily their looks and fame compete with books written by knowledgeable professionals whose goals are increased health and fitness. Spas and health clubs whose main objective appears to be selling memberships compete with legitimate establishments whose goal it is to serve the needs of the public well. You must choose sources of information, services, and clothing and equipment, all of which carry implications for social status. As with many products and services, the best-marketed fitness products usually prove to be the most successful. Unfortunately, these are not necessarily the products with the best overall quality.

As an illustration, if you decide to purchase a pair of running shoes you will need to choose from a tremendous assortment of styles and features, and the costs will range from the barely reasonable to the exorbitant. Is the most expensive pair the one to get?

A few generalizations can be made to help you in this selective process. First, make sure that you choose a running shoe and not a walking shoe, a basketball shoe, a court shoe, or a shoe designed for everyday use. If you are interested in activities other than running, your first consideration should be to choose a shoe that is designed for the type of activity you will engage in most frequently. Choose a shoe with a width that properly fits the width of your foot. The "last" of the shoe is the form on which a shoe is built, and is readily observable by looking at the sole. The straighter the last, the more support it will provide along the inner edge of the foot. If your experience tells you that you need such support, you should choose a shoe with such a straighter last. Then look for a shoe with a reputation for a durable midsole and a durable outsole. The *midsole* refers to the cushioning layers between the upper part of the shoe and the outsole, which is the part that hits the ground.

In addition to the above generalizations, the choice of which shoe to purchase depends on a number of other factors, including your height and weight, the number of miles you run per week, whether the shoes are to be used for training or racing, and most importantly, the nature of *your* foot mechanics as your foot strikes the ground. Technically, determining which shoe is best for you considering all such requirements would require that you have a running analysis done by a competent professional using slow motion photography while you wore each of the shoe models that fit. Only then could you determine which shoe is best for your needs. This method of choosing shoes is not generally employed, of course. The point of this example is to demonstrate that it is not a simple process to determine what is best for you.

As a consumer faced with a myriad of products and services, your best bet is to read consumer-oriented literature and be as educated as possible, to ask questions of those who seek to sell you a product, and to gauge the responses against what others have told you and against what you already know. In the case of services offered, it would be wise to ask about the training and experience of the service-giver, including a question as to whether he/she is certified and by what organization. Even the question of certification is a difficult one to answer satisfactorily since more than fifty organizations offer training and certification. Some of these are reputable and nationally recognized organizations; others are not. As the Latin phrase *caveat emptor* warns, "buyer beware"!

Common Problems Relating to Exercise

It is not uncommon for an individual to begin an exercise program with good intentions, only to develop some type of injury due to improper exercise techniques. This can be very discouraging. If properly treated and responded to, however, many injuries can be overcome without major inconvenience. This next section will discuss several common injuries and their treatments. Common postural problems that may be aggravated by improper exercise will also be discussed.

Muscle Soreness

The muscular pain that you feel a day or two after doing some form of strenuous exercise to which you are not accustomed is by far the most common fitness-related injury. Muscle soreness gradually subsides and in most cases is gone within 4-6 days. Recent evidence suggests that such soreness is caused by damage to the muscle cells and/or connective tissue that runs through muscle. The ways in which this damage alters the normal physiological activity within the muscle is not understood, but in one way or another nerve endings are stimulated and pain results.

Muscle soreness is not to be confused with the weakness and "burning" feeling you may experience when you exercise a muscle heavily and become fatigued. This immediate muscle fatigue itself is not fully understood, but it seems to be partly related to the build-up of a by-product of heavy exercise called *lactic acid*. Lactic acid does not seem to be implicated in the muscle soreness that appears 1–3 days following exercise, however, since it disappears from the muscles during the recovery period, usually within 1–2 hours.

Since both fit and unfit individuals become sore following any form of strenuous exercise to which they are not accustomed, it appears that muscle soreness cannot be avoided. However, an adequate warm-up before and cool down after engaging in vigorous activity should reduce its severity. Another suggestion for minimizing muscle soreness is to build up slowly in your exercise program, never subjecting your muscles to an excessively large strain to which they are not accustomed. Fortunately, once muscles begin to adapt to the stress of vigorous exercise, they do not become sore again unless they are used in different ways, in which case they are subject to new areas of soreness.

Once you are sore, the best method to reduce the severity appears to be gentle static stretching and low level muscular activity. Unfortunately, the pain will not totally disappear following exercise. As with most musculo-skeletal injuries, damp heat—as in a hot bath or whirlpool—can be used to stimulate local circulation, which will also hasten healing time.

Muscle Strains

Muscle strains are severe tears to the muscle fibers and surrounding tissues. They often occur in the quadriceps and hamstring muscles on the front and back of the leg respectively, or in the muscles of the groin, probably because of the large forces that these muscles are able to generate. They also occur in the muscles of the back due to improper lifting techniques and inadequate strength. The treatment for such an injury is rest and intermittent application of ice and pressure to the affected area to minimize hemorrhage. After a few days, providing there is no pain during activity, a gradual rehabilitative exercise program can begin. The program should emphasize full range of movement following application of cold to the affected area. Medical assistance should certainly be sought if the injury is severe and/or recovery does not occur in the expected manner. Adequate rest and the avoidance of vigorous activity until recovery is complete are vital if reinjury is to be avoided.

Tendinitis

Whenever a muscle is overused and/or overstretched, the connective tissue that attaches the muscle to the bone can become irritated and inflamed. This inflammation is called *tendinitis,* and the usual symptoms are pain during movement, tenderness to touch, and weakness, particularly when stretching. Tendinitis commonly occurs in the Achilles tendon in runners and in the shoulders of swimmers. Treatment includes rest and repeated applications of cold, moist heat, and gradual stretching 2–3 times per day. Cold can be applied by using icepacks for 15–20 minutes at a time. Moist heat can be applied through a warm shower, a hot tub or bath, or a damp, warm cloth under a hot-water bottle, for up to 20–30 minutes.

Postural Problems

Exercise can aggravate chronic strain that arises from postural problems. In correct posture the segments of the body (head, spine, pelvic girdle, upper leg, and lower leg) are aligned vertically one over the other as shown in Figure 4.6. If the normally occurring curvature of the spine becomes exaggerated, the additional stress of exercise can aggravate the strain of gravity on the affected muscles, tendons, and vertebra, particularly if the exercise is weight-supported, as in running or jogging.

Several common postural problems are illustrated in the panels of Figure 4.7. Such problems can be detected through a posture evaluation performed by a trained technician, which will indicate whether you have postural deviations similar to those depicted in Figure 4.8. In Chapter 6 we present several postural enhancement exercises that are designed to help strengthen key muscles in regions of common postural deviation. Since posture is also a matter of practice, another treatment for postural problems is to practice maintaining correct alignment and learn to do so continuously, a tactic that may be difficult but can lead to the prevention of much greater problems at a later date.

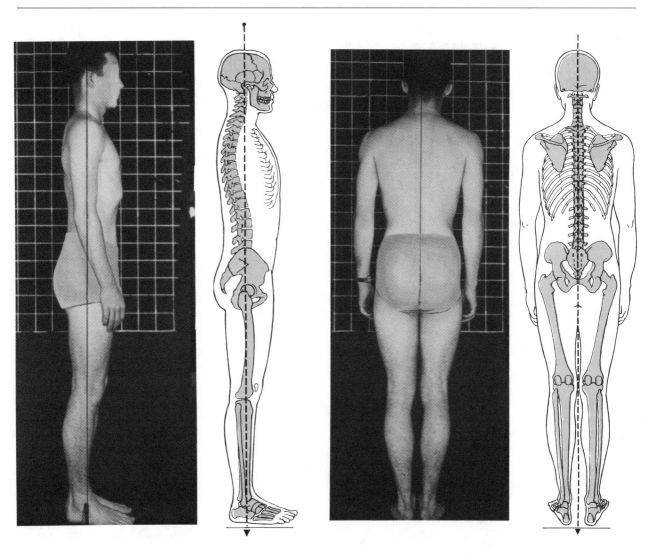

Lateral View   **Posterior View**

FIGURE 4.6
The skeletal form of a
person with good
standing posture.

Used with permission from
Kendall, H. D., Kendall, F. P.,
and Wadsworth, G. E.
Muscles, Testing and Function,
2nd Ed. Baltimore: Williams
and Wilkins, 1971.

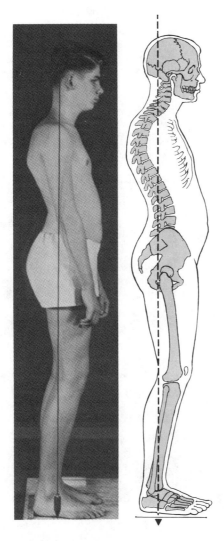
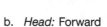
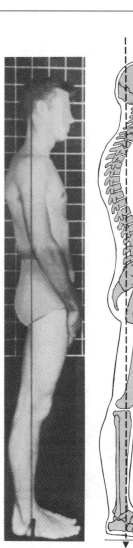

FIGURE 4.7
Four examples of common postural problems.

Used with permission from Kendall, H. D., Kendall, F. P., and Wadsworth, G. E. *Muscles, Testing and Function*, 2nd Ed. Baltimore: Williams and Wilkins, 1971.

a. *Head:* Forward

    Cervical vertebrae: Hyperextended

    Thoracic vertebrae: Increased flexion

    Lumbar vertebrae: Hyperextended

    Pelvis: Forward tilt

    Hips: Flexed

    Knees: Flexed

    Ankles: Dorsiflexed due to knee flexion causing leg to incline forward from ankle.

b. *Head:* Forward

    Cervical vertebrae: Hyperextended

    Thoracic vertebrae: Added flexion and increased curvature

    Pelvis: Backward tilt

    Hips: Hyperextended

    Knees: Hyperextended

    Ankles: Neutral

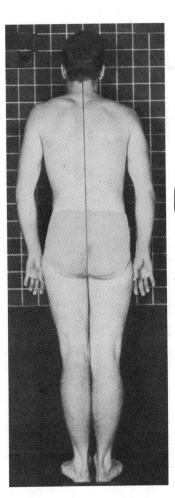
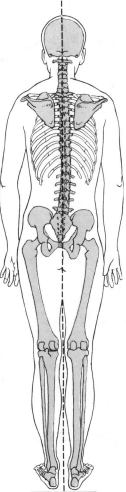
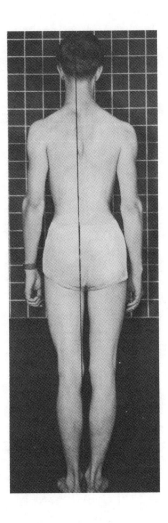
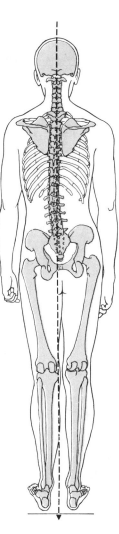

c.   *Head:* Proper alignment, not tilted or
rotated

Cervical vertebrae: Vertically aligned

Shoulders: Hunched or elevated

Shoulder joints: Rotated inward as
indicated by position of hands facing
backwards

Thoracic and lumbar vertebrae: Lateral
flexion of vertebral column toward left

Pelvis: Slightly higher on left

Hips: Left, shifted toward midline; right,
shifted away from midline

Feet: Slightly pronated

d.   *Head:* Good alignment, not tilted or
rotated

Cervical vertebrae: Vertically aligned

Shoulders: Lower on right

Scapulae: Lower on right

Thoracic and lumbar vertebrae: Lateral
flexion of vertebral column toward right

Pelvis: Higher on right

Hip joints: Right, shifted toward midline;
left, shifted away from midline

Lower extremities: Proper alignment

Feet: Both slightly pronated

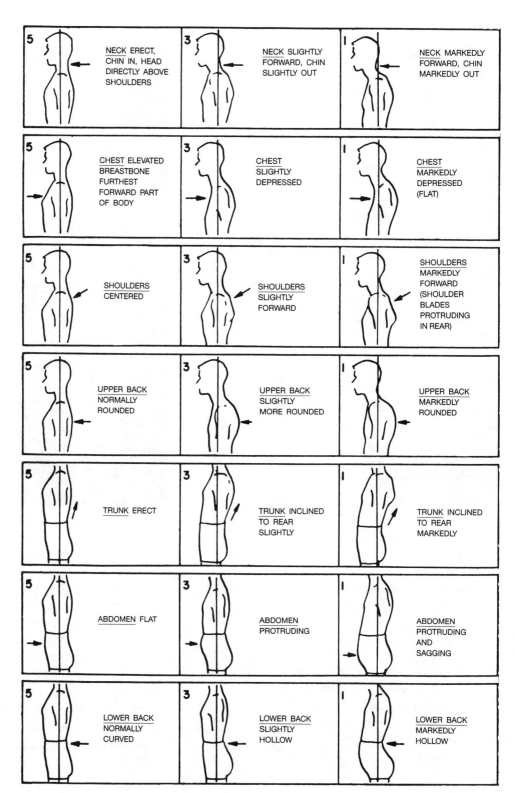

FIGURE 4.8
Posture evaluation chart.

Used with permission of Random House, Inc. & Alfred A. Knopf, Inc. Figure from: Wiseman, D.C. *A Practical Approach to Adapted Physical Education*. Reading, MA: Addison-Wesley, 1982.

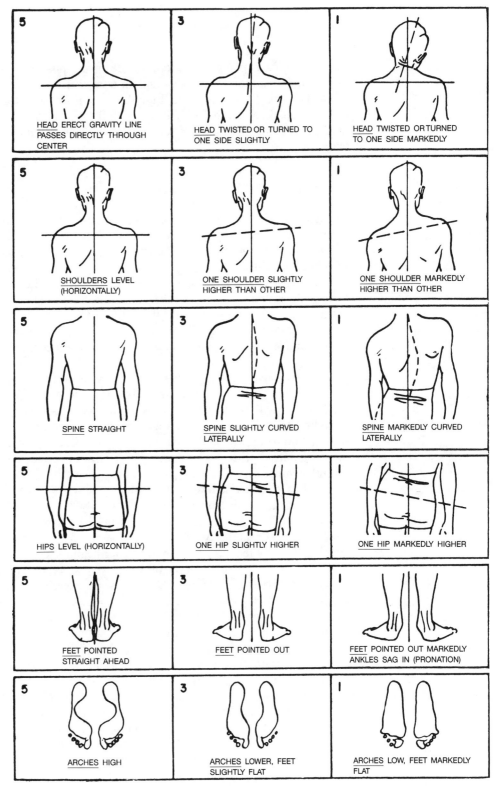

FIGURE 4.8
Posture evaluation chart.
(continued)

Environmental Considerations

The environment plays an important role in the pursuit of fitness since it is a rare luxury to find a mild, sunny day and an attractive setting in which to exercise. More often than not, it is cold, wet, humid, hot, or smoggy and you must adapt to the environmental conditions at hand. In the following section we will offer some general guidelines about what to do in such conditions, including the selection of clothing for exercise.

Heat, Humidity, and Fluid Requirements

The control of body temperature is one of the vital functions that must be closely regulated within narrow limits for health to be maintained. Exercise causes core temperature to rise, particularly if the exercise is vigorous and sustained for long periods of time. This effect is accentuated dramatically if the exercise is performed in a warm or hot environment. The immediate effect of this rise in temperature is for the body to initiate several heat loss mechanisms, including: (1) redirecting blood toward the surface of the body, causing the skin to appear red or flushed, and (2) the secretion and evaporation of sweat. This evaporative process cools the surface of the body and the blood passing through it, and this helps maintain core temperature within tolerable limits.

Several factors influence the evaporative process, including air currents, environmental temperature, humidity, and clothing. The greater the air currents, the more easily sweat will evaporate. Also, as temperature goes up during the day, the relative humidity drops. These two changes tend to offset each other to some degree: as temperature increases the thermal load on you will rise, but as relative humidity drops the evaporative process is enhanced. The overall effect on you depends on which change is greatest.

Unless you choose to exercise inside an air-conditioned gym, you cannot control the weather; but both temperature and humidity are still partly under your control as an exerciser. You can choose to exercise in places and at times of the day when the temperature and humidity are least hostile, such as in the early morning or in the evening, thereby reducing the threat to your health and well-being. You can choose to reduce the intensity or duration of your exercise or both. You can also choose the amount and type of clothing you wear while exercising. Any time that you are in danger of becoming overheated you should adjust your clothing appropriately to allow for the greatest possible heat loss. This includes taking off clothing and/or choosing clothing that "breathes" (i.e., allows water vapor to pass outward through it). Cotton is a good example of a material that breathes well.

Any garment that prevents or restricts the passage of air over the large surfaces of the body and head should never be worn during exercise in the heat or even in mild temperature because of the danger of overheating. This is especially true of rubber suits, which are still used occasionally as a means of losing weight rapidly. Such suits effectively eliminate evaporation; in an attempt to counteract this, the body releases excessive amounts of sweat. The effect is a dehydration of the body that can be a major threat to health if carried to extremes.

To offset the evaporative water loss, fluids must be replaced irrespective of thirst sensations. Under extreme conditions, waiting for thirst to dictate when to drink can be dangerous because thirst mechanisms are very slow to respond. Ideally, fluids should be replaced as they are lost in the form of cool water. While some commercially prepared drinks are satisfactory as replacement fluids, others contain sugar, which is detrimental when replacing fluids in the heat. Sugar slows the passage of fluid from the stomach into the intestine, thereby delaying its reabsorption. It is unnecessary to replace lost electolytes such as sodium and potassium during exercise as they can be replaced adequately later. All in all, commercially prepared drinks are unnecessary and some may even be counterproductive; the most important goal is to replace lost water and the best way to achieve this is to drink cool water.

If core temperature rises too high because of inadequate cooling, heat exhaustion and an even more dangerous condition called heat stroke can result. Both are very dangerous and first aid should be administered immediately. Proper first aid includes: (1) resting the individual in a cool environment with clothing removed; (2) administering cold fluids to drink; (3) in the case of heat stroke where body temperature is dramatically elevated, immediately cooling the individual by whatever means are available—e.g., cold shower, hose, cool water, pool; and (4) notifying an emergency vehicle and local hospital of a possible heat casualty.

Cold

Cold temperature, particularly if accompanied by wind that exaggerates the wind-chill factor, presents another problem for the exerciser. Just as excess heat must be eliminated so that core temperature does not rise precipitously, the core temperature must also be protected from dropping when the body is threatened by heat loss. Because exercise creates a warming effect, you can tolerate colder temperatures while exercising; however, certain body parts tend to be more vulnerable than others and they warrant protection. These include the hands and head, the latter giving off a large proportion of the total heat that is lost. It is important to keep these parts of the body covered adequately in cold temperatures. The remainder of the body should be covered with one or more layers of clothing that can be removed as comfort dictates. If wind is a factor, a garment that is impermeable to wind with sleeves and a collar that can be cinched up is particularly helpful. There seems to be no danger to the lungs from exercising in cold temperatures. Comfort should always be considered, however.

Air Quality

The majority of people live in an urban environment where air pollutants are emitted into the air in large quantities. Some pollutants such as carbon monoxide limit the ability to do aerobic exercise by reducing the oxygen-carrying capacity of the blood, an effect that is evident in smokers, whose lungs are exposed routinely to large quantities of this pollutant. Other pollutants such as ozone cause eye irritation, chest tightness, and pain that interfere with aerobic exercise. The effect of many such pollutants is dependent on their concentration and on the length of time you are exposed, with the impact being partly a function of how heavily you breathe. Therefore, it is wise on high-pollution days to avoid those times of the day when pollutants are likely to be highest and exercise at times when the levels are likely to be lowest. Often, but not always, pollution is highest in mid to late afternoon and lowest in early morning.

Individual Differences:
The Decision Process and Fitness

What would it take to be physically prepared for all eventualities? Is it cost effective in terms of time, effort, and the probability of an unusual and taxing event occurring? How much exercise should you get to avoid gradually increasing fatness or greater risk of cardiovascular disease? What would it take to be able to backpack without excessive fatigue, or ski without having to pace yourself or quit early? The behavior patterns that make up your current lifestyle are partly determined by the answers you have given to questions such as these in the past. The answer you give today and tomorrow will determine your behavior on such issues in the future, for what becomes of you is very much a matter of personal choice.

For some people, the time required to train is not worth the gain. For others, the effort is too much to put themselves through on a regular basis. Many believe that a high level of fitness is not really necessary in day-to-day life. Or, they find that there are too many things to think about on the issue of health and fitness and so they avoid dealing with any of it.

Should you decide to engage actively in the development and maintenance of fitness, the range of choices open to you is wide. It encompasses not only the different components of fitness, but also differences in what form of exercise to do as well as how long, how hard, and how often to exercise.

Attaining a high level of fitness at one time in your life does not protect you from the negative effects of sedentary living *unless you maintain your fitness by working on it regularly.* The pursuit of fitness requires ongoing commitment. Even for those who are diligent in this regard, there are no guarantees of health because aging is unavoidable and many chronic diseases have multiple causes, some of which you can make choices about and some of which you cannot.

It is a fair generalization to say that those who are most successful at developing a lifestyle that includes a commitment to fitness are people who have incorporated fitness activities into their interests and individual circumstances. If their daily schedule requires them to rise and depart early, they make time for exercise during the day, perhaps at the lunch hour or right after work. If they find it difficult to exercise very regularly during the week, they do so on the weekends and pick up the slack by doing one or two workouts during the work week. If they enjoy tennis or racquetball more than jogging, they join a club that offers such facilities and make arrangements for games with suitable partners ahead of time. They take opportunities to engage in exercise, such as walking instead of driving short distances, or choosing the stairs instead of the elevator, or working in the garden on a nice day. In short, they seek out rather than avoid exercise whenever and wherever the opportunity presents itself, and they do so in ways that bring enjoyment into their lives in keeping with their interests and preferences.

In the final analysis, it comes down to a personal choice. People who are fit made a decision to engage regularly in the development and maintenance of fitness, and they continue to reaffirm that decision on a regular basis. That decision may change at any time, for a variety of reasons. However, those who are committed find ways to follow through, to stay with it over the long haul.

As you consider what is being discussed in this book on the topic of exercise you should formulate your own decision. If you decide to attain and maintain fitness, the specifics of tailoring the forms of exercise to your needs and interests will follow. You are encouraged to do what works for you, to find the particular mix of activities you find pleasurable and satisfactory. The role of enjoyment in exercise should not be underestimated since it is difficult to sustain the commitment to anything if it does not bring you pleasure.

Only you can know what is best for you, only you can make the decision of whether you want to be fit, and only you can muster the necessary commitment to follow through. Perhaps you already have made a commitment to fitness, or perhaps you are considering making such a decision. The next few chapters will present the tools and basic knowledge that can be used to individualize a fitness program in light of your personal needs.

Summary

The capacity to meet the demands of modern day life with little strain is what is meant by physical fitness in its most general terms. More specifically, physical fitness can be broken down into components, some of which are more closely related to health and others which are more closely related to physical performance. The components of health-related fitness include cardiorespiratory fitness, body composition, strength, muscle endurance, and flexibility of the lower back and hip region. Performance-related fitness components include flexibility in other regions of the body, power, speed, and agility. Physical performance is also strongly influenced by the health-related components of fitness.

By taxing yourself within appropriate limits you can improve any of the fitness components. Such an overload must be regular and must include progressive increments in workload if improvements are to occur. Maintenance of any improvements that you achieve requires continued exercise without further increments in workload. The degree of improvement is partly determined by genetic factors but is also influenced by how hard you are willing to work and your initial level of fitness. To achieve a specific goal relating to exercise or to physical performance requires training in ways that specifically mimic the intended outcome.

Exercise sessions should always begin with a 5–10 minute warm-up and end with a cool down of sufficient length to allow substantial recovery. Injuries such as muscle soreness, muscular strains, tendinitis as well as many relating to poor posture often can be prevented. If they occur a prompt and specific therapeutic response should be made. Excessive heat and humidity can accelerate the fluid losses of the exercising person. Adjustments in clothing, fluid replacement, and how much exercise you do should be made to prevent heat exhaustion and heat stroke. When exercising in the cold, appropriate clothing should be used to prevent excessive heat loss, especially from the hands and head. Avoid or reduce the amount of exercise if the air pollutant levels are high. Individualizing your exercise to fit your talents, circumstances, and interests, especially if you find ways to make it bring you joy, will assist you in adopting and maintaining regular exercise habits. The decision rests with you.

References

Armstrong, R. B. 1984. Mechanism of exercise induced delayed onset muscular soreness: A brief review. *Medicine and Science in Sports and Exercise* 16:529-538.

Barnard, R., Gardner, G., Diaco, N., MacAlpin, R., and Kattus, A. 1973. Cardiovascular responses to sudden strenuous exercise—heart rate, blood pressure, and ECG. *Journal of Applied Physiology* 34(6):833-837.

Barham, J. N. and Wooten, E. P. 1973. *Structural kinesiology.* New York: Macmillan.

Brumick, T. 1986. On your feet. *Runners World* 21:13-15.

Fox, E. L., and Mathews, D. K. 1981. *The physiological basis of physical education and athletics.* 3rd Ed., 270-273. Philadelphia: Saunders College.

Hickson, H. C. 1980. Interference of strength development by simultaneously training for strength and endurance. *European Journal of Applied Physiology.* 45:255-263.

Kendall, H. O., Kendall, F. P., and Wadsworth, G. E. 1971. *Muscles: testing and function.* 2nd Ed., Baltimore: Williams and Wilkins.

Klafs, C. E. and Arnheim, D. D. 1981. *Modern principles of athletic training.* 5th Ed., 283-293. St. Louis: C. V. Mosby.

Paffenbarger, R. S., Hyde, R. T., Wing, A. L., and Hsieh, C. 1986. Physical activity, all cause mortality, and longevity of college alumni. *New England Journal of Medicine.* 314:605-613.

Nash, H. L. 1985. Instructor certification: Making fitness programs safer? *Physician and Sportsmedicine.* 13(10):142-155.

Raven, P. B. 1980. Effects of air pollution on physical performance. In *Encyclopedia of physical education, fitness, and sports: Training, environment, nutrition, and fitness,* ed. G. A. Stull and T. K. Cureton, Jr., 201-216. Salt Lake City: Brighton Publishing Co.

Wiseman, D. C. 1982. *A practical approach to adapted physical education.* Reading, Mass.: Addison-Wesley.

5

The Heart of the Matter: Cardiorespiratory Fitness

Why is cardiorespiratory fitness said to be the most important component of fitness for good health?

Do you know what your cardiorespiratory fitness is? What tests can you use to determine your level of cardiorespiratory fitness, and what precautions should you take?

To improve your cardiorespiratory fitness, what type of exercise do you need to do? How often, how hard, and how long should you exercise?

How do factors such as initial fitness and age affect the degree of improvement you will experience from training? What about genetic differences?

How can you motivate yourself to exercise regularly?

Introduction

If you wish to optimize your health status, regular exercise offers a variety of benefits. This chapter begins with evidence linking cardiorespiratory fitness to health, cardiovascular disease, and aging. Methods to assess your cardiorespiratory fitness status are then presented, followed by an overview of the guidelines to follow in developing and maintaining this type of fitness.

The Relation of Cardiorespiratory Fitness to Cardiovascular Disease (CVD)

Regular aerobic exercise has been shown to have a number of favorable effects on the cardiorespiratory system in healthy individuals. Some of these important benefits are summarized in Table 5.A. Improvements in the functional status of the cardiorespiratory system can be thought of as leading toward improved health. Included in Table 5.A are benefits that have been documented to occur in older individuals with mean age greater than 60 years.

Evidence linking CVD to lack of exercise (low cardiorespiratory fitness) is both direct and indirect. Epidemiological evidence has long indicated that active persons have a considerably lower risk of developing cardiovascular disease, and if they do develop the disease, it is less severe and there is a lower mortality rate. This has been demonstrated in persons who are more active on the job (as with manual labor) as well as in persons with sedentary occupations who are active in leisure-time pursuits, such as a personal fitness program.

Exercise yields positive effects for several reasons. For one, regular aerobic exercise has been shown to have a favorable effect on plasma lipids and lipoproteins. Cross-sectional studies comparing aerobically trained individuals to untrained individuals and longitudinal studies of people undergoing cardiorespiratory training have demonstrated that endurance training slightly lowers the forms of cholesterol that are harmful (VLDL and LDL), and raises the form of cholesterol that is helpful (HDL). (Refer back to Chapter 3 for a discussion of these forms of cholesterol.) Total cholesterol concentrations may be lowered by exercise, but for unknown reasons this does not always occur. The ratios of total plasma cholesterol to HDL cholesterol and plasma LDL cholesterol to HDL cholesterol are reduced. In addition, plasma triglyceride concentrations tend to be low as well. All of these changes are favorable and in line with a reduced risk of cardiovascular disease.

Although the above generalizations are supported by the sum of evidence to date, for reasons that are as yet unclear, not all studies have found such favorable changes. Further research is needed before firm conclusions can be reached. For example, some of the above-noted changes may not be the direct result of exercise but rather the result of changes that accompany regular exercise (such as a reduction in body fat, which has been suggested as a potential mechanism for inducing such changes). Recent evidence tentatively suggests that a threshold for achieving such favorable changes in lipid profile is as low as 10 miles of running/jogging per week.

Table 5.A   The effects of endurance training on physiological functions.

ORGAN/SYSTEM	CHANGES IN YOUNGER AND MIDDLE-AGED ADULTS	CHANGES IN OLDER ADULTS
Resting values		
oxygen consumption	unchanged	
blood pumped from heart/min	unchanged	
heart rate	decrease	decrease
blood ejected from heart/beat	increase	
blood pressure	unchanged/decrease	decrease
work of heart	decrease	
muscle capillary density	increase	
size of deepest breath	increase	increase
Submaximal values*		
oxygen consumption	unchanged/decrease	
blood pumped from heart/min.	unchanged	unchanged/increase
heart rate	decrease	decrease
blood ejected from heart/beat	increase	unchanged/increase
blood pressure	decrease	
work of heart	decrease	decrease
Maximal values		
oxygen uptake	increase	increase
blood pumped from heart/min.	increase	
heart rate	unchanged/decrease	unchanged
blood ejected from heart/beat	increase	
oxygen unloaded to tissues	increase	
ventilation capacity	increase	increase
blood pressure	unchanged	
work of heart	unchanged	
ability to do endurance exercise	increased	increased

*Measured at the same absolute workload before and after training.

Pollock, Wilmore & Fox, 1984; deVries, 1980; Fox & Mathews, 1981.

Several other factors may help explain the favorable effect of exercise on the cardiorespiratory system. First, hypertension seems to be reduced modestly by regular aerobic activity. Endurance activity has also been associated with reductions in stress and anxiety and with facilitating recovery from mild depression. Cigarette smoking tends to be reduced in smokers who adopt a physically active lifestyle. Exercise increases the body's tendency to break down clots that form in the blood. Obesity, which is a secondary risk factor for cardiovascular disease, is also favorably influenced by aerobic activity.

Cardiorespiratory training has been found to result in an enlarged and stronger heart, particularly in the left ventricle, which pumps blood into the aorta. A stronger heart can work harder and pump blood more efficiently at all levels of exercise. Figure 5.1 depicts the heart and circulatory system. Research on animals, which cannot be done on humans for obvious reasons, suggests that aerobic training brings about a growth in the number of capillaries feeding the heart, a positive effect. Also, changes in the coronary circulation have been documented, including an increase in total size and increased cross-sectional area in the main coronary arteries.

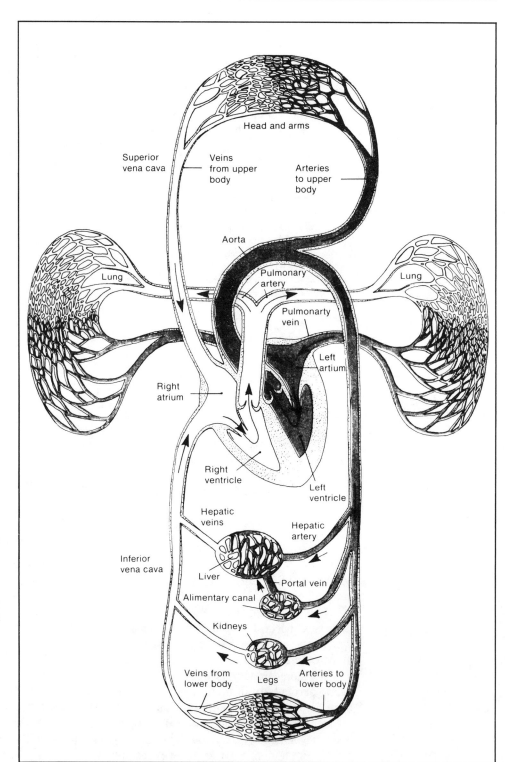

FIGURE 5.1

A schematic diagram of the cardiovascular system, which consists of the heart and the blood vessels leading to and from the lungs and other tissues. The dark shading indicates the oxygen-rich arterial blood, while the white areas indicate the paler, partially deoxygenated venous blood.

Used with permission from McArdle, W. D., Katch, F. I., and Katch, V. L. *Exercise Physiology,* 2nd Ed. Philadelphia: Lea and Febiger, 1986.

Regular aerobic exercise can also be of benefit in the health management and treatment of people who are known to suffer from cardiovascular disease. For example, supervised exercise is often prescribed for persons following bypass surgery or a heart attack. Aerobic exercise is also being used more and more in the management of diabetes, one of the risk factors of cardiovascular disease. Many of the favorable results of training that occur in healthy individuals have not been found to occur regularly in patients with cardiovascular disease, but nonetheless the work capacity of these patients has been shown to improve consistently before chest pain or other difficulties arise. This enables the ill person to return to a more normal lifestyle, which makes a big contribution to his/her quality of life. Recent evidence suggests a 25–30 percent improvement in mortality rates among exercisers engaged in a cardiac rehabilitation program compared to those who do not exercise. The effect of physical activity appears to be greatest during the first two years after a coronary event.

The Relation of Cardiorespiratory Fitness to the Effects of Aging

As noted in Chapter 3, a number of important physiological changes relating to cardiorespiratory fitness occur as we grow older. In the circulatory system, the maximum heart rate declines as does the heart's ability to pump blood at all levels of exercise. Breathing becomes less efficient because of a loss of elasticity in the lungs and chest wall, causing older people to breathe more heavily at all levels of exercise. The net effect of such changes is a lowered ability to consume and deliver oxygen to exercising muscles. The ability to consume oxygen is a good indicator of physical work capacity, which helps to explain why older people are unable to maintain the same level of work as when they were younger. Another reason for a gradual lowering of work capacity is the loss of muscle mass and the accompanying increase in fat mass that typically occurs with age. Resting blood pressure tends to rise with increasing age as well.

It should be noted that while the losses described above are generally related to aging, such changes may also occur because of a decline in exercise habits with increased age. True age changes cannot be avoided for the most part; however, you can exercise control over those changes that occur due to a poor environment or to poor stimulation, such as inadequate exercise, should you decide to take some preventative action.

Regular exercise by older people can have a number of beneficial effects on the physiological functions involved with cardiorespiratory fitness, as indicated earlier in Table 5.A. Though we do not have as much information to draw upon as we do with other age groups, nearly all the changes documented in older people are similar in kind to those changes that occur in adults of younger ages. The changes appear to occur more slowly, and the degree of improvement on an absolute scale is less. However, when expressed as a percent of initial capacity, the improvement in older individuals seems to be about the same.

Some longitudinal evidence on training in middle-aged adults is particularly worth noting. Over a ten year period, persons who regularly engaged in a moderate amount of aerobic exercise did not experience the usual 9–15 percent decline in standard measures of cardiorespiratory fitness that otherwise would have occurred during this time period. While it would be foolish to conclude from such findings that so long as you maintain a regular aerobic exercise program you will never decline, the data do illustrate that much can be done to maintain high levels of cardiorespiratory fitness at all ages.

A recent epidemiological study indicates that regular physical activity is also associated with decreased mortality rates from all causes. The benefits were proportional to the amount of activity, independent of hypertension, cigarette smoking, extremes or gains in body weight, and early parental death. Physical activity was defined as mild exercise such as walking, stair climbing, or sports play, suggesting that relatively low levels of activity can make significant contributions to longevity. At the present time, however, researchers are not in agreement as to how vigorous the exercise has to be for beneficial effects to be observed.

Though the exact relationship of cardiorespiratory training to overall *health* in older adults is difficult to establish, we can certainly verify that such training helps our overall fitness and thus helps us to function better. Presumably everyone would like to be able to function to his/her fullest capacity. It has been demonstrated that a 50-year-old person who maintains his/her cardiorespiratory fitness through regular exercise can attain the fitness status equivalent to that of many sedentary persons who are 25–30 years younger. As you contemplate your lifestyle and assess your personal goals, you might consider that while the evidence to date does not unequivocally indicate that maintaining a high level of cardiorespiratory fitness will enable you to live *longer*, it will certainly enable you to live more *fully*.

Assessing Your Cardiorespiratory Fitness

Before embarking on a training program designed to improve your cardiorespiratory fitness, it is wise to determine your current fitness status. This will enable you to measure the degree of improvement you experience from your training by charting your progress along the way. Such a record can provide considerable motivation! A complete assessment of your current health status is important for another reason: people are sometimes unaware of preexisting conditions that might put them at risk when doing vigorous exercise, and a thorough examination should reveal any possible problems.

What preexisting conditions should concern you? If you have symptoms of cardiovascular disease, such as chest pain or shortness of breath, or a previous history of CVD, you are strongly advised to complete a medical evaluation before beginning an exercise program. Such an evaluation would include having both a resting and exercise electrocardiogram (ECG) on a "graded exercise test." Such a medical evaluation is also recommended if you have one or more of the primary risk factors for CVD: cigarette smoking, resting blood pressure above 145/95, and/or a total cholesterol/HDL cholesterol ratio above 5. Still other risk factors that should prompt a preliminary medical evaluation include diabetes, an abnormal resting ECG, or a family history of artherosclerotic disease prior to age 50. If such conditions as those listed above are not present, the risks for most apparently healthy persons under the age of 45 are relatively low. This means an elaborate and expensive evaluation is probably not necessary, even though under ideal conditions undergoing such tests would be the safest for all concerned.

In males, the risk for CVD increases rapidly after the age of 45. Recent evidence suggests that it would be prudent for any previously sedentary male this age or older to have a preliminary medical evaluation such as the one described above before beginning an exercise program. This is true even if there are no symptoms or risk factors. For females, a test is recommended for those 50 and older.

The term *graded exercise test* (GXT) refers to a test in which the individual is required to exercise in gradual increments on a treadmill or a bicycle ergometer (which is a tool for measuring work capacity) until he/she is unable to continue or until symptoms warrant terminating the test. Normally, the individual has chest electrodes attached to an electrocardiograph, which monitors the electrical events of the heart at all levels of exercise to determine whether it is safe to exercise at similar levels on the field. Occasionally, the amount of oxygen the individual consumes is also measured during a GXT by analyzing the contents of the exhaled air. By measuring the amount of oxygen consumed under conditions of maximal exercise, the *maximum oxygen intake* of the individual can be determined. This is commonly referred to as the individual's *aerobic capacity* or $\dot{V}O_2$ *max*. Most authorities agree that an accurate measure of aerobic capacity is the best single measure of cardiorespiratory fitness.

Detailed descriptions of GXT procedures and how to measure $\dot{V}O_2$ max will not be given here, but we will describe those tests of cardiorespiratory fitness that can be administered easily and without expensive equipment. Should you need further information about the more technical tests, your personal physician can refer you to a place where you can obtain a GXT. Many well-equipped human performance or exercise physiology laboratories can complete a test of your $\dot{V}O_2$ max.

Tests of Cardiorespiratory Fitness

Submaximal Tests

There are several methods of estimating your cardiorespiratory fitness submaximally. The term *submaximal* refers to a test that does not require you to push yourself to the limits of your exercise tolerance. Submaximal testing is often used in field conditions for a variety of reasons: (1) the tests can be administered in a short period of time; (2) they are safer to the participant; (3) they do not require instruments that are unusually sophisticated and/or expensive; and (4) in some cases they can be administered to large groups of people all at the same time, making them convenient and inexpensive. The most common tests require you to repeatedly step up and down on a bench under controlled conditions or to ride a bicycle ergometer under standard conditions.

Such tests do not provide direct or exact measurements of aerobic capacity; instead they allow you to *estimate* your cardiorespiratory fitness. These tests require you to count how many times your heart beats in response to a standard amount of exercise, which allows you to *predict* your aerobic capacity. While such predictions are accurate when applied to large groups of individuals, they are not exactly accurate when applied to each individual (i.e., you). Error can also result if the testing procedure is not followed accurately. The size of the error is commonly described by computing the *standard error of the estimate* when the test is first developed and/or validated. Since there is no easy way of determining the actual degree of error for you personally, it is safest to recognize that such tests provide only a rough approximation of your aerobic capacity. If you require a more exact determination, you will need to go to a laboratory that can directly measure $\dot{V}O_2$ max.

Despite the error problems discussed above, such general testing can be very useful to you. If you compare your results *now* to your results *at a later date*, then whatever improvements you make will be just as visible as if you had completed a more sophisticated testing procedure. Your results may be off to an unknown degree in absolute value, but the error will remain constant over time and in a sense will be cancelled out when you determine the degree of change that has occurred.

Step Tests.   There are several types of step tests. Two of the more commonly used ones include the *Queen's College Step Test* and the step test used in the *Canadian Test of Fitness*. Specific details of how to administer each are found in Appendix 1, "Tests of Cardiorespiratory Fitness." These two tests are presented because they have been widely used and are easy to administer. The Queen's College Step Test involves stepping up and down at a fixed rate for three minutes; the Canadian step test involves 3 sequential 3 minute trials of stepping up and down from a 2-step bench.

The Queen's College Step Test is particularly useful because it uses as the step the standard bleacher found in most schools and gymnasiums. The standard error of estimate for this test is $\pm$ 8%. Standards against which to compare yourself are also provided in Appendix 1. The norms and prediction equations used to compute aerobic capacity are based on data from college-age men and women and will be accurate only if you fall into this category. If applied to middle-aged or older individuals, the predicted aerobic capacity would likely be overestimated on this test. One way to understand how to interpret the standard error for this or any other test is to examine some simple numbers. An example is provided in Table 5.B for this purpose. It should be obvious from Table 5.B that such predictive tests do not permit you to estimate your true $\dot{V}O_2$ max with great accuracy. Again, they provide only a rough estimate of your aerobic capacity, which can be useful for screening or as a reference point when used on a periodic basis.

It should be noted that on occasion an individual taking this test will find that he/she falls above the 100th percentile without being particularly active or fit. Assuming there is no measurement error, this usually means that compared to others this

---

Table 5.B   Sample calculations illustrating use of standard error of estimate in making predictions.

Given:	John's predicted $\dot{V}O_2$ max on Test A = 46.7 ml/kg/min Standard error of estimate for this test = 8%
Interpretation:	With a standard error of estimate of 8%, this means that there is a 68% chance that John's true $\dot{V}O_2$ max falls within $\pm$ 8% of his predicted score and a 95% chance that it falls within $\pm$ 16% of his predicted score. Translating this into units of oxygen:

$$.08\,(46.7) \;=\; 3.7\,\text{ml/kg/min}$$
$$.16\,(46.7) \;=\; 7.4\,\text{ml/kg/min}$$

Therefore, the probability is that John's true $\dot{V}O_2$ max is

(at the 68% level)	=	46.7 $\pm$ 3.7 ml/kg/min
	=	43.0 – 50.4 ml/kg/min
(at the 95% level)	=	46 $\pm$ 7.4 ml/kg/min
	=	39.3 – 54 ml/kg/min

individual has been genetically endowed with a big, strong heart which does not have to beat very often to do a given amount of exercise. Such a person is simply more able to do aerobic exercise with ease and, like anyone else, will experience a further drop in exercise heart rate if he/she begins an aerobic fitness program.

The Canadian step test provides standards for computing the predicted aerobic capacity for persons of all ages, thus making it the step test of choice for middle-age and older persons. Norms are also provided in Appendix 1.

Bicycle Ergometer Tests.   There are several bicycle ergometer tests that enable you to predict aerobic capacity. Recently a new protocol was developed by the American College of Sports Medicine. Procedures for completing this test and instructions for predicting your aerobic capacity are found in Appendix 1. It should be noted that the test cannot be completed on any exercise bicycle; it requires that you use an ergometer that can be calibrated and which measures the amount of work done. Most well-equipped human performance or exercise physiology labs have such ergometers.

Maximal Field Tests

The purpose behind a maximal field test is to determine the level of performance you can attain when pushed to your limits. The most commonly used test is the Cooper 12 Minute Run, in which the greatest distance that you are able to cover in 12 minutes is measured. (The Cooper 1.5 Mile Run test is virtually the same test except that the time taken to cover 1.5 miles is measured.) This test evolved initially from research showing a high correlation between $\dot{V}O_2$ max as determined in the laboratory and the ability to run distances. Continued research has determined that this correlation is not as high as originally thought. One reason for this is that while the ability to run distances is strongly related to aerobic capacity, it is also dependent on factors such as skill, a sense of the pace you can maintain, motivation, body composition, and the ability to avoid the rapid buildup of exercise-induced wastes or other by-products that interfere with performance. In other words, people who can run long distances at a fast pace are not able to do so simply because of a high aerobic capacity; they can do so for a variety of reasons. Nevertheless, because of its ease of administration to large groups and because it can be self administered on a repeated basis and with relatively little equipment, this test continues to be widely used as a screening test for cardiorespiratory fitness.

Such tests should only be given to healthy people who have had a few weeks of preliminary training to precondition themselves. If you have not had the necessary preconditioning, you should defer taking this test until you do. Certainly if you have any of the major risk factors or other contraindications for cardiovascular disease described earlier, you should have a thorough medical evaluation before taking this test. Specific instructions and norms are provided in Appendix 1.

How Fit to Be?

No single level of cardiorespiratory fitness is desirable for all persons to attain. This is particularly true since people score differently on most tests due to genetics alone. If you wish to compare yourself to others, norms are available that simply describe what category or percentile ranking you hold in relation to the sample of people on which the norms were based (Table 5.C). It is unlikely that everyone can attain the

Table 5.C Aerobic capacity classification based on sex and age.

	MAXIMAL OXYGEN CONSUMPTION (ml/kg•min)				
AGE	LOW	FAIR	AVERAGE	GOOD	HIGH
Women					
20–29	28	29–34	35–40	41–46	47
30–39	27	28–33	34–38	39–45	46
40–49	25	26–30	31–37	38–43	44
50–65	21	22–27	28–34	35–40	41
Men					
20–29	37	38–41	42–50	51–55	56
30–39	33	34–37	38–42	43–50	51
40–49	29	30–35	36–40	41–46	47
50–59	25	26–30	31–38	39–42	43
60–69	21	22–25	26–33	34–37	38

Used with permission from Katch, F. I. & McArdle, W. D. (1983), *Nutrition, Weight Control, and Exercise.* Philadelphia: Lea & Febiger.

"90th percentile" or the "excellent" category on a given test—even by training hard—simply because of inherent individual differences. Therefore, one suggestion might be to score as high on the norms as permitted by the time and interest you are willing to put into regular exercise.

As has already been pointed out, on some tests the norms pertain only to certain segments of the population, such as college-age adults. None of the norms have been developed from randomized samples taken from all segments of society, including the various ethnic groups; none consider education, socioeconomic, or demographic differences. Therefore, even if you are a college-age adult, for example, the norms for a given test may not truly describe where you fall relative to all others of your same age. Perhaps the safest generalization is that if you follow the recommended guidelines for developing cardiorespiratory fitness described in the next section of the book, then whatever level of fitness you attain on a given test is appropriate for you.

In your quest for fitness, comparisons between yourself and others are really irrelevant under most circumstances. The only person who matters is you. True, most of us like to know where we stand compared to others, particularly if we think we're better than most. But unless you are competing as an athlete or have some other job-related performance requirement that requires you to achieve a certain standard of fitness, the best comparison you can make is to yourself. By knowing your fitness status at a given point in time and then rechecking it periodically, you can determine how well you are doing, whether you are making progress, holding your own, or losing ground. This is analogous to the comparisons we make in other areas of our lives: we step on the scale periodically as a check of our body weight or go to the doctor periodically to check our health status. Imagine how silly it would seem if Carl Competitive asked his physician every time he had a check-up whether his cholesterol count, blood glucose, or blood pressure were in the 90th percentile compared to others and, upon discovering they were not, pushed himself competitively toward such an achievement within a few months.

It is true that comparisons to others provide a basis for determining what is normal. That is why cholesterol counts, blood pressure, and blood glucose tests are flagged if they fall outside the normal range. But in the case of cardiorespiratory fitness (and all other components of fitness for that matter), people tend to be overly concerned with where they fall when compared to others. Ironically, given the relatively low fitness status of most contemporary adults, the present norms may not even reflect a truly desirable level of fitness from the standpoint of optimal health!

Developing Cardiorespiratory Fitness

General Guidelines

When beginning an exercise program, several preliminary considerations should guide your behavior. In accordance with the principle of progression discussed in Chapter 4, your preliminary efforts should not abruptly raise your activity level well above what you have been doing previously. Experience has shown that such abrupt approaches to activity are counterproductive and may also lead to musculo-skeletal injuries, excessive fatigue, or in very extreme cases to increased risk of heart attack. (This latter risk applies mostly to middle-aged and older individuals who have not had appropriate medical evaluation and clearance before beginning an exercise program.)

When choosing an activity you should consider your interests, abilities, objectives, and circumstances. Setting realistic goals for yourself, both short-term and long-term, will help you adhere to the program you set up. The activities you choose should be compatible with your lifestyle and your financial means. Enlist the assistance of others who can help you. This includes choosing exercise leaders who are knowledgeable and who can help motivate you, as well as companions who have similar interests and capacities for exercise. Social support is a powerful stimulus for successfully beginning and maintaining regular exercise habits.

One very important component of any exercise program designed to improve cardiorespiratory fitness and/or assist with weight control is the amount of energy expended during the exercise program. For most people who are successful in maintaining an adequate level of fitness and body weight, the total caloric expenditure from exercise amounts to 900–1500 calories per week or 300–500 calories per exercise session. To assist you in determining the caloric cost of various activities, Appendix 6 contains a list of common activities and exercises. Instructions for how to compute caloric costs and more information on the role of exercise in weight control are found in Chapter 7.

A general description of warm-up and cool-down procedures was provided in Chapter 4. However, with particular respect to beginning endurance exercise, your warm-up should be specific to the type of exercise you plan to do during your training and should gradually increase in intensity. It may include light stretching exercises (see Chapter 6). The total duration of warm-up should be between 5–10 minutes. Your cool-down period should also be at least 5–10 minutes, depending on how hard and long you exercised, and should consist of light exercise that gradually tapers off in intensity toward full rest. You should avoid standing still immediately, particularly if you have been doing upright exercise with your legs. This is because of the danger of blood pooling in your lower extremities, creating a lightheaded feeling or worse effects. Following your cool-down is a good time to do strengthening exercises and more extensive flexibility exercises because your body parts and joints are very warm and will be more responsive to such stretching.

For the healthy, non-athletic individual who is interested in developing and maintaining a sufficient degree of cardiorespiratory fitness, the essential ingredients of an exercise program must take into account the type of exercise (the mode), the frequency of exercise (how often), the intensity of exercise (how hard), and the duration of exercise (how long). A summary of the generalizations that can be made from the completed research on these topics can be found in Table 5.D.

Table 5.D Guidelines for developing and maintaining cardiorespiratory fitness.

PARAMETER	GUIDELINE
Mode of Exercise	Any large-muscle, rhythmic exercise (e.g., walk, jog, run, swim, cycle, row, hike, cross-country ski, endurance games)
Frequency of Exercise	3–5 days per week
Intensity of Exercise	60–90% of heart rate reserve
Duration of Exercise	15–60 minutes per day

Source: American College of Sports Medicine Position Statement on the Recommended Quantity and Quality of Exercise for Developing and Maintaining Fitness in Healthy Adults, 1978.

Mode of Exercise

Evidence suggests that any *large-muscle, rhythmic exercise* is appropriate for improving your cardiorespiratory fitness. Large muscles need to be involved because this form of exercise places a large overload on the cardiorespiratory system. Small-muscle exercise, such as working with the upper body in carpentry, will cause the heart rate to increase modestly but will not put a sufficiently large overload on the heart to force it to increase its ability to pump blood. The exercise should be *rhythmic* because *static exercise*—exercise in which there is little or no movement, as in carrying a heavy load with the arms—puts an excessive strain on the heart. (While static exercise is safe for persons with healthy hearts, it puts anyone with potential heart disease at greater risk than rhythmic exercise because it raises blood pressure and heart rate.)

Examples of appropriate rhythmic activities are walking, jogging, running, swimming, cycling, rowing, cross-country skiing, aerobic exercises, rope skipping, and hiking. Intermittent activities or activities of low energy cost have little effect on increasing cardiorespiratory fitness. These include activities such as moderate calisthenics, golf, gardening, and weight lifting, Depending on how they are played, many games such as tennis, basketball, racketball, handball, and soccer can also be appropriate for developing cardiorespiratory fitness. Under most circumstances such games have frequent breaks in them, which reduce their potential usefulness as a tool in this regard, but by modifying these games the range of appropriate activities from which you can choose is widened considerably.

For example, imagine Bjorn Bigserve is a 35-year-old former college tennis player who has been a part of the business world for the last 12 years, only to find himself overfat and underfit. Having long ago discovered that if he has to jog/run to keep in shape, he doesn't keep it up because he dislikes running, Bjorn decides to take up tennis again. To assure himself of an adequate workout, he and his regular tennis partner agree to play tennis on a competitive level, and they also agree to continue moving actively between rallys. For example, instead of walking to pick up the balls, they both jog easily as necessary, in effect keeping themselves in motion. By modifying their game-playing in such a manner, Bjorn and his partner have made their game of tennis more aerobic than it otherwise would have been. In effect, they have ensured that they are involved in continuous large-muscle, rhythmic exercise for the 45–60 minutes that they play each day.

Frequency of Exercise

The relationship between the frequency of exercise and improvements in cardiorespiratory fitness (holding all else constant) is illustrated in Figure 5.2. As you can see, optimal benefits are obtained when exercise is performed regularly 3–5 days per week.

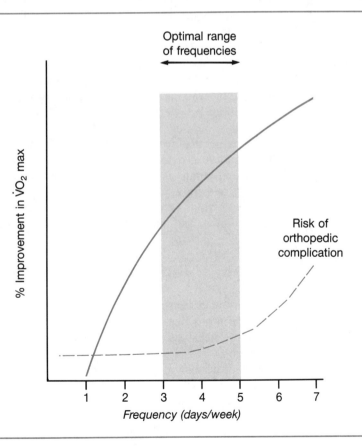

FIGURE 5.2
Improvement in $\dot{V}O_2$ max and the risk of orthopedic complication as a function of different *frequencies* of exercise, holding mode, intensity, and duration of exercise constant.

Modified from Hellerstein and Franklin, 1978.

It should be noted that benefits can be attained from as few as 2 days per week of exercise, but this requires exercising harder than when you exercise more frequently. Evidence indicates that in some cases—running, for example—exercise done in excess of 5 days per week results in a greater incidence of injury than exercise done less frequently. These data are depicted by the dashed line in Figure 5.2.

Most people who exercise 3 days per week choose to space out the exercise sessions to every other day. Though this is not absolutely necessary, allowing a day between exercise sessions permits you to recover fully and distributes the exercise relatively evenly throughout the week. However, exercise sessions performed three days in a row seem to be just as effective at improving cardiorespiratory fitness as sessions spread throughout the week. Therefore, don't worry if your particular schedule is such that you need to exercise both weekend days plus one additional day during the work week. This information should also be of help to you if you have a regular exercise schedule that has to be interrupted temporarily; for instance, many regular exercisers feel distressed when they miss their usual activity on vacation days, and fear that they will lose some of their hard-earned fitness or will not expend enough calories. One simple solution is to exercise a few additional days before and after the trip to make up the difference.

Depending on your initial state of fitness, the intensity at which you plan to exercise, and the total duration of exercise, increasing the frequency of exercise is one way to ensure that you expend additional calories. Perhaps more importantly, by exercising frequently you address what is perhaps the most important issue of all, namely, *establishing regular exercise habits*. For example, suppose Jason Barelyfit wishes to begin an exercise program. His initial state of fitness being relatively low, he begins with a walking program instead of a jogging program, initially walking for 15 minutes 2 days per week and progressing up to ½ hour per day 5 days per week within 4 weeks. (An alternative for Jason might be to walk for 15 minutes twice each day if that fit his schedule better.) Depending on how fast he walks and how much he weighs, by walking 5 days per week for 30 minutes Jason may expend as much as 750 calories per week of energy in his activity program. This is less than the recommended amount of 900–1500 calories per week mentioned earlier, but certainly closer to that target than when he was remaining sedentary. And despite his low fitness, Jason has demonstrated to himself that he can begin to exercise regularly without undue stress and strain. As his fitness improves, Jason may eventually progress with his activity, perhaps adding periods of walk-jog-walk into his routine and eventually moving into periods of continuous jogging as he is able, all of which will increase his fitness further and add to his total caloric expenditure.

Intensity of Exercise

Intensity of exercise refers to how hard you need to work to obtain some benefit. In practical terms that can be measured in the field, research indicates that the optimal range of intensities for developing cardiorespiratory fitness is to maintain a heart rate between 60% and 90% of your *heart rate reserve* (Figures 5.3 and 5.4). Heart rate reserve is defined as the difference between your *resting heart rate* and *your maximum heart rate*. Resting heart rate is the rate at which your heart beats under truly resting conditions. Maximum heart rate is defined as the fastest rate that your heart can attain under conditions of maximal exercise. In Table 5.E, the method for calculating a *target heart rate* at 60% and at 90% of your heart rate reserve is described.

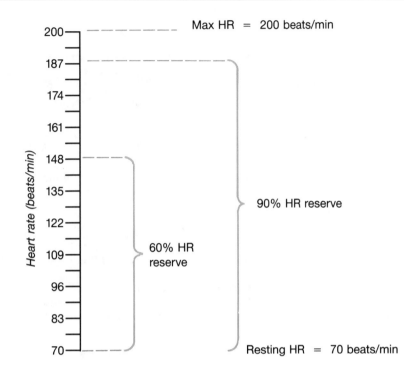

FIGURE 5.3
60% and 90% of heart rate (HR) reserve for an individual with resting HR = 70 beats/min and max HR = 200 beats/min.

Modified from Pollock, Wilmore, and Fox, 1984.

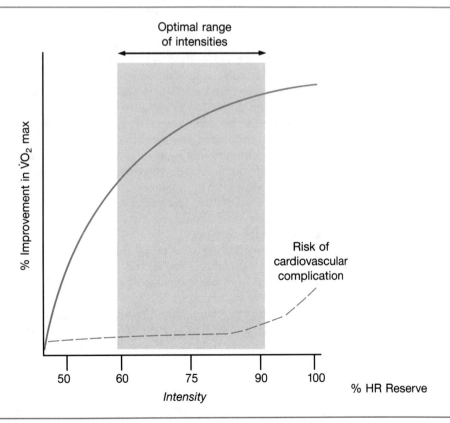

FIGURE 5.4
Improvement in $\dot{V}O_2$ max and risk of cardiovascular complication as a function of differing *intensities* of exercise, holding mode, frequency, and duration of exercise constant.

Modified from Hellerstein and Franklin, 1978.

Table 5.E   Calculating your target heart rate at 60% and 90% of your heart rate reserve.

Step 1.   Calculate your heart rate (HR) reserve as follows:
$$\text{HR reserve} = (\text{max HR}) - (\text{resting HR})*$$

Step 2.   Compute 60% and 90% of your HR reserve.

Step 3.   Compute your 60% target HR and your 90% target HR by adding the results in step 2 to your resting HR.

Example: Assume max HR = 200 and resting HR = 70

    Step 1.   HR reserve   = 200 − 70 = 130

    Step 2.   60% of HR reserve   = .60 (130) = 78
                     90% of HR reserve   = .90 (130) = 117

    Step 3.   60% target HR   = 78 + 70 = 148
                     90% target HR   = 117 + 70 = 187

*Max HR is defined as the highest heart rate (in beats/min) that you can achieve during heavy exercise. If it is not known, it can be estimated as follows: Max HR = 220 − age. Resting HR is defined as the heart rate (in beats/min) under truly resting conditions, as for example on arising in the morning.

A few words should be included about how to measure your heart rate: Each heart beat causes blood to be ejected by the heart, giving rise to a pulse wave that is transmitted throughout all arteries. It is this pulse wave that is commonly measured because of the direct correspondence between pulsations and heart beats. Many people measure their pulse at the carotid artery by pressing their fingers near their throat, just under their jaw (Figure 5.5a). However, recent evidence suggests that your heart may actually slow down due to pressure at this location; therefore, a better method is to find your pulse by pressing gently with your fingers and not your thumb at the radial artery near your wrist (Figure 5.5b). By counting the number of pulsations in 10 seconds and multiplying by 6 to convert it to a minute rate, you will obtain a good indication of your heart rate. You can also count your pulse at the temple (Figure 5.5c).

The easiest time to measure resting heart rate is before getting up in the morning, making sure, of course, that your heart rate has not been elevated by an abrupt alarm. This measure should be taken several times and averaged to determine the most representative value for you.

When measuring your pulse after exercise, it is very important not to wait too long to begin counting. You should start your counting within 5 seconds of stopping because your heart rate immediately begins to decline; if you wait longer your measurement will not accurately reflect how fast your heart was beating during exercise. If you do begin counting within 5 seconds of stopping and measure for only 10 seconds, evidence has shown that you can obtain a very accurate estimate of the rate at which your heart was beating during exercise. A 10-second count is superior to a 6-second count because it allows for a lower error should you miss a beat.

There are several methods for determining your maximum heart rate. If you have completed a maximal exercise test to evaluate your fitness status, then the highest heart rate value you achieved on this test is usually a good estimate of maximum heart

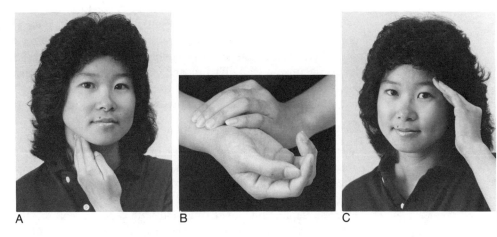

FIGURE 5.5
Measuring your pulse. You should not measure your pulse at the carotid artery (a) because it may slow your heart rate. Instead, you should measure at either the radial (b) or the temporal (c) artery.

A   B   C

rate. Another method is to measure your heart rate immediately after a bout of very heavy exercise (e.g., after the 12 minute run). Heart rate under such conditions can give a good indication of your maximum heart rate, but unless you are fit enough to take such a test safely, you should not do so. If neither of the above conditions apply to you, then the most common procedure is to predict maximum heart rate as follows:

predicted maximum heart rate = 220 − age

For example, the predicted maximum heart rate of Penelope Avidexerciser, aged 23, is: $220 - 23 = 197$ beats per minute. Although this will enable you to obtain a rough estimate of your maximum heart rate using average values obtained on people of differing ages, research has shown that there are considerable individual differences using such an estimate. The standard deviation is approximately ± 10 beats per minute, which means 68% of the individuals of any age have a true maximum heart rate within 10 beats of their predicted maximum heart rate. Another 27% may fall only within 20 beats per minute of their predicted maximum heart rate. Simply said, this prediction formula gives only a rough approximation of true maximum heart rate. It should be used only until you are able to obtain a more accurate measure of your true maximum heart rate using one of the other methods described above.

The reasons why exercise intensity is often monitored using *heart rate* is worth mentioning. Earlier, we mentioned that the most widely accepted measure of cardiorespiratory fitness is your maximum ability to consume oxygen (your $\dot{V}O_2$ max). Evidence indicates that the optimal overload to elicit improvements in fitness is for you to repeatedly tax yourself at a level of 50–85% of your $\dot{V}O_2$ max. When in the field, however, it is difficult to measure $\dot{V}O_2$ max since to do so requires expensive equipment, and considerable skill and time. Therefore, a different approach is used to determine whether you are working hard enough: Since your heart rate is directly related to oxygen consumption during exercise and heart rate *can* be measured in the field, this measurement is used instead. The values of 60–90% heart rate reserve, which correspond to the 50–85% of $\dot{V}O_2$ max, are used as the target heart rate zone.

The region of heart rates that falls between these two limits is often referred to as the *training sensitive zone* (see Figure 5.6). In effect, training at any intensity that causes your heart rate during exercise to fall within your training sensitive zone is appropriate if you wish to improve and/or maintain cardiorespiratory fitness.

Since maximum heart rate declines with age, target heart rates at the 60–90% levels decline as well. This means that as you get older you do not have to raise your heart rate as high during exercise to obtain a training effect. This declining target heart rate zone is illustrated by the downward slant of the training sensitive zone in Figure 5.6.

You may wonder what will happen if you do not achieve these limits for one reason or another. If you exercise in such a way that your heart rate does not reach your 60% target heart rate level, you simply will not receive as much of a training effect as if you had worked harder. This may be an entirely appropriate strategy for you if you are trying to gradually develop regular exercise habits and you find vigorous exercise unpleasant. Over time and with practice you are likely to find yourself able and willing to exercise harder, thereby bringing your heart rate into the training sensitive zone. A gradual approach toward improving your fitness is always preferred to an abrupt approach, and you should feel encouraged to set your own pace toward achieving such a goal.

At the other end of the spectrum, if you exercise so hard that your heart rate exceeds the 90% level, probably nothing will happen except that you will be placing all your bodily systems under greater strain and your fitness will not improve any

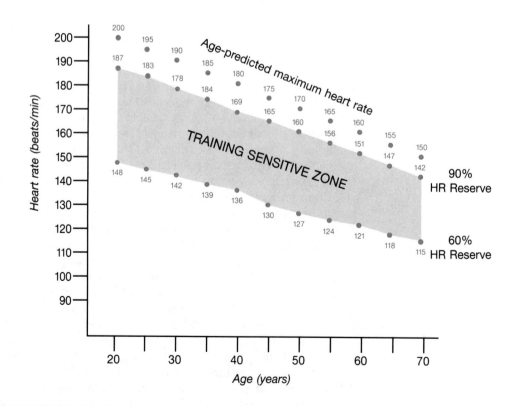

FIGURE 5.6
The Training Sensitive Zone as a function of age. Maximum heart rate and heart rates within the training sensitive zone decline with age. Resting heart rate does not.

Modified from Katch, Katch, and McArdle, 1983.

faster. If you are healthy, you may become more fatigued and less inclined to adhere to such an exercise routine. You may even be less inclined to exercise the next day. If you have risk factors or latent cardiovascular disease, such exercise will put you at greater risk for an injury or a heart attack.

Is it better to work closer to the 60% or the 90% target heart rate level? It appears that as long as you exercise within the training sensitive zone, you will receive optimal benefits. However, you will have to push yourself harder to achieve the 90% target heart rate than if you worked at the 60% level. The best strategy depends on your initial state of fitness and on the total duration of the exercise session; for example, exercise at the lower level of intensity if you are less fit and/or if you plan to exercise for a longer period of time. More will be said about both of these topics later.

Another way to monitor the intensity of exercise involves measuring your *rate of perceived exertion* (RPE) during exercise. In fact, this method is close to what many regular exercisers do naturally once they become experienced: they exercise at a pace that feels comfortable and that they know is sufficiently vigorous to accomplish their goals. The rate of perceived exertion is a measure that is based on all the sensory information you receive from your muscles, joints, and the various internal organs, as they all affect you at the same time. Some evidence suggests that RPE is an even better predictor of your maximum work capacity than is heart rate.

The scale for measuring RPE is seen in Figure 5.7. To use this scale, simply determine the number that best describes how hard the exercise feels using the scale of 6 to 20 and the adjectives adjacent to the scale. For example, if while swimming the crawl steadily for 20 minutes you felt like it was mildly vigorous, you might rate the exercise as a 12 or a 13 (i.e., "somewhat hard" or below). On the other hand, if it was very difficult to maintain your pace, your RPE score might have been a 17 or an 18 (i.e., "very hard" or above). A guideline for using perceived exertion that is roughly equivalent to your training sensitive zone is to exercise at a pace that falls between 12 and 16 on the RPE scale (i.e., between "somewhat hard" and "hard").

FIGURE 5.7
The Borg Perceived Exertion Scale allows you to rate the difficulty of an exercise according to your perceptions.

Used with permission from Borg, G. A. V. *Medicine and Science in Sports* 5, 1973:90–93.

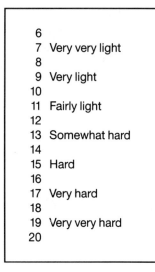

6	
7	Very very light
8	
9	Very light
10	
11	Fairly light
12	
13	Somewhat hard
14	
15	Hard
16	
17	Very hard
18	
19	Very very hard
20	

Duration of Exercise

Evidence suggests that for optimal improvements in cardiorespiratory fitness, exercise should last between 15 and 60 minutes per day. The time refers to exercise time—don't include the time it takes you to enter the locker room or to finish dressing after your shower! The relationship between the duration of exercise and improvements in $\dot{V}O_2$ max, holding intensity and frequency of exercise constant, is seen in Figure 5.8. Exercise that lasts less than 15 minutes, while not likely to cause as much of an increase in $\dot{V}O_2$ max, will nevertheless cause some improvement. In fact, evidence suggests that as little as 6 minutes of aerobic exercise per day can be beneficial. Exercise lasting longer than 60 minutes per day results in additional benefit but to a diminished degree.

It should be noted that, at least for people involved in jogging/running programs (which are the programs for which there is data), the rate of injury rises sharply after 45–60 minutes of exercise. The dotted line in Figure 5.8 represents this phenomenon.

It is important to note that intensity and duration are directly related to one another. That is, the harder you exercise, the less time you have to spend to achieve a given benefit. Or, if your exercise intensity is lower, then by working longer you can achieve the same benefit. This is important for anyone beginning an exercise program since what it means is that you do not have to exercise extremely hard to do yourself some good. You can accomplish your goals by working submaximally for a longer period of time. In fact, by working intensively for a short period of time, you

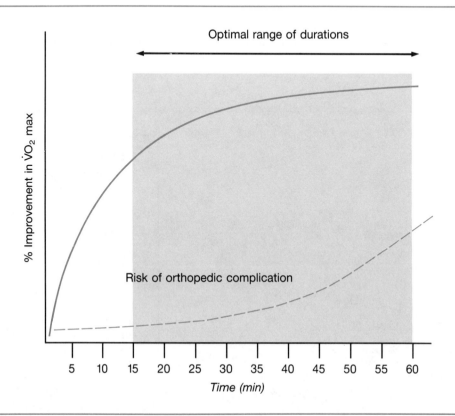

FIGURE 5.8
Improvement in $\dot{V}O_2$ max and risk of orthopedic complication as a function of differing *durations* of exercise, holding mode, frequency, and intensity of exercise constant.

Modified from Hellerstein and Franklin, 1978.

may even be doing yourself some harm in the long run: the psychological stress of intensive exercise (similar to that experienced by many athletes during competitive training) is so much greater than in submaximal exercise that most people will not continue the pace very long— certainly not over the course of a lifetime. So, even discounting the potential injury problems and other risks, it seems likely that gentle exercise of longer durations is most appropriate.

Does exercise need to be continuous to be effective? Although the evidence suggests that the total duration of exercise time needs to conform to the range of 15–60 minutes per day, it does not indicate that this exercise must be done all at one time. In fact, when the total caloric expenditure is held constant, continuous exercise is no different than 2 or 3 shorter bouts of slightly more intensive exercise. So, for example, you could jog twice a day for 10 minutes and expect approximately the same benefit as if you jogged once a day for 20 minutes.

It is important to remember that total caloric expenditure is a critical variable in determining the effects of an exercise program on cardiorespiratory fitness. Caloric expenditure is a function of the total work accomplished, which itself depends on a number of factors such as body weight, intensity, and duration of exercise. The greater the total work (i.e., the greater the caloric expenditure), the greater the improvement in fitness will likely be. For more on the caloric cost of exercise and related topics, see Chapter 7.

Guidelines published by the American College of Sports Medicine for developing and maintaining fitness in healthy adults suggest that as a minimum an exercise program should cause you to expend 300 calories per session.* If you wish to achieve this goal, some rough generalizations regarding how hard and how long you would have to exercise are as follows: (1) 40–50 minutes of moderate intensity exercise at 60–80% heart rate reserve; (2) 20–30 minutes of moderately high intensity exercise at 80–90% heart range; or (3) 15–20 minutes of high intensity exercise at greater than 90% heart rate reserve. As we mentioned earlier, high intensity exercise is not recommended for the average person. Again, exercise of moderate intensity and longer duration is a very satisfactory, and even preferred, method of improving cardiorespiratory fitness.

When beginning an exercise program, do not feel bound by the guidelines of 15–60 minutes of exercise per day. At first the duration of your exercise should be lower—perhaps as low as 5 minutes per day—and then slowly progress upward. It depends on what you can do comfortably. An alternative would be to begin with a longer duration but keep the intensity of exercise relatively low. Again, by progressing slowly and in small steps, your chances of maintaining a regular exercise routine are enhanced.

*The recommended guideline of expending at least 300 calories of energy in your exercise program is based largely on data in which males served as subjects. Since men on the average are taller and heavier than women, and energy expenditure in exercise is partly a function of body weight (the greater the weight, the greater the energy expenditure), then we can estimate that the number of calories an average woman should expend to accomplish the same gains, assuming all else is equal, will be less. A tentative guess might be 250 calories. Remember, however, that these are just generalizations based on averages; if you know that you are noticeably different than your peers in weight, for example, then you need to adjust these estimates upward or downward accordingly, regardless of your sex.

Integrating Mode, Frequency, Intensity, and Duration of Exercise

Having discussed each of these aspects of training separately, it is important to emphasize again their interrelationship. All the different aspects of training (mode, frequency, intensity, and duration) must be present to a sufficient degree for noticeable improvements in cardiorespiratory fitness to occur. If a given training program is inadequate in one area or more, the effect will be to reduce the total benefit drastically, even if all other aspects are adequate.

An example will illustrate this point more clearly. Suppose Henry Hurryup and Lester Laggard are college roommates. Henry always has too many things going for him and he never seems to have enough time to do anything he starts. Lester on the other hand is very methodical, almost plodding in his approach to life. Henry and Lester sign up for a college fitness class together, but as soon as the term gets underway it becomes clear that each is approaching the class in his own unique way. Henry figures that he can just as easily work out on his own time as come to class, so he schedules a chemistry lab on two of the three afternoons that the fitness class meets. After two weeks of missing class and not fitting in his alternative workout, he decides that he'll just run a little harder and longer on the one day that he does come to class, thereby making up the difference. Lester on the other hand always gets to class late. He feels he has to fold his clothes before he changes, and he has a hard time remembering his locker combination because his mind is always filled with dreams of adventure. Accordingly, by the time he finishes his warm-up on a typical day in class, usually less than 5 minutes of actual exercise time remains before he has to cool down and (slowly) move on to his next class.

Henry and Lester have both failed to include all the components of exercise to a sufficient degree to achieve a marked improvement, even in a 15-week term. Both used an appropriate mode of exercise (jogging); Henry worked out with sufficient intensity and duration to do himself some good, but he failed to do so frequently enough to achieve the improvements he desired. Lester's problem was not the frequency or the intensity of his exercise—it was the short duration. As a result, he improved only to a small degree, again much less than would have been the case had he met the recommended levels in all areas. For optimal (or even modest) improvements in cardiorespiratory fitness to occur, you must meet the recommended guidelines in mode, frequency, intensity, and duration *together*.

Maintaining Cardiorespiratory Fitness

Once a satisfactory level of cardiorespiratory fitness is achieved, how much exercise is required to maintain that status? Certainly one option is to simply continue at the same exercise level thereafter. As we discussed earlier, there is some indication that less exercise is required to maintain your cardiorespiratory fitness than is needed to improve it. Thus, if you have been exercising 5 days per week, if you drop down to only 3 days per week, all else remaining the same, your fitness status may not decline substantially. Unfortunately, very few longitudinal studies have followed individuals for more than a few months after such reductions in regular exercise; this means it may eventually be shown that if such a reduction were carried out over a year or more, a small loss in fitness would indeed occur. Therefore, the wisest conclusion at the present time is to maintain your exercise habits within the guidelines discussed previously for achieving an improvement. In other words, so long as you continue using an appropriate mode, frequency, intensity, and duration of exercise, the only reason for your fitness to decline will be from true aging. If the amount of exercise you do declines substantially, however, your cardiorespiratory fitness will decline as well.

Factors Affecting Performance and Improvement

Initial Fitness

The rate of improvement you are likely to experience when beginning an exercise program is dependent on your initial state of fitness (Figure 5.9; see also Figure 4.5). The lower your cardiorespiratory fitness when you begin, the more easily you will be

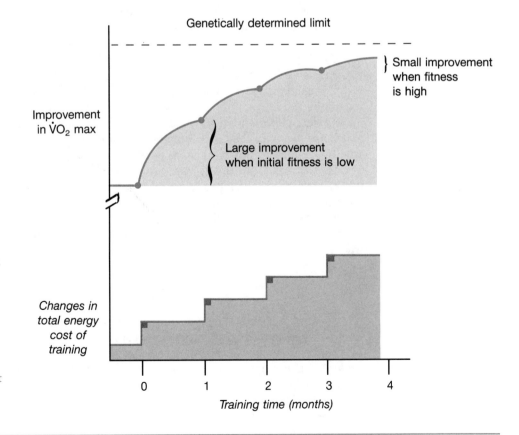

FIGURE 5.9
Improvements in $\dot{V}O_2$ max as a function of *initial fitness and genetics.* As a result of hypothetical monthly increments in training, larger improvements occur the lower the initial state of fitness. Smaller improvements occur the closer you get to your genetically determined limit.

able to achieve noticeable improvements, all else remaining the same. If your ability to do endurance exercise is low to begin with, you will be able to improve without undue effort and will likely be reinforced for your efforts. On the other hand, if your initial state of fitness is higher to begin with, not only will your improvements likely be smaller, but they will come only through more intensive, longer, and/or more frequent exercise.

Genetics

In cardiorespiratory or any type of fitness, the role that initial fitness plays is partly connected to the role of genetics. Whatever your genetic endowment is, the farther you are from achieving your limits the more easily you will improve. But as you approach your limits, it becomes successively more difficult to elicit further improvements as shown in Figure 5.9. Certainly this is not encouraging news, but it appears to be a fact of life.

The role of genetics is poorly understood at the present time, but it appears that the differences between people in terms of cardiorespiratory fitness are due to genetic endowment to a much greater extent than they are due to training. For example, let's suppose there is a 100 percent difference in $\dot{V}O_2$ max between an elite athlete and an average, sedentary individual. Since evidence indicates that through training you can improve your $\dot{V}O_2$ max by about 15–25%, this means that the remaining differences between elite and average are probably due to genetics.

Because of the differences due to genetic endowment, having a high $\dot{V}O_2$ max in itself does not provide an accurate picture of one's fitness status. Results of any testing—for cardiorespiratory fitness or another component of fitness such as body composition, strength, or flexibility—must be interpreted with respect to your genetic makeup as well as how much exercise you do.

For example, it is possible for someone with "great genes" to have a high $\dot{V}O_2$ max or even a high ability to perform endurance exercise easily (e.g., a former endurance athlete performing a 12 minute run test), and yet be unfit. That is, *compared to their own potential* they may be unfit because they do not exercise sufficiently, but when compared to others of more average potential, they may score near the top in norms. The reason for this is that most norms that allow you to compare yourself to others have been developed by measuring heterogeneous samples of people. Since most heterogeneous samples do not contain many persons who are genetically gifted, when those who are gifted compare themselves to these norms they are at the top of the scale, sometimes with no training at all. This is another example of "unfair but true"!

Age

As we have indicated, a given amount of training in older individuals results in improvements in cardiorespiratory fitness similar in *relative value* to those experienced by younger individuals. The improvements are smaller when expressed on an *absolute scale*, however. In addition, the rate of improvement is slower: the improvements that become visible in a young adult after several weeks of training might be seen in an older individual only after several months of training. This may be partly attributable to a more gentle approach to training used for older, sedentary individuals, particularly those over age 60.

As we noted earlier, cardiorespiratory training can make drastic improvements in the functional status of older individuals, enabling them to perform at a level similar to that of many sedentary individuals who are 20–30 years younger. However, evidence does not indicate that fitness can stop the aging process. Although the level of function can be raised by training, the rate of decline appears similar in the sedentary and the well-trained. Such declines appear to accelerate after age 60, but again it is not clear whether this is a result of true aging or a decline in the total amount of regular exercise. Even for the most active, the amount of exercise seems to decline more rapidly after age 60.

Sex Differences

Unfortunately, most of the research that has led to the generalizations regarding mode, frequency, intensity, and duration of exercise has been done using men as subjects. This is because until the last 10–15 years the number of women participating in such exercise was considerably smaller than the number of men. Although an equal volume of information on such topics is lacking for women, those studies that have been done indicate that women tend to adapt to cardiorespiratory training in a manner similar to men. However, there are numerous sex differences in performance and physiological function, changes that become apparent after puberty. Data comparing the sexes on several variables are seen in Table 5.F. Reasons why females have a lower $\dot{V}O_2$ max than males include smaller heart volume, smaller blood volume, lower oxygen carrying capacity in blood, and a lower ability to pump blood at maximum.

Disability

Developing and maintaining an adequate level of cardiorespiratory fitness is also of concern to those who are disabled, either permanently or temporarily. Depending on the cause of the disability and on how long it will last, fitness strategies will vary. For someone who is temporarily in a leg cast that allows them to walk on crutches, for example, the mere task of walking from here to there to meet the normal needs of

Table 5.F Sex differences in the circulatory and oxygen transport systems (50th percentile).

| | REST | | | | | | MAXIMUM | | | |
| | HEART RATE (BEATS/MIN) | | SYSTOLIC BLOOD PRESSURE (MM HG) | | DIASTOLIC BLOOD PRESSURE (MM HG) | | HEART RATE (BEATS/MIN) | | MAX $\dot{V}O_2$ (ESTIMATED) (ML/KG/MIN) | |
AGE	MALE	FEMALE	MALE	FEMALE	MALE	FEMALE	MALE	FEMALE	MALE	FEMALE
20–29	63	65	121	112	80	75	194	188	39.1	30.2
30–39	63	68	120	114	80	76	189	184	37.0	30.2
40–49	62	66	121	118	80	80	182	177	35.7	26.7
50–59	63	67	128	122	82	80	173	170	32.9	24.5
60+	62	64	131	130	81	80	162	153	29.0	21.8

Data from the Cooper Clinic Coronary Risk Factor Profile Charts. Source: Pollock, M. L., Wilmore, J. H. & Fox, S. M. *Exercise in Health & Disease*. Philadelphia: W. B. Saunders, 1984.

contemporary living is usually sufficient physical stress to the upper body to provide sufficient exercise. Concerning those with more permanent disabilities, it is no longer uncommon to see people engaging in wheelchair activities. Road races often have paraplegic competitors whose upper bodies are superbly developed from miles of aerobic wheelchair training. A number of activities that can be done in the water, from simple swimming to water exercises and water games, provide an alternative medium for engaging in physical activity while weight supported. In effect, if you find yourself in a disabled state and you wish to develop and maintain your cardiorespiratory fitness, you should be able to achieve positive results through one of many means.

Motivation

For one reason or another, many people do not exercise regularly. Many among these would like to exercise and may frequently dedicate themselves to, and later abandon, new exercise regimes. If this description fits you and you would like to follow through on a lasting exercise/fitness program, then the issue of motivation is of paramount importance. Throughout this chapter, a number of suggestions have been given that address the issue of motivation. These included a suggestion to feel free to exercise at a lower intensity of exercise when beginning rather than feeling like you must achieve a target heart rate at the 60% to 90% level right at the start. The goal is to develop some form of regular exercise, regardless of how hard or how long it is, that you will be motivated to continue for the rest of your life. Another suggestion was to modify endurance games you enjoy (e.g., tennis, basketball, and so on) so that you can do what pleases you and develop and/or maintain cardiorespiratory fitness at the same time. The bottom line is to do whatever is necessary when beginning an exercise program to make your exercising experience *as comfortable and pleasant as possible*. Once you achieve regular exercise habits, continue to attend to this issue.

Someone once described an exercise program as "something that a mesomorph thinks up for an endomorph" (translation: "something that a person with a muscular, fit body thinks up for a person with a round, fat body"). Although that may have been the case at one time, *your exercise program should be designed by you and for you*. If exercising with others makes it easier for you to keep at it, then look for some way to create those conditions for yourself. If you like the outdoors and the time alone, then choose such an exercise setting. Certainly you should enlist the assistance of others as it seems appropriate. The point is that only you know how you feel. With careful personal choices you can make your exercise as pleasant as possible and help yourself move from the ranks of the sedentary to the ranks of the fit.

Summary

Regular aerobic exercise has been shown to bring about a number of favorable effects in adults of all ages, including several that reduce the risk of cardiovascular disease. Regular activity is also associated with increased longevity, independent of other influencing factors. When first beginning an aerobic exercise program, it is wise to determine whether you have any medical condition that might put you at greater risk during exercise. Your initial fitness status can be assessed in a variety of ways. Some of these ways are sophisticated and expensive; others are relatively simple and just as effective if used on a periodic basis for comparing yourself to yourself. To improve cardiorespiratory fitness, a healthy adult should engage in any form of large muscle, rhythmic exercise, 3–5 days per week, for 15–60 minutes per day, at an intensity of 60–90% of heart rate reserve. The methods of building up to such a level of exercise depend on individual differences, including initial fitness, genetics, age, and sex. Specific warm-up and cool-down procedures should be followed. Most importantly, making your exercise experience as comfortable and pleasant as possible will greatly help with motivation.

References

American College of Sports Medicine guidelines for exercise testing and prescription. 3d ed., 1986. Philadelphia: Lea and Febiger.

American College of Sports Medicine position statement on the recommended quantity and quality of exercise for developing and maintaining fitness in healthy adults. 1978. *Medicine and Science in Sports* 10(3):vii–ix.

Blair, S. N. 1985. Physical activity leads to fitness and pays off. *Physician and Sportsmedicine.* 13(3):153–157.

Boone, T., Frentz, K. L., and Boyd, N. R. 1985. Carotid palpitation at two exercise intensities. *Medicine Science in Sport and Exercise.* 17(6):705–709.

Borg, G. A. V. 1973. Perceived exertion: a note on "history" and methods. *Medicine and Science in Sports* 5:90–93.

Cooper, K. H. 1982. *The aerobics program for total well-being: Exercise, diet, emotional balance.* New York: M. Evans.

deVries, H. A. 1986. *Physiology of exercise.* 4th ed. Dubuque, IA: W. C. Brown.

Drinkwater, B. L. 1984. Women and exercise: physiological aspects. *Exercise and Sports Sciences Reviews* 12:21–51.

Fox, E. L. and Matthews, D. K. 1981. *The physiological basis of physical education and athletics.* 3d ed. Philadelphia, PA: Saunders College.

Haskel, W. L. 1984. Exercise induced changes in plasma lipids and lipoproteins. *Preventative Medicine* 13:23–36.

Hellerstein, H. K. and Franklin, B. A. 1978. Exercise testing and prescription. In *Rehabilitation of the coronary patient.* N. K. Wenger, ed. New York: John Wiley and Sons.

Jetté, M., Campbell, J., Mongeon, J., and Routhier, R. 1976. The Canadian home fitness test as a predictor of aerobic capacity. *CMA Journal* 114:680–682.

Kasch, F. W. and Wallace, J. P. 1976. Physiological variables during 10 years of endurance exercise. *Medicine and Science in Sports* 8:5–8.

Katch, F. I. and McArdle, W. D. 1983. *Nutrition, Weight Control, and Exercise.* 2d ed. Philadelphia: Lea and Febiger.

LaPorte, R. E., Dearwater, S., Cauley, J. A., Slemenda, C., and Cook, T. 1985. Physical activity or cardiovascular fitness: which is more important for health? *Physician & Sportsmedicine* 13(3):145–150.

McArdle, W. D., Katch, F. I., and Katch, V. L. 1986. *Exercise Physiology.* 2d ed. Philadelphia: Lea and Febiger.

Moffat, R. J., Stamford, B. A., and Neill, R. D. 1977. Placement of tri-weekly training sessions: importance regarding enhancement of aerobic capacity. *Research Quarterly* 48:583–591.

Morris, J. N., Chave, S. P. W., Adam, C., and Sirey, C. 1973. Vigorous exercise in leisure-time and the incidence of coronary heart disease. *The Lancet* 1:333–339.

Paffenbarger, R. S., Hyde, R. T., Wing, M. B. A., and Hsieh, C. C. 1986. Physical activity, all cause mortality, and longevity of college alumni. *New England Journal of Medicine* 314:605–613.

Paffenbarger, R. S., Wing, A. L., and Hyde, R. T. 1978. Physical activity as an index of heart attack risk in college alumni. *American Journal of Epidemiology* 108:161–175.

Paffenbarger, R. S. and Hyde, R. T. 1980. Exercise as protection against heart attack. *New England Journal of Medicine* 302:1026–1027.

Pollock, M. L., Wilmore, J. H. and Fox III, S. M. 1984. *Exercise in health and disease.* Philadelphia: W. B. Saunders.

Shephard, R.J., Bailey, D. A., and Mirwald, R. L. 1976. Development of the Canadian home fitness test. *CMA Journal* 114:675–679.

Shephard, R. J. 1983. The value of exercise in ischemic heart disease: a cumulative analysis. *Journal of Cardiac Rehabilitation* 3:294–298.

Smith, E. L. & Zook, S. K. 1986. The aging process. Benefits of physical activity, *JOPERD* 57:32–34.

Canadian standardized test of fitness: Operations manual. 1985. Hull, Quebec, K1AOS9: Fitness and Amateur Sport.

6

Able Bodies: Flexibility, Strength, and Muscle Endurance

How do adequate flexibility, strength, and muscle endurance enhance quality living?

How can you tell if you have adequate flexibility? Strength? Muscle endurance? How can you increase these components of fitness safely and effectively? Are there methods that are superior? Unsafe?

Is there something you can do to improve your posture?

What effects, if any, do procedures such as circuit training and interval training have on fitness?

How should you train to improve your power, speed, and/or agility, which you may need for participation in a particular sport?

How can you build muscle? Is the use of anabolic steroids for this purpose safe?

Introduction

If you wish to attain optimum function, all-around fitness is necessary. Having good *flexibility* in all of your muscles and joints enables you to move freely without restriction. An adequate level of *strength* and *muscular endurance* will reduce the fatigue from daily tasks, and you will look better and feel better about yourself. You will also be better prepared in the event of an emergency. This chapter will discuss these components of fitness and the role they play in overall function, and provide guidelines for how to measure, develop, and maintain your status in each of these areas.

The Process of Degeneration

The term *hypokinetic degeneration* refers to a degenerative process that occurs because of too little movement. Many bodily functions deteriorate when movement is restricted. In extreme cases, such as with prolonged bedrest, the following have been documented to occur to some degree:

1. *Muscle atrophy:* This is a gradual loss of muscle tissue, resulting in loss of strength and loss of ability to do aerobic exercise. Such atrophy is dramatically visible when a limb such as the lower leg is casted for several weeks after a fracture, causing it to be immobilized. When the cast is removed, the affected calf is often noticeably smaller in circumference and the leg is weak from not being used and from the resultant loss in muscle. This demonstrates rather graphically that our muscles are designed for use and that their functional abilities deteriorate whenever they are not used sufficiently.

2. *Loss of flexibility:* Without regular movement, the connective tissue that makes up the tendons and ligaments shortens and becomes resistant to stretch. It is this connective tissue, and the connective tissue that holds muscle fibers together, that limits your flexibility to a large extent when you try to stretch.

3. *Osteoporosis:* This is the degenerative disease spoken of in Chapter 3 that involves the loss of proteins and minerals from bones. A bone weakened from osteoporosis is considerably more susceptible to fractures. Incidence of osteoporosis is dramatically increased in extremely sedentary individuals. In fact, weight-bearing exercise is necessary for proper maintenance of bone function.

4. *Cardiovascular and respiratory malfunctions:* In the bedridden, resting heart rate tends to rise while the ability of the heart to eject blood per beat drops. Aerobic capacity declines dramatically and the person is unable to maintain an adequate blood pressure when upright. Blood volume decreases and blood clots tend to develop in the veins. The lungs become congested with fluids and bronchial obstructions can occur. Pneumonia is also not uncommon in bedridden persons.

5. *Bladder and bowel malfunction:* Being immobile often leads to difficulty in voiding the bladder and bowel.

While such dramatic malfunctions have been observed to occur in persons who are confined to bed for prolonged periods of time, the same types of degenerative processes can occur to a lesser degree in people who remain seated day after day at their jobs. Often such a lifestyle includes only a minimal amount of walking to and from an automobile, where again the individual is seated; once home, the better part of the remaining hours before bed may also be spent seated. When added to 7–8 hours of sleep, such a lifestyle can closely approximate that of the bedridden. Most of us would not have to go far to find people who are suffering from hypokinetic degeneration. They're found wherever old people reside: in nursing homes and retirement communities. Many people of all ages suffer from this problem, and the problem is one that does not occur overnight. It can be prevented by engaging in regular amounts of exercise involving the whole body.

Working Against Degeneration

Virtually all the degenerative processes associated with hypokinetic degeneration can be alleviated by engaging in regular exercise. Muscles can regain their strength through continual use. Flexibility can be regained by properly following a gradual stretching program. Loss of bone mass and bone density can also be reduced by regular exercise. Evidence suggests that regular exercise throughout one's life and especially during the rapid growth periods of youth are particularly important in minimizing the degree of bone loss. The losses in cardiorespiratory, bladder, and bowel function can be eliminated through minimal exercise. In recent years post-surgical patients were usually kept bedridden for days or weeks; today, however, such people are encouraged to get up and move as soon as they are able since experience has demonstrated that people respond better when they move around. *People who are active on a regular basis are healthier.* They feel better, look better, and perform better. Regular exercise can and does play an important part in maintaining a high quality of living for most people.

An interesting illustration supports this point. As we get older, grip strength normally declines, particularly once we reach the age of 60. In a group of men whose job duties required them to use their hands vigorously on the job, this decline in grip strength was not evident. Even for the men who were in their 60s, grip strength was similar to that of their younger counterparts, presumably because they continued to use their strength. Imagine what the world would be like if people remained vigorously active all their lives? Now imagine what you will be like when you retire, and what you will want to do and to experience with your time.

Another health problem that affects a great number of adults is low back pain. This problem was previously discussed in Chapters 3 and 4. It has been estimated that nearly 80% of the American adult population has at one time or another suffered from simple backache, and some 16% (or 25–30 million Americans) suffer from classical low back pain syndrome. Back pain is said to be second only to upper respiratory infections as a cause of absenteeism from work. The total dollar cost of this condition has been estimated at $250 million in worker's compensation, and there is in excess of $1 billion in lost productivity from this problem on an annual basis in the United States. This accounts only for the dollar cost and does not take into account the pain and suffering that people experience.

Based on clinical evidence, fitness experts, physical and corrective therapists, and orthopedic surgeons have long linked the incidence of low back problems to a lack of exercise. The rationale is that weak muscles are easily fatigued and cannot support the spine and pelvis in proper alignment. In an upright position, the abdominal muscles and the spinal extensors in the lower back are designed to stabilize the spine and pelvis and keep it from tilting forward into the "sway-back" position (see Figure 4.2). If the abdominal muscles are weak, the pelvis tilts forward into the abnormal sway-back position, putting greater stress on the vertebral column and compressing the space through which nerves pass to and from the spinal cord. Other postural muscles also have to work harder to maintain the upright posture, causing them to fatigue more easily.

Another contributing factor to this problem is tight muscles at the back of the leg (hamstrings), which attach onto the lower pelvis. Tight hamstrings inhibit the natural forward tilt of the pelvis when bending forward at the waist or stretching, thereby reducing mobility and increasing the possibility of strain, spasm, and pain.

This raises the general question of posture and the role that flexibility and strength play in overall postural problems. Whenever one or another body part is out of alignment, greater strain is placed on other muscles to compensate against the pull of gravity and keep the body upright. As a result, these muscles are more susceptible to fatigue, spasms, and chronic pain. Over long periods of time, the muscles, tendons, and ligaments accommodate to such misalignment with more permanent changes in structure, which makes attempts at correction more difficult to accomplish.

Consider the example of Stanley Stiffneck who has a tilt in his shoulder girdle, his right shoulder being slightly lower than his left. The effect on his spinal column is a compensatory adjustment in his pelvic girdle and lower leg. See Figure 4.8 for an illustration of such a postural problem. Such postural deviations are not uncommon and can lead to problems in the future. The fact that Stanley may not experience much difficulty at the present time underscores the importance of early postural evaluation and the need for him to perform strengthening and stretching exercises in appropriate areas to help correct his problem. Another important corrective strategy is for Stanley to relearn how to maintain good posture. Many postural problems are ones of habit that have long ago become unconscious. Improvement requires conscious alteration of such poor habits, to be replaced by correct ones.

Flexibility

Measuring Flexibility

Being able to assess your current flexibility status in an accurate manner that can be repeated at a later date is important for several reasons. For one, you may wish to determine where you fall in relation to others. As we have stressed, it is a wise strategy to assess yourself when you first begin a fitness program so that you can monitor your progress periodically. This will help you gauge the appropriate level of progression to follow. Such a record will also be an important motivational tool since you'll be able to see how much you have improved (assuming, of course, that you have!).

The most commonly used test of flexibility is the *sit and reach test*. There are many versions of this test, all of which provide essentially the same type of information, namely your ability to bend forward from the waist. Although the test is designed to measure flexibility of the lower back and posterior leg regions, recent evidence suggests that it may not truly measure flexibility in the lower back. However, until a simple alternative test is developed, the sit and reach test continues to be useful as a field test.

In the version of the test developed by the national YMCA for use in their fitness programs, no specialized equipment is needed, although special sit and reach benches make it easier to evaluate yourself. Using a home-equipped set-up, you simply sit down on the floor with your feet extended in front of you and your legs slightly apart as indicated in Figure 6.1. Your heels should be positioned on a line on the floor. Place a yardstick between your legs so that the 15-inch mark is on the line and the 36-inch mark is away from you. By bending forward at the waist, keeping your legs straight, and moving your hands along the yardstick you can measure how far you can reach. This should be done after you have done some light stretching to loosen up. Your forward movement should be slow and your final position should be one that you can sustain for 2–3 seconds. Age and sex specific norms from the YMCA are found in Table 6.A.

Although the sit and reach test is the only flexibility test for which there are standardized norms for both sexes and all ages, the range of motion of all the moving body parts (limbs, trunk, etc.) can be measured using either a goniometer or a flexometer. Both are specialized pieces of equipment that require some experience to use properly; thus, they are not generally useful for self-testing. Most well-equipped exercise science or therapeutic exercise labs can provide you with the expertise to do so, should the need arise.

As an alternative, the Nicholas Overall Body Mobility Test provides you with a series of easily administered self-tests in which you score yourself in one of three categories: loose, average, or tight. Such self-testing can provide useful information. For example, evidence suggests that persons who tend to be "tight" in a specific region are more prone to muscle and tendon pulls than people who are not. Similarly, persons who are "loose" in a particular region are not as prone to muscle or tendon pulls but

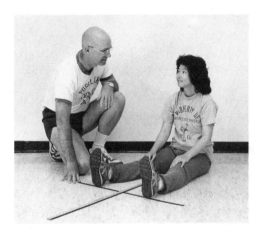 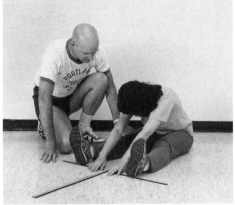

FIGURE 6.1
The sit and reach flexibility test.

Table 6.A Norms for the YMCA Sit & Reach Test.

| | | AGE (YRS) | | | | | |
| | | 35 & YOUNGER | | 36-45 | | 46 & OLDER | |
PERCENTILE	RATING	MALES	FEMALES	MALES	FEMALES	MALES	FEMALES
95	Excellent	21	23	22	23	20	22
85	Good	19	21	19	21	17	19
75	Above avg.	17	20	16	19	15	18
50	Average	15	18	14	17	13	15
30	Below avg.	12	15	12	14	11	14
15	Fair	9	14	10	12	8	11
5	Poor	7	11	5	10	5	9

Adapted from Golding, L. A., Myers, C. R., & Sinning, W. E. (Eds.), *The Y's Way to Physical Fitness (Revised)*, Rosemont, IL: YMCA of the USA, 1982.

are more likely to experience injuries of the ligaments in that region. The test items and related instructions for the Nicholas Overall Body Mobility Test are included in Figure 6.2. If you find that you are loose or tight in one or more regions, then you would be wise to include some strengthening and/or stretching exercises respectively to help correct your tendency. Methods for doing so are discussed later in this chapter.

Developing and Maintaining Flexibility

Stretching Principles

To improve your flexibility, you should use exercises that cause you to move through your whole range of motion. There are two common means of accomplishing this. One involves doing exercises that are dynamic or bouncy, such as jumping jacks, alternate toe touches, and side bends. This is called *ballistic* stretching. *Static stretching* involves exercises in which you stretch by holding yourself in a fixed position. An example is reaching forward to touch your toes while sitting on the ground with your feet extended ahead of you.

Evidence suggests that both ballistic and static stretching techniques are effective methods for improving your flexibility. However, caution should be used when stretching ballistically because there is the possibility of overstretching, which may cause soreness and/or injury. For this reason static stretching is currently considered to be the safer technique. Ballistic exercises are probably safe if they are done easily and not vigorously, as in a gentle warm-up routine in which you move around easily to loosen up your muscles and joints.

When using static stretching techniques, begin by holding each stretch for 5–10 seconds; then with practice, eventually work your way up to 15–30 seconds or more for each stretch. Each stretch may be repeated 1–5 or more times depending on time and interest, and the overall routine should be done 3–5 days per week. You should never stretch to the point of pain or burning discomfort. Rather, you should move to the limits of your range of motion using comfort as a guide, and then stretch slightly beyond and hold it there. You should try to relax when stretching, particularly those

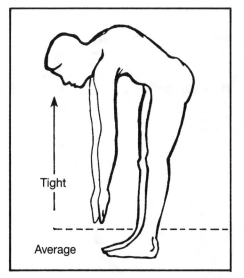

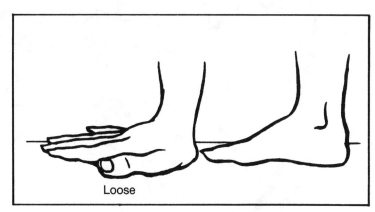

a. *Instructions:* Attempt to touch floor keeping knees straight.

b. *Instructions:* Stand
as you normally
stand and evaluate
knee position;
evaluate knees on
both sides of body.

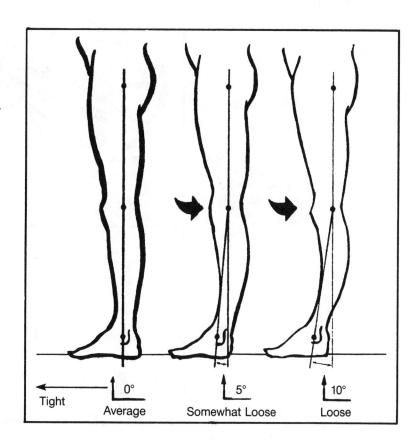

FIGURE 6.2
Nicholas Overall Body
Mobility Test.

Used with permission of J. A.
Nicholas, Lenox Hill Hospital,
130 E. 77th St., New York, NY
10021.

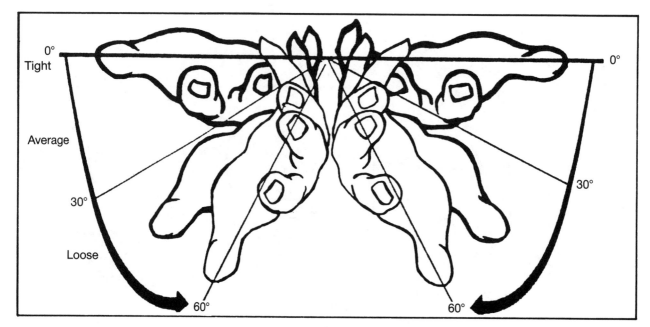

c. *Instructions:*
Keeping elbows
straight, rotate your
hands outward in
one movement as
far as possible.

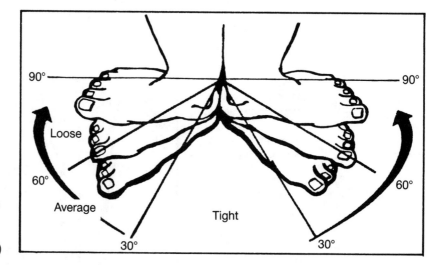

d. *Instructions:* In one
movement, turn
feet outward (you
must keep balance)

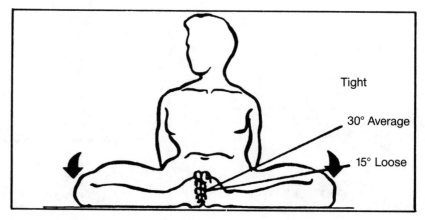

e. *Instructions:*
Determine how far
you can extend
knees downward.

muscles which are being stretched. It is important to note that for most effective results and least likelihood of injury, *you should be adequately warmed up before doing any stretching*. Stretching when not warmed up, or using vigorous stretching as a warm-up procedure, may be injurious to your muscles and joints and should not be done.

Factors That Limit Flexibility

The resistance you feel when stretching comes predominantly from connective tissue. Connective tissue binds muscle fibers together into bundles, surrounds muscles in sheaths, connects muscles to bones (i.e., via the tendons), and connects bones together (i.e., via the ligaments). This connective tissue has elastic properties that resist stretching. With time and practice it will stretch in response to applied pressure. Within reasonable limits, this deformation is the desired goal when undertaking a flexibility program.

Other factors can also limit flexibility. For example, resistance from skin, excessive fat, large muscles that interfere with a full range of motion, and even bone can serve as limiting factors to flexibility improvement. As with any type of training, the longer you work at stretching, the greater the changes will be. A word of caution, however: excessive flexibility may serve as a hindrance in some cases, particularly if the support structures are weakened or loosened so as to not protect the joint from injury from the normal stresses that occur in vigorous activity. Therefore, it would be wise to avoid working on flexibility if a particular joint and the surrounding muscles and tendons already provide great range of motion.

A Sample Stretching Routine

A series of mild to moderate stretches that focus on enhancing the range of motion of the shoulder region, the trunk, the hip region, and the ankle are seen in Figure 6.3a-j. We mentioned earlier that clinical evidence suggests that low back pain is related in part to poor flexibility in the hamstring muscles at the back of the upper leg. The hamstring stretch exercise (Figure 6.3i) should be of particular interest in preventing and treating this condition. It should be noted that many commonly practiced stretching exercises, when done repeatedly for long periods of time, have been linked to structural injury and/or chronic pain (see the section "Exercises to Avoid," below). Therefore, it is wise to do only those exercises that have been proven to be safe, such as those in Figure 6.3.

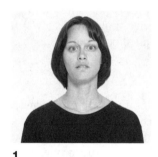 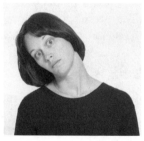 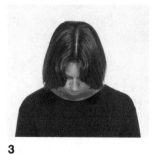 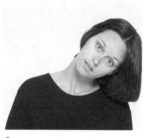

1   2   3   4

a. **Neck Stretch**

Position one: Head erect, eyes looking forward.

Position two: Roll head to the right side, then return to position one.

Position three: Roll head forward, then return to position one.

Position four: Roll head to the left side, then return to position one.

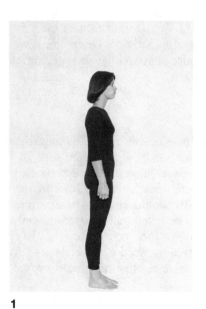 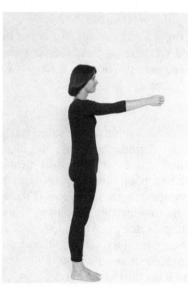 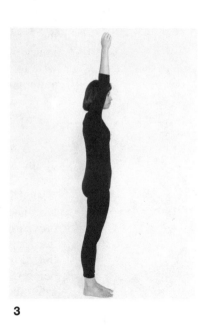

1   2   3

b. **Forward Arm Raise:**

Position one: Standing, fists slightly clenched, thumbs forward, body relaxed.

Position two: Raise arms forward slowly level with shoulders.

Position three: Continue to raise arms forward and upward to a point above head.
Return arms to position 1.

FIGURE 6.3
Flexibility exercises:
Mild to moderate
stretches.

Photos courtesy of
Kinesiotherapy Laboratory,
Portland State University,
Portland, OR.

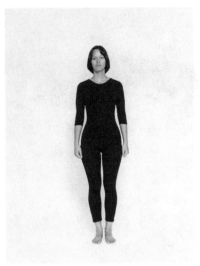 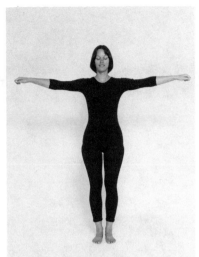 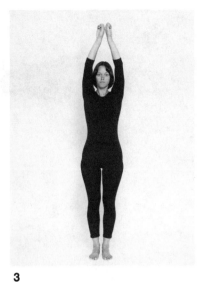

1   2   3

c. **Side Arm Raise:**

Position one: Standing, fists slightly clenched, thumbs forward, body relaxed.

Position two: Raise arms to the sides to shoulder level.

Position three: Continue to raise arms to the side and up until backs of hands touch. Return to position 1.

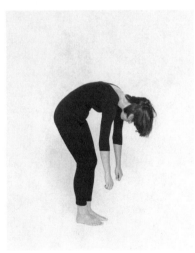 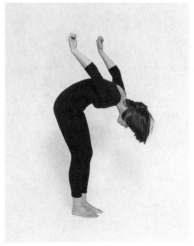

1   2

d. **Back Arm Raise:**

Position one: Body bent forward, arms hanging down from shoulders, fists lightly clenched, palms facing backward, bending at hips and knees, back rounded.

Position two: Arms pull back.

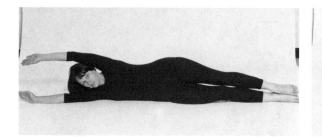

1

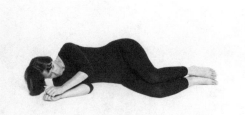

2

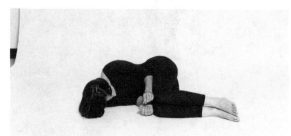

3

e. **Body Curl Extension:**

Position one: Side lying, both arms overhead, head neutral.

Position two: Head, torso and hips bending toward mid tuck position.

Position three: Full tuck position, then return to position 1.

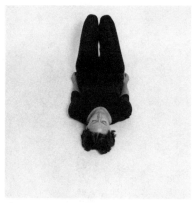

1

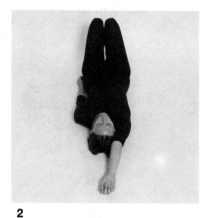

2

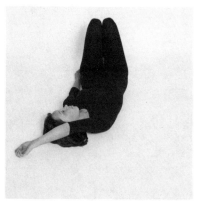

3

f. **Upper Back Stretch:**

Position one: Back lying, legs bent at knees, arms by side.

Position two: Sweep right arm up right side to the above head position.

Position three: Continue right arm sweep with lateral bending of trunk to left. Repeat with left arm and lateral bending of trunk to right.

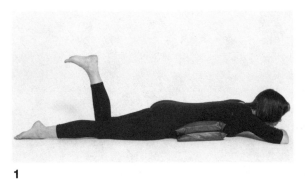 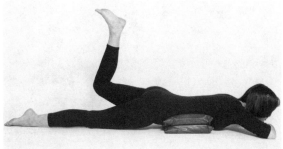

1   **2**

g. **Hip Extension:**

Position one: Lying face down, pillow support under stomach, one leg bent at knee at a 90° angle, arms folded under chin, body relaxed.

Position two: Raise bent leg towards ceiling, lower, repeat with opposite leg.

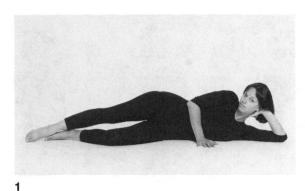 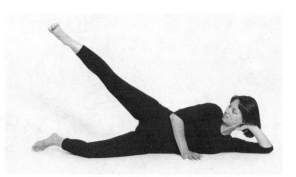

1   **2**

h. **Hip Abduction:**

Position one: Side lying, bottom leg bent for balance, top leg straight, bottom arm supporting head, top arm supporting body.

Position two: Elevate top leg to approximately a 45° angle while keeping pelvis forward, ankle position is neutral. Repeat on other side.

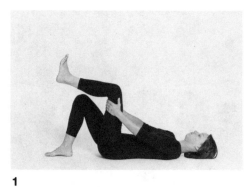 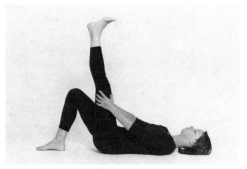

1   **2**

i. **Hamstring Stretch:**

Position one: Back lying, one leg bent with foot on floor, other leg bent at 90° with hips at 90°, support bent leg at thigh with hands.

Position two: Straighten leg slowly, and return extended leg to starting position. Repeat with other leg.

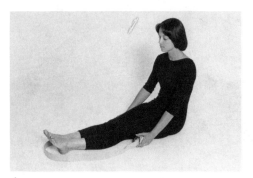 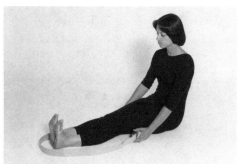

1   **2**

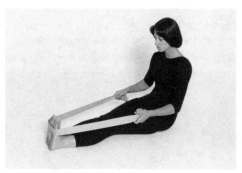

3

j. **Heel Cord Stretch:**

Position one: Long-sit position, feet relaxed, strap unattached.

Position two: Pull toes back toward shins, as far as possible.

Position three: Hold previous position, attach strap to balls of feet and apply additional stretch.

Exercises to Avoid

The exercises shown in Figure 6.4a-h have recently been associated with chronic pain and the likelihood of developing exercise-related injuries. While many books and exercise leaders still advocate use of some or all these exercises, it would seem prudent to avoid their use and substitute the safer flexibility exercises just presented in their place. The exercises are arranged in order of decreasing relative danger.

a. The *yoga plow* and related exercises are particularly dangerous because they can overstretch the cervical region of the spine, possibly resulting in disc injuries. Such exercises can also restrict the carotid artery, which supplies blood to the brain.

b. The *hurdler's stretch* and related exercises should not be done because they can lead to an overstretching of the muscles and ligaments in the groin region, making them more susceptible to a groin pull. In addition, such exercises overstretch the medial collateral ligament, which stabilizes the inner side of the knee. This can lead to instability of the knee. The sciatic nerve may also be stretched, leading to back pain.

c. The *deep knee bend* and *duck walk* put great pressure on the lateral meniscus of the knee. (The meniscus is the cartilage within the knee joint on the outer side that acts as a cushion between upper and lower leg bones.) This can damage the meniscus resulting in permanent disability and/or surgery.

d. *Toe touching* puts excessive stress on one of the main supporting ligaments in the spine and can also put undue stress on the spinal discs, possibly leading to their rupture. Such exercises also stretch the sciatic nerve, often leading to back pain.

e. *Ballet stretches* put excessive demands on the hips, knees, ankles, and feet. They overstretch the sciatic nerve and are a common cause of back and leg pain.

f. *Stiff leg raises,* especially if they are done with added weights on the feet, put excessive stress on the hip flexor muscles. Also, most people cannot do them without arching the lower back region. This arching puts great strain on the structures in the lower back and should be avoided for this reason.

g. *Knee stretches* can cause the range of motion of the knee to be exceeded; they can overstretch the patellar and collateral ligaments of the knee, leading to reduced stability in this region. As the knee is one of the joints that is most easily injured, such exercises should be avoided as they serve no useful purpose.

h. *Straight legged sit-ups* are generally recognized to put undue strain on the lower back and can lead to nerve elongation. By bending the legs (knees up) into the "hook lying position," the strain on the sciatic nerve is lessened, making the exercise more safe.

Note also that doing the *Sit and Reach* exercise, while safe enough to do as a test on an occasional basis, stretches the posterior longitudinal ligament and elongates the sciatic nerve, which can lead to back pain.

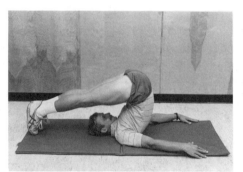
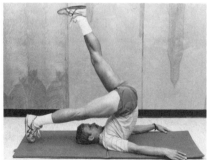

a. Yoga "plow" and variation

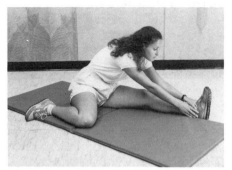
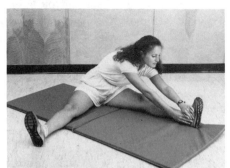
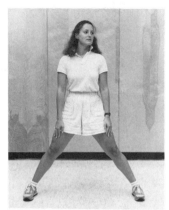

b. Hurdler's stretch and related exercises

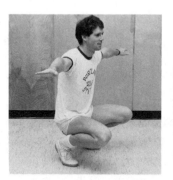
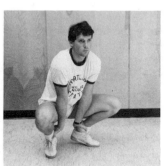

c. Deep knee bend and duck walk

FIGURE 6.4
Exercises to avoid.
 See text discussion for
explanation of these
exercises.

Adapted from Domingues and
Gajda, 1982.

EXERCISES TO AVOID

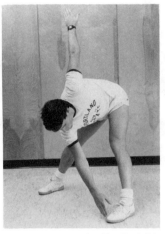 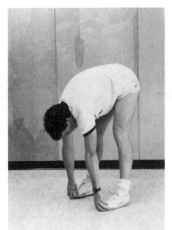 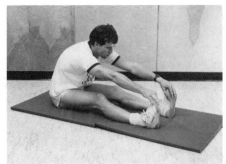

d. Toe touching

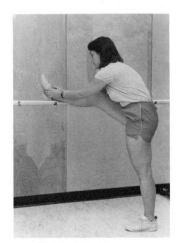

EXERCISES TO AVOID

e. Ballet stretches

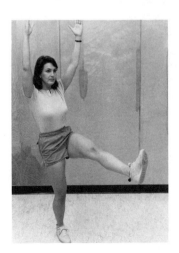

f. Stiff leg raises

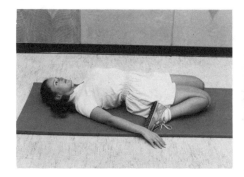
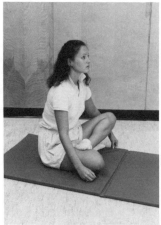
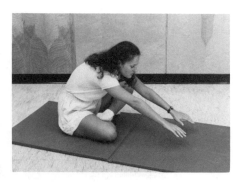

g. Knee stretches

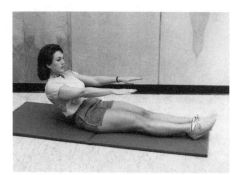

h. Straight leg sit-ups/sit and reach

EXERCISES TO AVOID

Strength and Muscle Endurance

Measuring Strength

Strength is defined as the capacity of a muscle or muscle group to exert force under maximal conditions. Several methods can be used to measure strength, all of which are very different from one another. As a result of these differences, strength is defined operationally in different ways, depending on the measurement procedure that is used.

    Static Strength. Static strength is measured using special devices called *dynamometers* and *tensiometers,* which you push or pull against in a fixed position. The most common example is to measure static grip strength using a grip dynamometer (Figure 6.5). After adjusting the grip size to fit your hand comfortably, simply squeeze as hard as you can for 1–2 seconds and your strength score will be registered on the device. Norms for combined right- and left-hand grip strength are found in Appendix 2. Tests of static leg extension strength or static strength of most other muscle groups require specialized equipment and techniques that are not as widely available. It should be noted that a measurement of static strength is of somewhat limited value because it has been shown that static strength varies within the same muscle group according to the joint angle. In other words, you do not have just one static strength in a given muscle group, you may have many, depending on the position in which you measure the strength. Taking a single measurement of static strength will not provide an overall indication of your strength status because no single measurement is highly representative of the large number of strength scores you could determine should you take the time to do so.

    Isokinetic Strength. Isokinetic strength is defined as the peak force (or "peak torque" as it is called) that you are able to exert while pushing against an isokinetic machine. To measure your strength, you push against a movable lever on the machine with a body part such as your lower leg, moving it through the full range of motion.

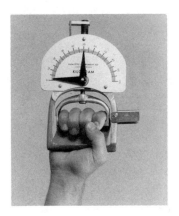

FIGURE 6.5
A grip dynamometer for measuring static grip strength.

The isokinetic machine is set to allow only one speed of movement at a time regardless of how hard you push against it. Because such machines are very expensive, they are not widely available and are found mostly in rehabilitation clinics. No widespread norms have been developed using isokinetic machines, so if you have a chance to be measured, the best method is to compare your strength score to a score recorded for you at an earlier or later date.

Dynamic Strength.   Dynamic strength is defined operationally as the heaviest weight that you can correctly lift just one time. This is called your 1 *repetition maximum* (1 RM). Since weights are widely available in most gyms and fitness establishments, determining your 1 RM is the most practical way of measuring your strength. Typically, a trial and error approach is used to determine your 1 RM. After a sufficient warm-up—including a warm-up of the specific muscle group you are about to measure—using easy repetitions with a light weight, you simply guess at a weight that you think is close to your maximum. If you find you can lift it easily, then after a rest period of a few minutes adjust the next trial upward accordingly and try again. Making adjustments upward or downward as necessary, you will be able to determine your 1 RM in a few trials.

It should be noted that you may use free weights or weight machines for this measurement. There are many different types of weight machines; no one brand is particularly better than another and the technique for measuring strength is the same on all.

Recommended standards for dynamic strength in several different muscle groups are seen in Table 6.B. These standards may not be representative of all segments of the population (e.g., athletes), but they are suggested as appropriate goals for the average person. It is recommended that all the tests in Table 6.B be used to assess your strength status, since an overall strength profile is preferred; however, if there is time for only one test it should be the bench press exercise, which has been shown to

Table 6.B Strength standards recommended for four weight-lifting exercises. (Data based on the 1-RM test.)

BODY WEIGHT (LB)	BENCH PRESS		STANDING PRESS		CURL		LEG PRESS	
	MALE	FEMALE	MALE	FEMALE	MALE	FEMALE	MALE	FEMALE
80	80	56	53	37	40	28	160	112
100	100	70	67	47	50	35	200	140
120	120	84	80	56	60	42	240	168
140	140	98	93	65	70	49	280	196
160	160	112	107	75	80	56	320	224
180	180	126	120	84	90	63	360	252
200	200	140	133	93	100	70	400	280
220	220	154	147	103	110	77	440	308
240	240	168	160	112	120	84	480	336

Note: Data collected on Universal Gym apparatus. Information collected on other apparatus could modify results. Data expressed in pounds.

Reprinted with permission of Macmillan Publishing Company from *Health and Fitness Through Physical Activity* by Pollock, M. L., Wilmore, J. H., and Fox, S. M; originally published by John Wiley & Sons, Inc (New York: Macmillan, 1978).

have the highest correlation to the whole battery of tests. The bench press exercise is pictured in figure 6.10(d), later in this chapter.

Unfortunately, for those who wish to determine where they fall relative to standardized norms, at the present time such data exist only to a limited degree and in some cases only for college-age persons. These norms and instructions for their use are included in Appendix 2.

It should be noted that whenever you compare yourself to standards or to norms, you must measure yourself using the same apparatus. For example, the standards listed in Table 6.B were collected on the Universal gym and not using free weights. Your 1 RM on a Universal gym may not be the same as one determined using free-weights because of calibration and design differences.

Measuring Muscle Endurance

Typically, *absolute* muscle endurance and/or *relative* muscle endurance are measured dynamically using either free weights or weight machines.

Absolute muscle endurance is determined by counting the number of correctly completed repetitions you can do with a standard weight before being unable to continue. For example, suppose you decided to count the number of lifts you could do of the arm-curl exercise (in which you lift a weight upward to your chest with your arm flexors) using 40 pounds. If you could do 15 repetitions before being unable to continue, that would be your muscle endurance score. As you might surmise, muscle endurance measured in this manner is highly related to your dynamic strength; in other words, the greater your strength, the greater your absolute muscle endurance. The YMCA fitness test battery includes a test of absolute muscle endurance for the bench press exercise using free weights. Norms for both sexes and all ages are seen in Table 6.C.

Relative muscular endurance is measured by taking some fraction of your 1 RM score (usually 70%) and determining the number of correctly executed repetitions you can do. For example, if your 1 RM score is 110 pounds for a particular exercise, then

Table 6.C Norms for absolute muscular endurance on the bench press.

PERCENTILE	RATING	35 & YOUNGER MALES	35 & YOUNGER FEMALES	36-45 MALES	36-45 FEMALES	46 & OLDER MALES	46 & OLDER FEMALES
95	Excellent	35	30	30	29	28	30
85	Good	29	24	24	21	22	22
75	Above avg.	24	20	19	18	19	18
50	Average	20	16	17	15	16	14
30	Below avg.	15	13	14	11	12	9
15	Fair	11	10	10	7	8	5
5	Poor	7	5	3	4	3	2

AGE (YRS)

Women use 35 lb. barbell; men use 80 lb. barbell. Score equals number of successful repetitions.

Adapted from Golding, L. A., Myers, C. R., & Sinning, W. E. (Eds.), *The Y's Way to Physical Fitness (Revised)*, Rosemont, IL: YMCA of the USA, 1982.

the sum of .70(110), or 77 pounds, is the weight you would use to determine your relative muscular endurance. If you cannot adjust the weight this accurately, you can use a 70 or 75 lb. weight as an alternative. Standards for measuring muscular endurance using this method have not been developed, but on the basis of limited experience a rough goal for the recreational exerciser is to be able to do 12–15 repetitions in a given exercise with this method. For the competitive athlete, 20–25 repetitions is a reasonable goal.

Relative muscle endurance may also be measured by taking a fraction of your body weight to determine the load with which to measure yourself. In this case, muscle endurance is said to be relative to body weight rather than relative to strength. For example, you might take 40 percent of your body weight and count the number of repetitions you can do with this load. Alternatively, you might count the number of repetitions you can complete in a specific period of time, such as 60 seconds.

Calisthenics are another common method of measuring muscular endurance relative to body weight. Calisthenics are defined as exercises in which your body weight serves as the resistance. Push-ups, sit-ups, and pull-ups are examples. If you use a calisthenic exercise as a test of muscular endurance (e.g., a push-up test), you are actually lifting a fraction of your body weight. In the case of the push-up, for example, the resistance is your body weight acting as if it were pivoting as a lever around your toes. The effect of the leverage in this case is to reduce the resistance to less than it would be if you had to lift your entire body.

Two commonly used calisthenic tests of muscle endurance are the push-up and sit-up tests. The push-up test is administered using the standard push-up starting in the "up" position with hands pointed forward and positioned directly under the shoulders (Figure 6.6). You lower yourself, using your toes as a pivotal point, until your chin touches the mat and then push up to return to the starting position. Your back must be kept in a straight line throughout the test. The maximum number of correctly executed push-ups is your score. Women should perform this test using the bent-knee position (Figure 6.7). Norms and percentiles for age and sex are provided in Table 6.D.

The sit-up test actually involves a modified curl-up motion (Figure 6.8). In this test, you begin by lying on your back with your hands behind your head and fingers interlocked (see caution advisory below Figure 6.8, page 152). Your heels should be 12 inches from your buttocks and knees bent about 90 degrees. The testor should hold your feet down and count the number of times in 60 seconds that you can curl up, touch your elbows to your knees, and return down to the full lying position before repeating. Standards for age and sex are provided in Table 6.E. To ensure that your

FIGURE 6.6
The standard or full push-up.

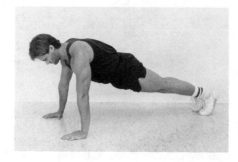 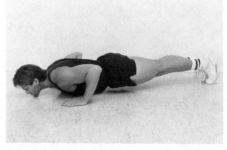

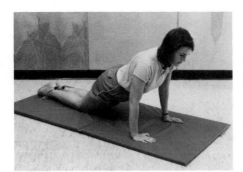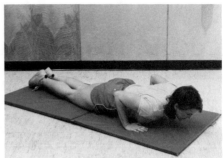

FIGURE 6.7
The modified push-up, which uses the bent knee position.

Table 6.D   Norms and percentiles by age groups and sex for push-ups.

AGE (YRS).	15–19		20–29		30–39		40–49		50–59		60–69	
SEX	M	F	M	F	M	F	M	F	M	F	M	F
Excellent	≥ 39	≥ 33	≥ 36	≥ 30	≥ 30	≥ 27	≥ 22	≥ 24	≥ 21	≥ 21	≥ 18	≥ 17
Above avg.	29–38	25–32	29–35	21–29	22–29	20–26	17–21	15–23	13–20	11–20	11–17	12–16
Average	23–28	18–24	22–28	15–20	17–21	13–19	13–16	11–14	10–12	7–10	8–10	5–11
Below avg.	18–22	12–17	17–21	10–14	12–16	8–12	10–12	5–10	7–9	2–6	5–7	1–4
Weak	≤ 17	≤ 11	≤ 16	≤ 9	≤ 11	≤ 7	≤ 9	≤ 4	≤ 6	≤ 1	≤ 4	≤ 1

AGE (YRS).	15–19		20–29		30–39		40–49		50–59		60–69	
SEX	M	F	M	F	M	F	M	F	M	F	M	F
Percentiles												
95	50	46	48	37	36	36	30	32	28	30	25	30
90	43	38	41	32	32	31	25	28	24	23	24	25
85	39	33	36	30	30	27	22	24	21	21	18	17
80	35	31	34	26	27	24	21	22	17	17	16	15
75	32	28	32	24	25	22	20	20	15	15	13	13
70	31	26	30	22	24	21	19	18	14	13	11	12
65	29	25	29	21	22	20	17	15	13	11	11	12
60	27	23	27	20	21	17	16	14	11	10	10	10
55	26	21	25	18	20	16	15	13	11	10	10	9
50	24	20	24	16	19	14	13	12	10	9	9	6
45	23	18	22	15	17	13	13	11	10	7	8	5
40	22	16	21	14	16	12	12	10	9	5	7	4
35	21	15	20	13	15	11	11	10	8	4	6	3
30	20	14	18	11	14	10	10	7	7	3	6	2
25	18	12	17	10	12	8	10	5	7	2	5	1
20	16	11	16	9	11	7	8	4	5	1	4	—
15	14	9	14	7	10	6	7	3	5	1	3	—
10	11	6	11	5	8	4	5	2	4	—	2	—
5	8	4	9	2	5	1	4	—	2	—	—	—

Canada Fitness Survey 1981

From *Standardized Test of Fitness,* 2nd Ed., Fitness and Amateur Sport, Canada, 1981.

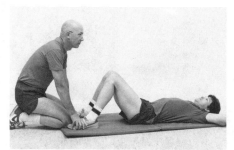 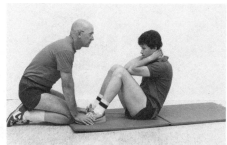

FIGURE 6.8
The modified curl-up, with feet held.

Placing the hands behind the head as depicted can put undue pressure on the cervical spine. To make use of the norms for this test, which are the best age and sex specific standards available, this position should be used during testing only. *Caution is advised*.

Table 6.E   Norms and percentiles by age groups and sex for curl-ups (no. in 60 seconds).

AGE (YRS).	15–19		20–29		30–39		40–49		50–59		60–69	
SEX	M	F	M	F	M	F	M	F	M	F	M	F
Excellent	≥ 48	≥ 42	≥ 43	≥ 36	≥ 36	≥ 29	≥ 31	≥ 25	≥ 26	≥ 19	≥ 23	≥ 16
Above avg.	42–47	36–41	37–42	31–35	31–35	24–28	26–30	20–24	22–25	12–18	17–22	12–15
Average	38–41	32–35	33–36	25–30	27–30	20–23	22–25	15–19	18–21	5–11	12–16	4–11
Below avg.	33–37	27–31	29–32	21–24	22–26	15–19	17–21	7–14	13–17	3–4	7–11	2–3
Weak	≤ 32	≤ 26	≤ 28	≤ 20	≤ 21	≤ 14	≤ 16	≤ 6	≤ 12	≤ 2	≤ 6	≤ 1

AGE (YRS).	15–19		20–29		30–39		40–49		50–59		60–69	
SEX	M	F	M	F	M	F	M	F	M	F	M	F
Percentiles												
95	53	47	49	43	42	34	36	28	34	26	26	20
90	50	43	45	39	38	31	33	26	28	22	24	18
85	48	42	43	36	36	29	31	25	26	19	23	16
80	46	40	41	34	34	27	30	23	25	17	21	15
75	44	39	40	32	33	26	29	22	24	16	19	14
70	43	37	38	31	32	25	27	21	23	14	18	13
65	42	36	37	31	31	24	26	20	22	12	17	12
60	41	35	36	29	30	23	25	18	21	11	15	10
55	40	34	35	28	29	22	24	17	20	10	15	9
50	39	33	34	27	28	21	23	16	20	7	13	5
45	38	32	33	25	27	20	22	15	18	5	12	4
40	36	31	32	24	26	18	21	13	17	4	11	2
35	35	29	31	23	24	17	20	12	16	3	10	—
30	34	28	30	22	23	16	19	10	15	—	10	—
25	33	27	29	21	22	15	17	7	13	—	7	—
20	32	25	27	19	21	13	16	5	11	—	2	—
15	30	23	26	17	20	11	14	3	10	—	—	—
10	28	21	24	15	17	7	11	—	8	—	—	—
5	23	15	20	11	14	—	6	—	—	—	—	—

Canada Fitness Survey 1981

From *Standardized Test of Fitness*, 2nd Ed., Fitness and Amateur Sport, Canada, 1981.

back returns to the starting position, your interlocked fingers must touch the mat before curling up again. Also you should exhale when curling up.

Recent evidence suggests that the above-mentioned curl-up test does not place optimal overload on the abdominal muscles and instead calls upon the hip flexor muscles to a considerable degree. An alternative test involving the type of motion pictured in Figure 6.9c, below, has been shown to focus more completely on the muscle endurance of the abdominal muscles. In the alternative test, your feet are not supported by the testor. Your hands lie at your side as depicted in the picture. The test involves curling your head and upper trunk upward only far enough to allow your hands to slide 3 inches forward on the ground and then returning to the down position. Your upper back must touch the mat each time but it is not necessary for your head to do so. Your finger tips must maintain contact with the mat throughout the test. Your score is the number of correctly completed curl-ups done in 60 seconds. Unfortunately, norms for this test have yet to be developed, so testing yourself in this manner will require repeated comparisons to your own scores over time.

Developing and Maintaining Strength and Muscle Endurance

General Principles

The general principles of warm-up, overload, and progression discussed in Chapter 4 are particularly applicable to this type of training because of the great stress it places on your muscles, joints, and related connective tissue. Both a general warm-up that raises your body temperature slightly and a specific warm-up of the muscles that you will be training should always be done for 5–10 minutes before beginning this type of training. General warm-up can be accomplished with walking and/or light calisthenics, followed by light jogging. Specific warm-up can be accomplished by beginning with much lower resistances at first. As with any type of training, properly applying the principle of progression will enable you to improve without subjecting yourself to excessive stress and potential injury. Your rate of progression will depend on your motivation to improve and how trained you are to begin with. A prudent and cautious approach is one in which you progress slowly rather than trying to set a world record in a few months. If you are training toward a specific goal such as improved performance in a specific athletic event, then you also need to pay attention to the specificity principle and train in ways that mimic or imitate your performance (or parts of it) as much as possible. Otherwise, a general all-around training program that emphasizes the major muscle groups and particularly those of the upper body is recommended for the average exerciser.

Exercises for Building Strength and Muscle Endurance

The exercises illustrated in Figure 6.9a–j, when done slowly, are safe exercises for persons of all ages and require little or no special equipment. For persons with low initial fitness, these exercises will contribute modestly to the development of strength and muscle endurance and can be used as a preconditioning program before moving on to more rigorous training.

If your initial fitness permits you to begin at a higher level of training, the most practical method to build strength and muscle endurance is through use of dynamic

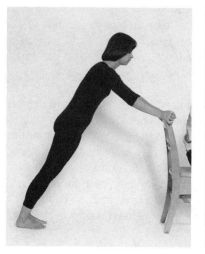 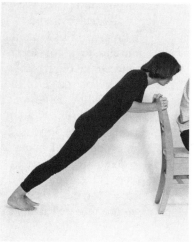

1   2

a. **Incline Press:**

Position one: Support the inclined body with the arms, body inclined at a 45° angle.

Position two: Keep body straight while bending arms to touch chin to support surface, then return to position 1.

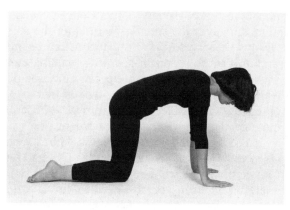 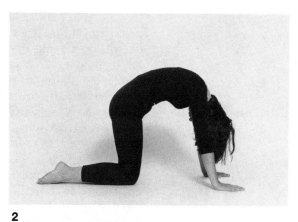

1   2

b. **Cat Curl:**

Position one: Begin on all fours, knees together, arms extended shoulder width apart, back and neck rounded, head forward, eyes looking between hands.

Position two: Tighten stomach muscles and arch back, head drops between elbows.

FIGURE 6.9
Mild resistive exercises for building strength and endurance in persons of all ages.

Photos courtesy of Kinesiotherapy Laboratory, Portland State University, Portland, OR.

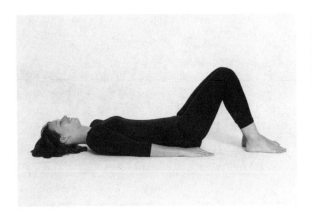
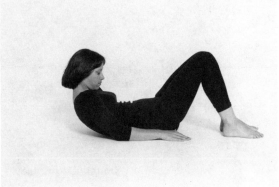

1

2

c. **Pelvic Tilt:**

Position one: Back lying, legs bent at knees, feet slightly apart, arms at sides, head on floor.

Position two: Curl head and trunk forward. Do not raise pelvis off floor.

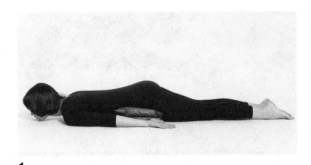
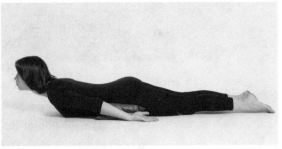

1

2

d. **Back Raise:**

Position one: Lying face down, pillow support under pelvis, legs straight and together, arms by sides, palms up, head neutral, chin resting on floor.

Position two: Head and upper back raise up, feet down, hold for ten seconds.

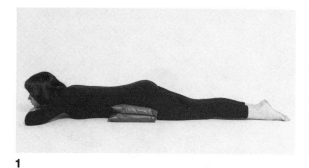
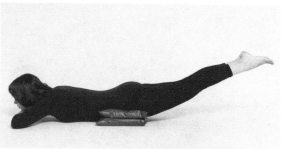

1   2

e. **Double Leg Raise:**

Position one: Lying face down, arms folded under chin supporting head, legs relaxed and straight.

Position two: Raise both legs upward and hold for ten seconds.

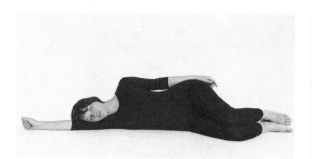
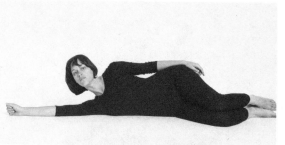

1   2

f. **Lateral Flexion of Neck:**

Position one: Side lying, legs comfortably bent, head supported by outstretched bottom arm, top arm resting on hip.

Position two: Raise left ear to left shoulder, hold for two seconds and return to position 1. Repeat on opposite side.

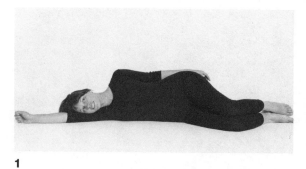
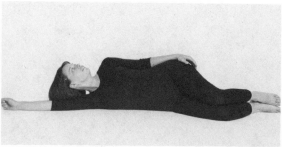

1   2

g. **Neck Rotation:**

Position one: Same position as in exercise f., eyes looking straight ahead.

Position two: Rotate chin so that eyes look up. Repeat on opposite side.

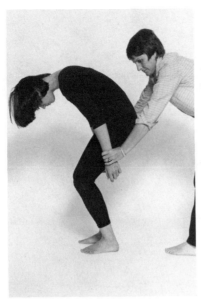
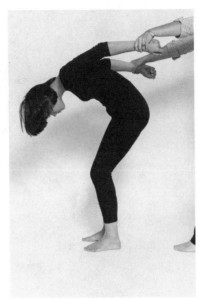

1   **2**

h. **Shoulder Extension:**

Position one: Standing position with legs bent, hips bent, back rounded, arms hanging
down. Partner supports wrists from the rear.

Position two: Maintain body position, pull arms slowly to the rear as partner offers
partial resistance to the motion.

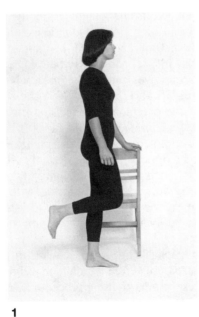
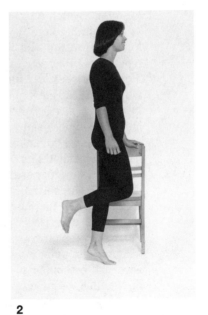

1   **2**

i. **Toe Raise-One Leg:**

Position one: Standing position, weight balanced on one foot, other foot in bent leg
position, one hand provides support.

Position two: Raise on toes, then return to position 1. Repeat with opposite leg.

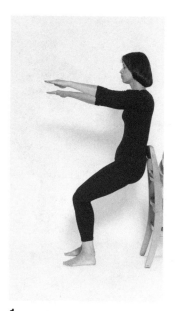

1

j. **Ski Squat:**

Position one: Stand in a partial squat position with hips against support, hips flexed at 45°, feet apart, arms parallel to floor. Hold this position for 30 seconds.

exercises, which typically involve lifting weights, although calisthenic exercises such as those in Figure 6.9a–j are also a form of dynamic exercise. Most beginners find it tolerable to start with loads that are about 50% of their 1 RM, doing a series of 10 repetitions of a given exercise in a set and slowly building up to 3–4 sets per workout, 3 days per week. As fitness improves you can begin slowly adding weight so that you work with loads that equal 60% 1 RM, and then 70% and 80% 1 RM. Figure 6.10a–k gives examples of some of the common dynamic and calisthenic exercises used for building strength and muscle endurance.

A special comment is warranted regarding abdominal exercises. Recent evidence has demonstrated that compared to the more traditional curl-up exercise in which you curl to the upright position to touch your knees (Figure 6.8), greater overload is placed on the abdominal muscles by doing a partial curl-up with the feet unsupported, the legs bent, and the hands at the side of the body, as illustrated in Figure 6.9c. This abdominal exercise is particularly recommended if you are interested in preventing low back problems.

Another point is worth emphasizing. Improvements in strength and muscle endurance will be similar whether you use free weights or weight machines like Universal or Nautilus, provided you use similar training procedures. Machines are handy in that the weights can be changed quickly to adjust to masses of people using the equipment in a small amount of time. However, they do not allow for significant adjustment in position to accommodate the different biomechanical needs of people of different sizes and leverage. Free weights can be used by anyone in any position, so they provide the greatest flexibility in this regard. However, since much time is required to change the weights on a barbell they are not as easily adapted to the needs of large groups of

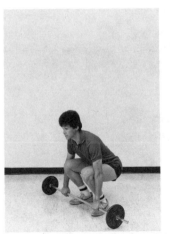 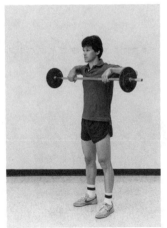 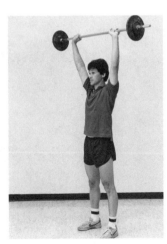

a. **Dead lift and vertical press:**

To do this exercise correctly, you must keep your back straight and hold the bar with an overhand grip. Lift the barbell to the chest level, drop your elbows, and then lift the barbell vertically. Reverse motions to return the barbell to the floor. This exercise can be used effectively with light weights as a warm-up since it involves many of the major muscle groups of the body.

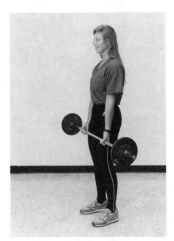 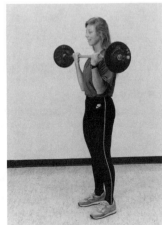

b. **Elbow curl:**

Keep your back straight when doing this exercise. Lift the barbell upward by flexing the elbows and return.

FIGURE 6.10
Dynamic exercises for building strength and muscular endurance.

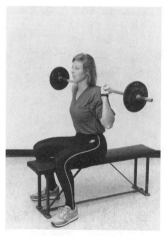 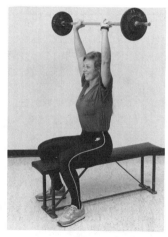

c. **Seated vertical press:**

This exercise can be done with the barbell placed behind the head as pictured or in front of the head. Lift vertically keeping the back straight and return.

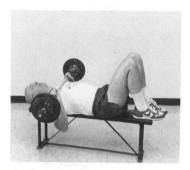 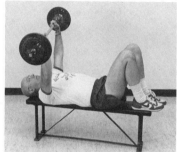

d. **Bench press:**

To keep the lower back flat, this exercise should be done with the knees bent as pictured. Lift the barbell vertically overhead and return.

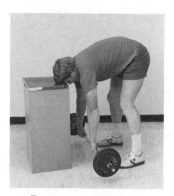 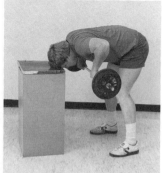

e. **Bent over row:**

In this exercise, the head should be supported as pictured. The barbell should be raised to the chest and then lowered.

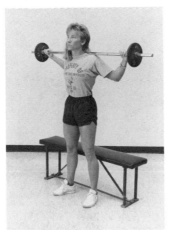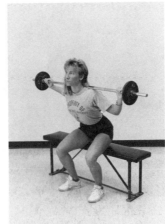

f. **Half squat:**

With the barbell supported on your shoulders, squat to a bench and return. Keep your back as straight as possible and do not bend your knees more than 90°.

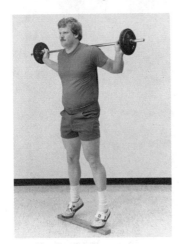

g. **Heel raises:**

With the barbell supported on your shoulder and your toes placed on a board as pictured, raise your heels as high as you can and return.

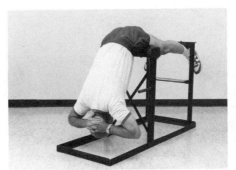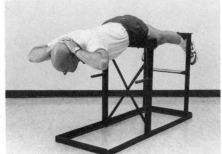

h. **Back extensions:**

With your feet supported, your hands placed behind your head, and your trunk bent at the waist as shown, lift upward until your spine is horizontal and return. Do not lift above the horizontal plane. Extra weights can be used behind the head if desired.

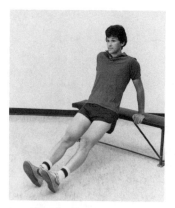
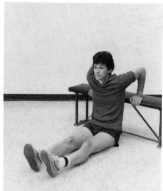

i. **Bench dip:**
    With your hands placed on a bench and your feet extended in front of you as shown, lower yourself to the floor and return.

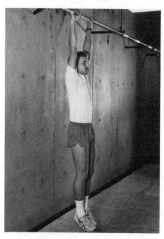
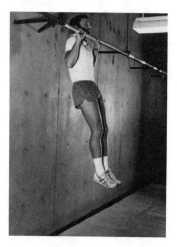

j. **Pull-up:**
    With your hands placed in the forward grip, hang from a bar as pictured and raise yourself upward until your chin is above the bar and return. If you are unable to do this exercise, an assistant can help you partially by lifting up on your legs.

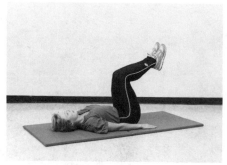
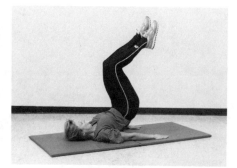

k. **Reverse curl:**
    Lying on your back with arms placed at your sides and with your legs elevated as pictured, lift your lower spine upward as far as you can and return.

people who all exercise in a short period of time. The point is that machines and free weights are equally effective in similar conditions, and your choice should be based on your preference and circumstances.

If your focus is to be strictly on building strength using dynamic exercise, you should do a few repetitions with very heavy resistances. Translating this into more specific terms, this means doing 3–4 sets with sufficiently heavy weights so that you cannot do more than 3–10 repetitions in a set. Such training is very rigorous and should be undertaken only by the well-conditioned and highly motivated individual. It also should not be done more than 3 days per week for a given muscle group.

Similarly, to build muscle endurance using dynamic exercise, you should do many repetitions with lower resistances. Specifically, this translates to 3–4 sets of 10–30 repetitions, each with loads you can lift only 10–30 times, 3 days per week. Again, such training is very rigorous and should only be done by those who are fit and highly motivated.

Gains in both strength and muscle endurance will occur from both types of training described above. However, strength is optimally developed with heavier weights and fewer repetitions while muscle endurance is optimally developed with lighter weights and more repetitions. If you are interested in developing both at the same time, a good compromise is to work with 3 sets of 10 repetitions with loads you can lift only 10 times, 3 days per week.

Preliminary evidence suggests that you can maintain your strength and muscle endurance gains with fewer training sessions per week than are needed for improvements. Whereas 3 training sessions per week are required for increasing strength and muscle endurance, as few as 1–2 training sessions per week may be required to maintain yourself at that level. This appears to be true over at least a 1–2 month period. Follow-up periods of longer duration using such a maintenance schedule have not been studied, however.

Before leaving the topic of building strength and muscle endurance, it is important to mention that two other training methods, *static exercise* and *isokinetic exercise,* can be used in this regard. For different reasons, neither of these is used as frequently as dynamic exercise.

Static exercise involves doing a maximal (or near maximal) contraction against an immovable resistance for 5–10 seconds. For example, you could stand in a doorway and press outward with your arms on the doorjam. Research into such training procedures has demonstrated that strength will improve dramatically with such a procedure. However, there is one liability: improvements occur only in the position in which you train. This means that in the example cited above, your strength in that position would improve quickly but your strength would not be much greater if you tested yourself in a slightly wider doorway, causing your arms to be farther apart. Such training is rather impractical since you would have to train a given muscle group in a variety of positions through its full range of motion to increase its overall strength in that range. Nevertheless, static exercises can be useful, particularly when equipment or time is limited or for reconditioning after an injury. Typical examples of static strength exercises are included in Appendix 3.

Static strength exercises can also be employed as an aid to dynamic strength. When lifting weights, it is not uncommon for one position or joint angle in the range of motion to be particularly difficult to move past. This is referred to as the "sticking point." Static exercise at this joint angle can be used to improve the strength at the sticking point and thereby increase the ease with which the weight can be lifted through its full range of motion.

Isokinetic exercise makes use of isokinetic machines. As mentioned earlier, isokinetic machines are designed to allow you to pull (or push) against them at a variety of speeds that are predetermined by setting the controls of the machine. Once the speed is set, no matter how hard you pull, the speed does not change. This type of training appears to combine the advantages of dynamic exercise (which allows you to move through your whole range of motion but does not equally overload your muscle in all positions; only the weakest position is overloaded optimally) and static exercise (which allows you to work maximally at all points in your range of motion but which does not involve movement). However, because of the high cost of isokinetic machinery, few people have opportunities to train in this manner. To reduce cost, some manufacturers have developed isokinetic-like machines which, although they do not hold speed of movement strictly constant, permit training that is similar to isokinetic training. When doing such training, 1–5 repetitions done at slow speeds are recommended for developing strength, although optimal training procedures have not yet been developed. Explosive repetitions at faster speeds are recommended when training for power.

Factors Affecting Strength and Endurance Gains

There seem to be large individual differences in the degree of improvement in strength and muscular endurance from training. In some, improvements in excess of 40 percent have been documented, with small increases continuing to occur even after several years of training. In others, the improvements are smaller. Reasons for the differences are not entirely clear. Improved strength has been shown to be partly related to changes in the cross-sectional area of muscle. Muscle fibers increase in size but not number as a result of strength training. Such changes result from increases in protein synthesis within these trained muscle fibers, causing them to increase in cross-sectional area. Muscle, connective tissue, tendons, and ligaments are also strengthened by heavy exercise.

Improvements in strength also appear to occur due to changes within the central nervous system. A number of lines of evidence suggest this conclusion, including the fact that the improvements in strength are proportionally larger than the increase in cross-sectional area of the muscle. Such mechanisms appear to be particularly significant in elderly persons, who experience improvement from strength training with little muscle hypertrophy.

Contraindications and Safety Precautions

Not only does strength and muscle endurance training put a high strain on muscles and joints, it also works the heart more than aerobic exercise does in one specific way. Exercises designed to build strength and muscle endurance tend to raise heart rate while also raising blood pressure to higher levels than during aerobic exercise. This combined effect of elevated heart rate and elevated blood pressure can put an excessive burden on anyone with a weak heart. This same effect definitely applies when training statically or doing any form of static contraction. It is also exaggerated when doing intensive exercise with the smaller muscles of the body such as those in the arms (e.g., chopping wood, pull-ups, etc.). Anyone with a weak heart because of past or continuing illness, and anyone with the primary risk factors for cardiovascular disease (hypertension, cigarette smoking, high serum cholesterol) would be wise not to put great emphasis on training for strength or muscle endurance. Even if the above conditions do not apply to you, whenever lifting weights you should avoid holding your breath and instead inhale and exhale slowly while exercising. Holding your breath under such circumstances is called the *Valsalva maneuver,* and the effect is to raise your blood pressure higher than otherwise. This accomplishes no benefit and may result in a lightheaded feeling afterward.

One last suggestion relates to the skill needed in working with heavy weights and some exercise machines. Lifts in which you raise anything above your head can be dangerous should you lose control. Lifts in which you use your lower back can increase the strain on this region and can cause injury should they be done incorrectly. We highly recommend that you seek instruction as to proper technique and make use of "spotters" to assist you in certain lifts.

The Role of Sex Differences in Training

While there are typical differences between the sexes in strength and muscle endurance, evidence suggests that the training procedures to develop these components of fitness are similar for both sexes. Because men tend to be larger in stature and body weight and because they tend to develop larger musculature during puberty than women, their strength and endurance tends to be higher, although many individual women, particularly athletes, can out-perform the average man in specific areas. In fact, the differences between the sexes are smaller in the legs than in the upper body, perhaps as a result of similar levels of habitual activity using the lower body. Nevertheless, dynamic training has been shown to create dramatic improvements in the strength and muscle endurance of many women, often without large changes in muscular size. Exercises that focus on improving the strength and muscle endurance in the upper body can be particularly useful as an aid in handling one's body weight.

A common fear among women is that by engaging in strength or muscle endurance training they will "bulk up" and develop large, unattractive muscles. The available evidence suggests this is not the case in most women. Muscle hypertrophy, referring to growth of muscle tissue in size, appears to be related to the amount of circulating male sex hormone, testosterone. Beginning at puberty, testosterone levels are much higher in males than females. This causes the typical increase in muscle mass and decrease in body fat at this age. Since testosterone levels continue to be much lower in females than males during adulthood, women appear to be able to engage in weight training exercises without fear of significant hypertrophy. There are individual differences, however, and therefore some women may increase their musculature size from such training. Practically speaking, women who already exhibit well-defined muscles are more likely to hypertrophy than those who do not.

Back Problems and Posture Enhancement Exercises

As a result of the widespread prevalence of backache and other back related problems, the National YMCA developed and implemented a program called *The Y's Way to a Healthy Back.* Over the years, this program has proved to be very successful and effective in reducing the chronic discomfort of thousands of persons. If you suffer from such an ailment, it would be wise to see your personal physician for possible referral. However, for purposes of prevention and treatment of mild backache, an abbreviated overview of the exercises used in the YMCA program is provided in Appendix 3.

Because postural asymmetries often result from muscular weakness in particular regions of the body, Appendix 3 also provides a number of beginning *postural enhancement exercises*. As was mentioned earlier, a postural deviation in one region of the body often is associated with deviations in other parts of the body. Therefore, if you discover you have a postural deviation it is recommended that you work on all the posture enhancement exercises as a set rather than merely focusing on the ones that pertain to the region of the body where you have the deviation. The set as a whole is designed to improve your total body alignment.

Other Types of Training

Circuit Training

Circuit training refers to a type of training in which several exercises are completed one after the other in a series. The exercises can vary from calisthenics, to weight training exercises, to running stairs or stretching, and so on. The term *circuit weight training* is used when weight lifting exercises are used. What distinguishes circuit weight training from traditional weight training is that each exercise is done only for a specified period of time (usually 20–30 seconds) and then the individual moves onto the next exercise "station" with only minimal rest. Usually the exercises are arranged in such a way that no one body part or muscle group is stressed in adjacent stations, thereby permitting some recovery to occur before the body part is taxed again.

Using circuit training you can easily develop a relatively taxing exercise program that serves your particular needs. Created circuits can be general, focusing on all the major muscle groups of the body for example, or specifically designed to focus on a particular goal, such as improving strength in the shoulder region. By varying the number of repetitions, the length of time you work at each station, the amount of time between each station, and the number of times you complete the whole circuit, you can determine how hard you wish to work. In recent years, *parcourse* facilities have become more widely available, usually adjacent to parks, golf courses, or other recreational areas. The parcourse is simply a variation of circuit training, and is usually a multi-station exercise apparatus, often built out of wood, offering a variety of self-directed strengthening/stretching exercises.

A helpful variation of circuit weight training is worth noting. Research has demonstrated that you can significantly improve your strength and muscle endurance using circuit weight training. However, evidence has also shown that even when persons trained for 20–30 minutes per day, 3 days per week, the improvements in $\dot{V}O_2$ max were only modest. This was true even though the participants remained almost continuously active throughout the training, allowing very little rest between stations. Also, their training heart rates were maintained within their target heart rate zones (see Chapter 4) throughout the training. One would think that such a training procedure would not only contribute to improved muscle function, which it did, but would also serve as sufficient stimulus for large improvements in aerobic capacity. Unfortunately, the improvements in aerobic capacity were much less than those that typically occur from an aerobic program of similar duration—for example, jogging.

Fortunately, an easy adjustment in this training procedure can be made simply by doing 30–60 seconds of aerobic activity between each exercise station. This aerobic activity can be as simple as riding a stationary bicycle, jumping on a mini-trampoline, jumping rope, or running in place. It is also possible to run/jog/walk between stations, as is often the case when parcourse stations are arranged at various locations around a park. This modification is called *super circuit weight training*. Research comparing super circuit weight training with traditional circuit weight training procedures has shown that it creates much larger improvements in aerobic function. Super circuit weight training has proven to be an excellent method for developing and maintaining an overall fitness program, one that is particularly useful for persons who find it difficult to exercise outdoors all year round. It can serve as an alternative for the winter months, when outdoor activities may be more difficult to do.

Interval Training

Interval training is a procedure involving periods of work interspersed with periods of rest or light exercise. It is often used as a means of gently increasing the total demands of exercise on an individual. A common example is a run/walk program. By running for 20 yards and walking for 20 yards, and so forth, for a given distance, an individual can raise his/her intensity of exercise compared to just walking the same distance. Gradually, as fitness improves, the running intervals can be increased in length, the walking intervals decreasing in a corresponding manner. Such a program is very useful when people wish to exercise frequently and for an adequate length of time, but cannot maintain a high level of intensity because of low fitness or other reasons. Of course, the same approach can be used in a pool, on an exercise bicycle, or with any form of aerobic exercise for that matter. Another application of interval training, discussed in the next section, is used for training athletes for maximal performances that require great speed, agility, and/or power.

Performance-Related Fitness

Power, speed, and agility were identified in Chapter 4 as components of performance-related fitness that are not directly associated with health. Some individuals may be inclined to improve these types of fitness, perhaps simply for the joy of reaching their limits in an all-around manner. This is particularly true of the athlete. Many sports and games require the performer to move herself/himself, an object, or an opponent rapidly, explosively, and with great power.

Power

Power involves the application of force and speed together. Those with the greatest power are not necessarily the strongest, although increasing strength helps improve power. Therefore, the strength training procedures described earlier in this chapter are one way to increase power. Since greatest power is achieved by maximizing both force and speed together, another method that can be used to improve power is to add light resistances as an overload and train explosively. For example, suppose Janis Jumpinggood is a Scandinavian exchange student trying out for the volleyball team. She wants to jump higher so she can spike the ball over the net and not into it. She may choose simply to jump a lot as a means of increasing her jumping skill as well as her leg power. In this case her body weight would serve as the overload resistance. She could also do rebound jumps by jumping off and back onto a 2-foot box or a bleacher. This is called *plyometric* training and is often used to increase the explosive leg power of sprinters, jumpers, and so on. (Creative variations could be explored to increase the explosive power of other parts of her body such as her arms and shoulders as well.) Another method Janis could use would be to do repeated squat-jumps while holding a light weight on her shoulder or using some other form of light resistance, such as a weight vest, as an overload. A squat-jump means jumping from a position with her legs bent slightly. The weight should not be so heavy that she cannot jump, however.

Speed and Agility

Speed usually refers to the capacity to move rapidly in a straight line, as in sprinting. Agility refers to the capacity to change directions of movement rapidly, as in tennis, where you must start, stop, and change directions of movement and body position in a variable manner. Both speed and agility are highly dependent on skill, meaning that an excellent way to improve is simply to practice doing the event in a realistic manner and force yourself to move rapidly. For example, if you are interested in improving your agility and speed in tennis, play a lot of tennis and push yourself to move rapidly, especially when you are tired.

Another training method involves the interval training discussed earlier. The basic principle behind interval training for speed and agility is to do repeated periods of near-maximal exercise interspersed with periods of rest or light exercise to facilitate partial recovery. The length of each exercise period and the length of each recovery interval can vary from 10 seconds to several minutes, depending on the intended application. For example, a sprinter might do 8 repetitions of a 200 yard run before taking a long recovery. Between each run, she/he would do light exercise like walking until she/he had recovered for 2–3 times as long as it took to run the 200 yards. This would be followed by another 200 yard sprint and so forth, until a set of 6–10 had been completed. The length of the recovery interval and the speed of running should be adjusted so that the performer can maintain a heavy rate of work and be working maximally or near-maximally by the end of the set. After a long rest of 10–15 minutes, a second and a third set may be done.

This type of training is very difficult to do, particularly if the individual is pushing herself/himself to maximum. It is not recommended for any but the highly fit and the highly motivated. Variations can be created to incorporate the types of agility movements required in a specific game (such as tennis, racquetball, basketball). The basic procedures are similar in that periods of rapid activity are broken up with periods of rest or light activity. Of course, the length of each exercise bout and related rest intervals should be determined by the intended application and the specificity principle described in Chapter 4.

Building Muscle

For a variety of reasons, many people are interested in building up the amount of muscle mass on their body. For some, this desire to build muscle becomes excessive and many positive health practices may be sacrificed to attain as large and well-defined muscles as possible. Little scientific attention has been focused on the matter of how to accomplish these results effectively and safely. However, it appears that any systematic overload to a muscle will result in some degree of muscle hypertrophy. The most commonly practiced method involves doing several sets of 10–20 RM loads. The greater the total amount of work done, the greater the overall gain that is likely to occur. The greatest gains will probably be seen in muscles that habitually experience the least amount of habitual overload. Also, larger muscles will likely experience greater improvements on an absolute level.

For unknown reasons there appear to be large individual differences in responsiveness to such training. For some, particularly young males at or soon after puberty, heavy resistance training results in greater gains in muscle while in others of the same age and sex it has a smaller effect. We mentioned previously that women in general experience much less hypertrophy from strength training than do men, probably due to lower levels of male sex hormone. It also appears that as men get older the ability to increase the size of muscle through training declines. One possible clue as to whether you are likely to be responsive to such training is to observe the degree of muscle development you have without training. If you are heavily muscled already, you may be more responsive than others, and vice versa.

Anabolic Steroids.   Many body builders and other athletes who require great strength, such as football players, shot putters, discus throwers, weight lifters, and so forth, take anabolic steroids to hasten and magnify the improvement they obtain from their training. Anabolic steroids are synthetically produced drugs that have growth-promoting properties similar to those of the male sex hormone testosterone. Research into the effectiveness of these drugs has demonstrated that for some, but not all, males the types of weight training procedures discussed in this chapter result in greater weight gain, particularly in fat-free tissue, and greater strength gain when the person is taking anabolic steroids than when not. It should be noted, however, that the dosages used in this research have been significantly lower (for ethical and safety considerations) than the dosages that are reportedly being taken by many athletes in the field. The research has also been conducted only over 1–2 month periods, which are relatively short time periods compared to the time spans during which many appear to be using these drugs.

A number of very significant negative health consequences are associated with anabolic steroids. These include liver dysfunction, liver cancer, lowered high density lipoprotein levels, high total cholesterol and triglyceride levels, hypertension, and testicular atrophy. Anabolic steroid use has also been shown to be associated with virilization in females, including deepening of the voice, increased facial and body hair, and clitoral enlargement. Some of these masculine changes are irreversible in women. Children are also particularly susceptible to the virilizing effects of these drugs. They may develop precociously on initial exposure to these drugs and later experience a premature closing of the growth centers of their bones, resulting in an overall stunting of growth. Long term use of anabolic steroids has also been implicated in the development of abnormal changes in the structure of muscle.

In view of the possible grave and life-threatening consequences of using anabolic steroids, use of these drugs is strongly discouraged. Athletes are prohibited from using anabolic steroids by most international amateur athletic organizations, although enforcement of such rules is difficult. Because the use of such drugs is so widespread, drug testing is becoming increasingly commonplace.

Summary

Maintaining a sufficient level of flexibility, strength, and muscle endurance is important in maintaining a high quality of life and in preventing hypokinetic degeneration and low back pain. You can determine your status in any of these fitness components using specific tests. The commonly available tests and related norms are provided in this book. Flexibility will improve with gentle, dynamic, range-of-motion activities or through static stretching for 15–30 seconds, 3–5 days per week. Examples are provided of both desirable and undesirable exercises for improving flexibility.

Strength and muscle endurance will increase through repetitively contracting your muscles against a relatively large resistance. Strength improvement requires performance of a small number of repetitions with very high resistances; muscle endurance improves from performance of a large number of repetitions against a lower resistance. Calisthenics, weight lifting, and working on exercise machines are the most common forms of activity for such training. Static exercises can also be used to increase strength and muscle endurance when equipment is not available. Common examples have been provided of all forms of strength and muscle endurance training, exercises designed to enhance posture, and general safety precautions for such training.

Training procedures should be similar for both sexes. Circuit training may be used to increase strength and muscle endurance in many areas of the body and, with proper adjustment of exercises, to improve aerobic capacity. Power, speed, and agility will improve from specific, high intensity training procedures.

Finally, though the use of anabolic steroids has become increasingly common in many athletic settings, such substances are banned and are known to have numerous harmful health consequences.

References

American College of Sports Medicine. 1984. The use of anabolic-androgenic steroids in sports. *Sports Medicine Bulletin* 19:13–18.

Clarke, D. H. 1973. Adaptations in strength and muscular endurance resulting from exercise. *Exercise and Sports Science Reviews* 1:73–102.

Corbin, C. B. and Noble, L. 1980. Flexibility: a major component of physical fitness. *JOPER* 51:23.

deVries, H. A. 1986. *Physiology of exercise*. 4th ed. Dubuque, IA: W. C. Brown.

Domingues, R. H. and Gajda, R. S. 1982. *Total body training*. New York: Charles Scribner's Sons.

Fox, E. L. and Mathews, D. K. 1981. *The physiological basis of physical education and athletics*. 3d ed. Philadelphia: Saunders College.

Gettman, L. R. and Pollock, M. L. 1981. Circuit weight training: A critical review of its physiological benefits. *Physician and Sportsmedicine* 9:44–60.

Gettman, L. R., Ward, P., and Hagen, R. D. 1982. A comparison of combined running and weight training with circuit weight training. *Medicine and Science in Sports* 14:229–234.

Golding, L. A., Myers, C. R., and Sinning, W. E., eds. 1982. *Y's way to physical fitness (revised)*. Rosemont, IL: YMCA.

Heyward, V. H. 1984. *Designs for fitness*. Minneapolis, MN: Burgess.

Jackson, A. W. and Baker, A. A. 1986. The relationship of the sit and reach test to criterion measures of hamstring and back flexibility in young females. *Research Quarterly for Exercise and Sport* 57:183–186.

Kraus, H., Melleby, A., and Gaston, S. R. 1977. Back pain correction and prevention. *New York State Journal of Medicine* 77:1335–1338.

Kraus, H., Nagler, W., and Melleby, A. 1983. Evaluation of an exercise program for back pain. *American Family Physician* 28:153–158.

Lamb, D. R. 1984. *Physiology of exercise*. 2d ed. New York: Macmillan.

Mayhew, J. L. and Gross, P. M. 1974. Body composition changes in young women with high resistance weight training. *Research Quarterly* 45:433–440.

Messier, S. P. and Dill, M. E. 1985. Alterations in strength and maximal oxygen uptake consequent to Nautilus circuit weight training. *Research Quarterly for Exercise and Sport* 56:345–351.

Nicholas, J. A. 1970. Injuries to knee ligaments. *JAMA* 212:2236–2239.

Nicholas, J. A. Nicholas overall body mobility test. New York: Institute of Sports Medicine and Athletic Trauma. Lenox Hill Hospital.

Petrofsky, J. S. and Lind, A. R. 1975. Aging, isometric strength and endurance, and cardiovascular responses to static effort. *Journal of Applied Physiology* 38:91-95.

Pollock, M. L., Wilmore, J. H., and Fox, III, S. M. 1978. *Health and fitness through physical activity*. New York: John Wiley and Sons.

Pollock, M. L., Wilmore, J. H., and Fox, III, S. M. 1984. *Exercise in health and disease*. Philadelphia: W. B. Saunders.

Robertson, L. D., Darville, D., and Magnusdottir, H. 1986. Abdominal fitness testing: A new approach. *Proceedings, VIII Commonwealth and International Conference on Sport, Physical Education, Dance, Recreation, and Health*. Glasgow, Scotland.

Sapega, A. A., Quendenfeld, T. C., Moyer, R. A., and Butler, R. A. 1981. Biophysical factors in range of motion exercise. *Physician & Sportsmedicine* 9:57–65.

Svoboda, M., Kauffman, L., Robertson, L., Gilbert, G., Heyden, M., Althoff, S., Davis, R., Lehman, A. E., and Schendel, J. S. (Ed.) 1985. *Health and fitness for life laboratory manual*. 2d ed. Scottsdale, AZ: Prospect Press.

Standardized test of fitness: Operations manual. 1985. Hull, Quebec, K1A0S9: Fitness and Amateur Sport.

Wilmore, J. H. 1974. Alterations in strength, body composition, and anthropometric measurements consequent to a 10-week weight training program. *Medicine and Science in Sports* 6:133–138.

Wilmore, J. H. 1982. *Training for sport and activity: The physiological basis of the conditioning process*. 2d. ed. Boston: Allyn and Bacon.

Y's way to a healthy back. 1976. YMCA of the City of New York and National Council of YMCA's.

7

The Weight Control Struggle

What is the relation between body composition and quality living?

How can you tell whether you are too fat? Are all methods of assessment equally accurate?

How can you determine how much energy you consume or how much energy you expend on the average?

How can you lose fat without losing weight from other parts of your body, such as from muscle tissue?

Why is regular exercise most effective if you wish to maintain your weight at a certain level over the long run? What type of exercise should you choose to achieve this?

Introduction

You do not need great deductive powers to discover the importance of weight control in contemporary American society. In any given week the top ten best-selling books will invariably include one or more on diet, exercise, nutrition, or related topics. Many of us tend to be preoccupied with body weight on a daily basis, and devote a great deal of money, time, and energy to modifying and regulating our weight. This preoccupation with weight is usually centered around the amount of visible fat on the body. In the ensuing sections of this chapter we will describe the nature, extent, and consequences of the problem of excess fat and describe methods of controlling and reducing fat.

Definition of Terms

The term *obesity* refers to having an excess amount of fat. Being able to determine the point at which obesity begins has been of considerable interest for researchers, health professionals, and consumers alike, but unfortunately no clear line of demarcation exists between the obese and non-obese states. Rather, fatness exists on a continuum and the point at which obesity begins is an arbitrary one that experts continue to discuss and debate.

Overweight describes the state of having excess weight relative to the average person of the same sex and stature. While being overweight is often the result of excess fatness, this is not always the case. For example, many professional football players are heavily muscled and weigh 30–40 pounds more than the average person of the same height.

The term *body composition* refers to the proportion of body weight that is composed of fat and the proportion that is composed of fat-free tissues (e.g., muscle, bone, connective tissue, etc.). Unfortunately, the most accurate methods for determining body composition are not generally available for use in population studies, making it difficult to determine accurate standards at the present time. Therefore, height/weight tables derived from the characteristics of life insurance policy holders (who may not be entirely representative of the American population as a whole) have come into use (Table 7.A). Ways to determine your own body composition will be discussed later in this chapter.

Two other terms also require clarification. *Weight loss* of course refers to the loss of weight. Many people find themselves continually trying to lose weight as a means of losing fat. Often those who are successful at losing weight are unable to maintain the loss permanently. This usually occurs because they are unsuccessful at transforming the method they used to lose the weight into a long-term plan that will enable them to maintain their weight at the new and lower level. *Weight control* refers to maintaining a stable body weight.

Table 7.A Desirable body weights (ages 25 and over).

	HEIGHT	WEIGHT (LBS.)		
		SMALL FRAME	MEDIUM FRAME	LARGE FRAME
Women	4'8"	88–94	92–103	100–115
	9"	90–97	94–106	102–118
	10"	92–100	97–109	105–121
	11"	95–103	100–112	108–124
	5'0"	98–106	103–115	111–127
	1"	101–109	106–118	114–130
	2"	104–112	109–122	117–134
	3"	107–115	112–126	121–138
	4"	110–119	116–131	125–142
	5"	114–123	120–135	129–146
	6"	118–127	124–139	133–150
	7"	122–131	128–143	137–154
	8"	126–136	132–147	141–159
	9"	130–140	136–151	145–164
	10"	134–144	140–155	149–169
Men	5'1"	104–112	110–121	118–133
	2"	107–115	113–125	121–136
	3"	110–118	116–128	124–140
	4"	113–121	119–131	127–144
	5"	116–125	122–135	130–148
	6"	120–129	126–139	134–153
	7"	124–133	130–144	139–158
	8"	128–137	134–148	143–162
	9"	132–142	138–152	147–166
	10"	136–146	142–157	151–171
	11"	140–150	146–162	156–176
	6'0"	144–154	150–167	160–181
	1"	148–159	154–172	165–186
	2"	152–163	159–177	170–191
	3"	156–167	164–182	174–196

*Based on the weights published by the Metropolitan Life Insurance Company in 1959 which were associated with the lowest mortality of those who were insured. They have been recalculated from the originally published tables to permit you to determine your height in bare feet and your weight without clothes. See text for further discussion. [Adapted from *Statistical Bulletin of the Metropolitan Life Insurance Co.* 40 (Nov.–Dec. 1959):1–4.]

Problems Associated with Obesity

It has been estimated that approximately 14% of adult males and 20% of adult females are obese. This represents some 30–40 million Americans. To illustrate this statistic, it was once estimated, based on the population estimates in 1975, that if all the excess fat in the U.S. adult population were added up it would amount to about 2.3 billion pounds. The energy saved by dieting to lose this excess fat would be equivalent to that contained in 1.3 billion gallons of gasoline. The savings in energy from people eating less thereafter to maintain their lower weights would be equivalent to 750 million gallons of gasoline per year, enough to cover the gasoline needs of 900,000 cars driving 13,000 miles per year and averaging 14 miles per gallon. Stated another way, this would be energy enough to meet the combined electrical needs of Boston, Chicago, San Francisco, and Washington, D.C. for a full year. We cannot make such utilizations of energy derived from weight loss, of course, but such figures graphically illustrate the extent of obesity in this country and its economic consequences. Some of the very real problems brought about by obesity in our culture are discussed below.

Social Problems

Collectively, our culture has evolved into a culture preoccupied with thinness, in which excessive fatness is viewed negatively. This national viewpoint is evident in a number of arenas. The mass media promote thinness and the cosmetic and clothing industries perpetuate the image: to be "with it," one must be lean. Socially, fat people are shunned in many ways, some overt and others more subtle. Prejudices may take the form of hostile and derisive jokes, lower rates of acceptance into employment or college, fewer job promotions, decreased interpersonal relations, and reduced social mobility. Such social rejection can of course affect the quality of life of the obese if it results in a poor self-image or social withdrawal for an individual. By no means is it suggested that such reactions happen to every individual. However, it is an accurate and unfortunate observation that as a whole the obese face a social handicap in contemporary American society that the lean do not, a handicap that acts as a burden or constraint to their being able to develop themselves fully.

Health Problems

Obesity is clearly implicated in a number of diseases. Evidence comes from large surveys of the U.S. adult population taken during the past 15 years. For example, for those who are in the top 15% of their weight category across all ages, the risk of hypertension is 2.9 times greater than in the overall population; in younger adults (ages 20–44) it is 5.6 times greater than average. Further, the risk of having a high total cholesterol count (i.e, in excess of 250 mg/dl) is 2.1 times greater, and the risk of diabetes is 2.9 times greater. All of these are primary or secondary risk factors for coronary heart disease (CHD), and as we might expect obesity puts a person at greater risk for this disease as well. (Research has not been entirely clear regarding whether the effect of obesity on CHD is directly linked to its effect on other risk factors or is independent of those factors. The reasons for the discrepancies are unclear at present.)

Other negative health consequences are related to obesity as well. The risk of cancer is higher. So also are the risks for gout, gallstones, respiratory insufficiency, congestive heart failure, and thromboembolic or vascular disease. Arthritis and low back pain are exacerbated by obesity. Obese persons are at greater risk in surgery, and their overall longevity is lowered. As you may surmise, the profile of obesity from the point of view of overall health is rather bleak. Clearly, obesity has a negative impact on the quality and the quantity of life.

Before leaving the health problems associated with obesity, two others that have become increasingly evident in recent years need to be discussed, namely *anorexia nervosa* and *bulimia*. Both conditions seem to occur predominantly in females, anorexia being most prevalent during the teenage years, bulimia occurring during the late teens and early to mid-twenties. Although they have several characteristics in common, these conditions are now recognized as separate and distinct health problems. Simply stated, anorexia is self-induced starvation. Persons suffering from anorexia nervosa are characterized by an intense fear of becoming obese. Anorectics have a disturbed body image and become so irrationally attached to having an emaciated figure that they refuse to maintain body weight within normal range and lose as much as 25% of their original body weight or more. Amenorrhea, meaning loss of menstrual function, is also common in anorexia nervosa.

Bulimia is a syndrome characterized by binge eating followed by purging, either through vomiting or excessive use of laxatives. Bulimic individuals are obsessively preoccupied with thoughts of food but do not exhibit abnormal body weights. Bulimics also exhibit fasting behavior and usually have frequent weight fluctuations of 10 pounds or more due to alternating fasts and binges.

Both anorectics and bulimics are often characterized by a poor sense of identity and a lack of competence and assertiveness. The more successful approaches to treating these conditions involve psychotherapy and/or behavior therapy that focuses on the underlying causes and behaviors that lead to the problems. In the case of anorexia, therapy usually involves the family and related interactions.

Methods of Measuring Body Composition

Before discussing the process of weight loss, the means of determining your body composition will be presented. *Body composition* refers to the makeup of your body — to the proportions of your body weight that are made up of fat or of fat-free tissues. Once you have determined your body composition you will be better able to make decisions regarding weight loss and exercising. *Hydrostatic weighing* and *skinfold fat measurement techniques* are the two most common methods of determining body composition.

Hydrostatic Weighing

In the research laboratory, the most widely used method for measuring body composition is called *hydrostatic weighing,* also referred to as "underwater weighing." In this technique, the individual is weighed both on land and under water, and then, using an equation, the percent of body weight composed of fat is calculated. Adjustment for the amount of air left in the lungs after a full exhalation is also required. The total technique normally requires a half-hour or more of time, making it impractical to use on a wide-scale basis. The standard error of estimate for hydrostatic weighing is approximately 3–4% fat units, which means that most people will fall within ± 3–4% fat units of their true fat content using this technique.

Skinfold Fat Techniques

Other measurement techniques have been developed for more widespread use. These typically involve taking measurements of skinfold fat thickness at various sites on the surface of the body. The procedures have evolved over the years because of difficult questions such as where to take measurements, what technique to use, the type of caliper needed, and so on. The more fundamental problem of determining whether a set of such measurements taken at standard sites can truly reflect the total fat content of all types of people, considering differences in age, sex, fitness status, fat content, body size, and shape is still being explored through research. At the present time, the best that can be said is that no *one* skinfold technique will be accurate given all the variations that exist between people. With the above qualification in mind, the best procedures to use for most adults are the generalized equations of Jackson and Pollock. The procedures for using this technique are described in Appendix 4. Included in the appendix is an example illustrating the computational procedures for hypothetical data on a young male named Curious George.

The standard error of estimate using these procedures is between 4–5.5% fat, meaning that most people will fall within approximately ±4–5.5% fat units of their true fat content. Greatest accuracy will be possible using such skinfold techniques if a trained technician using a reliable set of calipers takes the measurements. If you have occasion to be measured using this technique, inquire whether this is the case.

Other Methods of Measurement

In recent years a number of alternative procedures for measuring body composition have been developed. These include circumference, ultrasound, arm X-ray, bioelectrical impedence, and computerized tomography. Some are still in the development stage and/or are not readily available for widespread use. One in particular, the method of bioelectrical impedence, which involves measuring the resistance to a very low level of electrical current passing through the body, has been marketed recently as an easy and accurate alternative to other more standard technniques like hydrostatic weighing. Unfortunately, attempts to validate the technique have shown that it needs further research before it can be used to obtain accurate and reliable estimates of body composition.

Before leaving this topic, the *body mass index* (BMI) should be mentioned. This is an easily calculated index that is often used to determine relative risk from excess weight. The equation for determining body mass index is

$$BMI = \frac{Wt}{Ht^2} \text{ (where body weight is in kg. and height is in meters)}$$

Although BMI is not a measure of body composition, it is highly correlated to percent of fat as determined with hydrostatic weighing. Most adults have a BMI between 20–25, while adults in the top 15% of their weight categories have BMIs in excess of 26, the point at which the health risk from obesity begins to increase. Figure 7.1 illustrates an easy-to-use nomogram for calculating your BMI based on measurements of your height and weight.

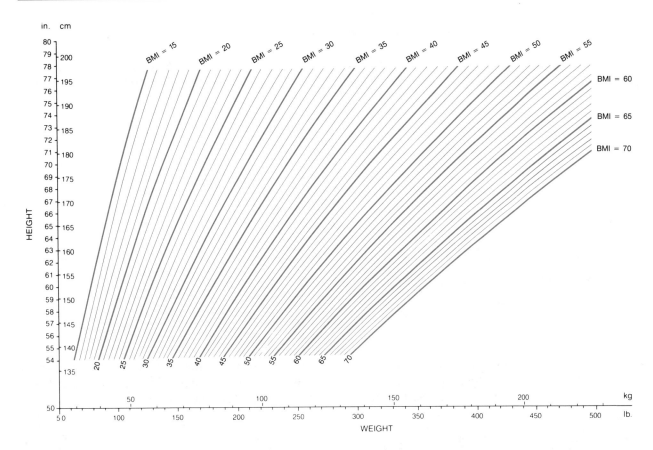

FIGURE 7.1 Body mass index (BMI) for specified heights and weights.

Used with permission of Frankel H. M.,
Portland Health Institute, Portland, OR.

The Components of Body Composition

Fat weight is simply how many pounds your fat weighs. Your fat weight consists partly of *essential fat,* which refers to the minimum amount of fat needed for optimal health. Essential fat levels are thought to equal 3% *fat for males* and 12% *fat for females.* (Females require a higher level of essential fat for reasons related to reproductive needs.) That part of your fat weight that is not essential is called *storage fat.* The amount of storage fat varies from individual to individual, and obesity is the state of having an excessive amount of storage fat.

   Fat-free weight is an estimate of how much all the other tissues in your body would weigh if all the fat were removed. Of course you should not aspire to attain a body weight equal to your fat-free weight. This is actually impossible, and efforts to achieve such a goal will severely compromise your health status. The lowest body weight you can strive to achieve is equal to the sum of your fat-free weight plus your essential fat (Figure 7.2). Considering the margin of error in measuring body composition, even this weight would probably result in your being too lean, particularly if

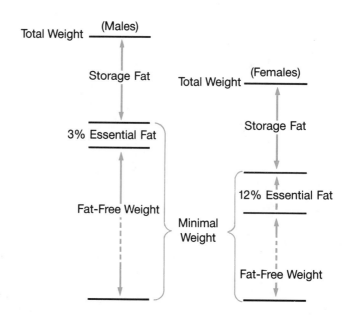

FIGURE 7.2
The components of body composition. Body weight is composed of fat-free weight, essential fat, and storage fat. Health risk increases if body weight falls below minimal weight (i.e., fat-free weight plus essential fat).

you were to get sick and need extra energy reserves. Methods for computing all these components of body composition are described in Appendix 4. Also included is a method for determining your target weight at different percentage fat levels.

Desirable Fat and Weight Standards

The following questions often occur to those considering body composition: "How much fat is desirable?" and "How can I tell if I am obese or not?" Unfortunately, there is not enough objective data on a large enough sample of individuals to determine the point at which the risk from obesity accelerates. All that can be said is that numerous studies of young American men and women indicate that on the average, women fall between 23–25% fat and men fall between 14–16% fat. As an arbitrary estimate of where obesity may be thought to begin, the young adults who are in the top 16% of their weight categories are those women who have in excess of 30% fat and those men who have in excess of 20% fat. Since there is no known reason why aging should cause an increase in body fat, some experts suggest that these values should be used to mark the beginning of obesity for persons of all ages. This line of demarcation is arbitrary, but it defines a cut-off point over which approximately the top 16% of the U.S. population is said to be obese.

Some further comments need to be made about the use of height/weight tables (as in Table 7.A). In 1983, the Metropolitan Life Insurance Company released a revised version of their 1959 Body Weight Tables. In all categories and for both sexes, the desirable weight for height increased in the 1983 Tables compared to the 1959 Tables, sometimes by as much as 12–14 pounds. From a point of view of optimal health, experts disagree as to whether desirable weight should have increased by this amount in the relatively short period of 24 years. Importantly, these tables do not reflect the mortality and illness-related risks of *all* Americans, but only those of policy holders, a sample that may not be representative.

A second qualification relates to recent evidence suggesting that with increasing age, the BMI associated with lowest risk of death slowly increases. Stated in other terms, this means that as you get older it may be healthier if you slowly gain weight. Mechanisms for such a phenomenon are unclear. Nevertheless, some researchers have argued that height/weight tables should be adjusted accordingly; and, since the trend is the same for both sexes, tables have been proposed that reflect age-related but not sex-specific changes (as in Table 7.B). For now, however, experts are not in agreement as to whether or not you should gain weight as you grow older. Further research is needed to resolve this issue.

The Role of Energy Balance in Weight Control

The *caloric balance equation* describes the relationship between the amount of energy you consume and the amount of energy you expend. When your energy intake equals your energy expenditure, you are in a state of energy balance, and as long as you remain in energy balance, your body weight will remain essentially the same. On a

Table 7.B   Age adjusted height–weight tables.

	WEIGHT RANGE FOR MEN AND WOMEN BY AGE (YEARS)				
HEIGHT	25	35	45	55	65
FT.–IN.			LB.		
4–10	84–111	92–119	99–127	107–135	115–142
4–11	87–115	95–123	103–131	111–139	119–147
5–0	90–119	98–127	106–135	114–143	123–152
5–1	93–123	101–131	110–140	118–148	127–157
5–2	96–127	105–136	113–144	122–153	131–163
5–3	99–131	108–140	117–149	126–158	135–168
5–4	102–135	112–145	121–154	130–163	140–173
5–5	106–140	115–149	125–159	134–168	144–179
5–6	109–144	119–154	129–164	138–174	148–184
5–7	112–148	122–159	133–169	143–179	153–190
5–8	116–153	126–163	137–174	147–184	158–196
5–9	119–157	130–168	141–179	151–190	162–201
5–10	122–162	134–173	145–184	156–195	167–207
5–11	126–167	137–178	149–190	160–201	172–213
6–0	129–171	141–183	153–195	165–207	177–219
6–1	133–176	145–188	157–200	169–213	182–225
6–2	137–181	149–194	162–206	174–219	187–232
6–3	141–186	153–199	166–212	179–225	192–238
6–4	144–191	157–205	171–218	184–231	197–244

*Values are for height without shoes and weight without clothes.

Adapted from Andres, R. et al. (1985). *Annals of Internal Medicine*. 103, 1030–1033.

daily basis, it is not uncommon for you to consume more calories than you expend or vice versa, but as long as your total intake over several days equals your total expenditure, you will not experience any net change in body weight or in body composition. If your caloric intake exceeds your caloric expenditure, then you are said to be in positive caloric balance and the extra calories will be stored, mostly in the form of fat. If your caloric intake is less than your caloric expenditure, then the additional calories are obtained from stored energy, again mostly in the form of fat.

Weight control is a process of achieving energy balance on a lifelong basis. For some, this is easy. For countless others, however, the task is very difficult, and very often the long term result is "creeping obesity" or a gradual increase in body fat as the person grows older. As we have discussed, this gradual fat gain can cause many health-related problems, not the least of which is the daily stress experienced by those who deal with the continual, nagging problem of being overfat.

Very often the degree of imbalance is no more than a few calories, perhaps less than 25 calories per day on the average; cumulatively, however, an imbalance of 25 calories/day would result in 2.6 pounds per year of added fat. Since most people who are overfat have perhaps 25–30 pounds of excess fat at most, and since in most cases this extra fat is put on over a period of 10–15 years rather than in one, the problem of achieving energy balance does not involve making significant changes. In other words, for most people the degree of imbalance is relatively small. Nonetheless, for many the task of achieving lifelong energy balance is difficult and often leads people into taking extreme weight loss measures such as fasting or going on very restrictive diets.

Before we discuss ways of losing weight and ways of achieving lifelong energy balance, you may find it useful to determine your energy intake and energy expenditure to see if you are currently in energy balance. The next section will describe methods of doing this, beginning with a discussion of energy.

Energy

Of all the functions of food, one of the most important is the energy it provides. To be useful to your body, the energy contained in food must first be broken down, transformed into forms that are useful to your cells, and then transported to those cells. Since food is typically eaten in three meals or less (with occasional snacks), the supply of energy coming from such digestive processes is not continuous. More energy than you can use at one time arrives in a big volume followed by periods without any additional intake, sometimes for as long as 12–18 hours. To compensate for this unsteady supply of energy, much of the food from a meal is converted into a usable form (fat) and stored in fat cells for later use as needed. (You can read about this process in more detail in Chapters 8 and 9.) Thus, throughout the day the cells of the body receive a mixture of foodstuffs coming both from the stomach and from various storage depots throughout the body. Foodstuffs from both sources serve the important function of providing energy for all life functions and for the rebuilding and replacement of cells.

The unit of measure used to equate energy from different foods is called the *calorie*. The definition of a calorie is the amount of heat required to raise one kilogram of water one degree centigrade in temperature. The term "kilocalorie" is sometimes used synonomously with calorie.

Caloric Intake

Caloric intake is defined as the number of calories of energy you consume in a 24-hour day, which means the sum of the caloric values of all the foods you eat in that period of time. In Table 7.C you will find step-by-step procedures for most accurately determining the total caloric values of two sample lunches. In brief, this process involves weighing and/or measuring all the foods you eat as precisely as possible and then using the caloric values for each food (found in Appendix 8) to determine your total caloric intake. This can become quite a chore, but it is necessary if you wish to achieve the greatest accuracy.

While Table 7.C describes the most practical method you can use to determine your caloric intake, it is not without error. Given the difficulty of obtaining accurate measurements of the volume and weight of the food you eat, given the seemingly infinite variations in the contents of most prepared foods, and given the large variations in calories in two samples of the same type of food (for example, the fat content of two 6-ounce steaks can vary considerably), such estimates require you to be meticulous if any reasonable level of accuracy is desired.

Caloric Expenditure

Your caloric expenditure is defined as the total number of calories you expend in the form of heat and work in a 24-hour day. This is also difficult to measure precisely, for

Table 7.C Computations illustrating how to determine caloric value of two sample meals.

FOOD	MEASURE	WEIGHT[1] (G)	TABLED CAL VALUE	UNIT CAL VALUE[2]	NET CAL[3]
Lunch No. 1					
Turkey Sandwich					
Italian bread	2 slices	60 g	85 Cal/30 g slice	2.83 Cal/g	170
lettuce	1 outer leaf	15 g	trace/leaf	—	—
mayonnaise (reg.)	1 teaspoon	5 g	100 Cal/15 g	6.67 Cal/g	33
turkey (light)	1 slice	60 g	150 Cal/85 g	1.76 Cal/g	106
Skim milk	1 glass	245 g	85 Cal/245 g	.35 Cal/g	85
Orange (peeled)	1 medium	120 g	65 Cal/131 g	.50 Cal/g	60
				TOTAL	454 Cal
Lunch No. 2					
Burger King whopper	1 complete				606
French fries	1 serving				214
Vanilla shake	1 glass				332
				TOTAL	1152 Cal

[1]See Appendix 5 for Table of Weights and Measures.
[2]Determined by dividing the tabled Cal value by the weight associated with that value.
   (E.g., Italian Bread: Dividing the 85 Cal by 30 g = 2.83 Cal/g)
[3]Determined as follows: (unit Cal value)(weight). E.g., Italian bread: (2.83 Cal/g)(60 g) = 170 Cal

a number of reasons. Most important, there is no easy way of accurately measuring how much physical activity you do on a particular day given the great variety of things you might do. In an hour, you may start and stop moving an untold number of times and change your pace a similar number of times. To calculate how much energy was expended, you would have to keep accurate records of the intensity and duration of each activity throughout a 24-hour period, and then be able to translate this into units of energy expenditure. This task would be easier if each hour was spent at a relative steady rate of physical activity, but of course this is not usually the case.

The method typically used to obtain an approximate estimate of caloric expenditure involves keeping accurate activity records throughout the hours you are awake. By computing the calories you expend during your daily activities and adding this to the calories spent due to your *basal metabolic rate* (BMR), you obtain an estimate of your total caloric expenditure. BMR is defined as the number of calories that your body spends in a 24-hour period simply to maintain bodily functions under resting conditions. It represents the number of calories you would need to maintain yourself in energy balance if you were able to lie in bed awake for a 24-hour period and were fed intravenously so that you didn't even have to spend the energy required to digest your food.

Since measuring BMR is impractical and expensive to do on a routine basis, a closely related measure called *resting metabolic rate* (RMR) is estimated indirectly instead. Directions for calculating your RMR and an example are provided in Box 1, below. Box 2 provides instructions for computing a 24-hour activity record and then translating the activities into an estimate of total caloric expenditure. Refer to Appendix 6 for estimates of the average caloric expenditure for a complete list of exercises and household and recreational activities.

It may be helpful at this point to clarify two terms that are often used interchangeably although they actually describe different concepts. *Physical activity* refers to any bodily movement produced by skeletal muscles that results in energy expenditure. Subcategories include household, occupational, recreational, and sport-related activities. *Exercise* is another subcategory of physical activity and refers to planned, structured, and repetitive physical activity which has as a goal the improvement or maintenance of physical fitness.

BOX 1 COMPUTING YOUR RESTING METABOLIC RATE (RMR)

RMR is similar to BMR except that RMR includes the energy needed for digestion of food. Instructions for predicting your RMR are as follows:

1. *Predict your surface area:* Use Figure 7.3 and line up a straight-edge between your body weight and your standing height. By reading to the middle column, you will obtain an estimate of your surface area in square meters.
2. *Determine the average resting metabolic rate (RMR) for your sex and age:* Refer to Figure 7.4.

3. *Determine your specific RMR:* Multiply the average RMR by your surface area to obtain an estimate of your RMR in calories per hour. When multiplied by 24, this will give you an estimate of your RMR over a 24-hour day.

A sample calculation illustrating this whole procedure on a step-by-step basis is seen below (Example A). Note that such techniques are at best only approximations; numerous factors including age, sex, the amount of fat-free tissue, emotions, food, fever, and of course, prior exercise cause individual differences in RMR.

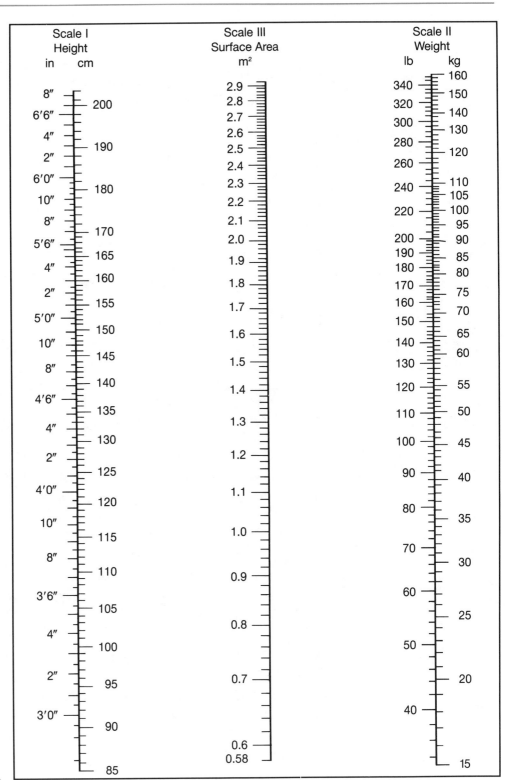

FIGURE 7.3
Nomogram to estimate body surface area from height and weight.

Used with permission from Katch, F. I. and McArdle, W. D. (1983) *Nutrition, Weight Control and Exercise,* 2nd Ed. Philadelphia: Lea and Febiger. Originally produced from *Clinical Spirometry* by Warren E. Collins, Inc., Braintree, MA, with permission. Nomogram prepared by Boothby and Standiford of the Mayo Clinic.

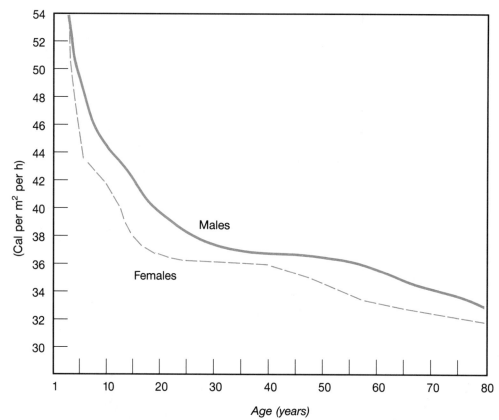

FIGURE 7.4
Resting metabolic rate for men and women as a function of age.

Used wtih permission from Katch, F. I. and McArdle, W. D. (1983) *Nutrition, Weight Control and Exercise,* 2nd Ed. Philadelphia: Lea and Febiger. Data are from Altman, P. L. and Dittmer, D. S. (1968) *Metabolism.* Bethesda, MD: Federation of American Societies for Experimental Biology.

Example A. Sample calculation for determining resting metabolic rate

Name: Napoleon Periwinkle

Age: 32   Height: 71 inches   Weight: 177 lbs.

1. Lining up a straight edge on Figure 7.5 between Napoleon's height and weight, his predicted body surface area is:

    1.96 m²

2. From Figure 7.5, the resting metabolic rate for a male aged 32 is:

    37 Cal / m² / hour

3. Resting metabolic rate = (1.96 m²) (37 Cal / m² / hr)

    = 72.52 Cal / hr

    or

    $\frac{(72.52 \text{ Cal})}{\text{hr}}$ $(24 \frac{\text{hr}}{\text{day}})$ = 1740.48 Cal / day

BOX 2   SAMPLE COMPUTATION OF 24-HOUR CALORIC EXPENDITURE

1. *Keep an activity diary:* You must keep an accurate diary of your activities throughout an entire 24-hour period. In fact, since a given day may not be typical, records averaged over three or more days will likely provide you with more accurate estimates of your average caloric expenditure. Such records should include (a) the type of activity, and (b) the duration of the activity.

2. *Determine your rate of energy expenditure for each activity:* Using the list of activities seen in Appendix 6, determine the average rate of energy expenditure in Cal/min/lb for each activity in your diary. If you cannot find an activity in Appendix 6 that describes precisely what you do, find one that is similar and estimate as best you can.

3. *Determine your total caloric expenditure:* Multiply the number of minutes that you spend in each activity

throughout the day by the rate of energy expenditure listed for that activity and also by your body weight. For example, in Appendix 6 the listed value for sitting quietly is .010 Cal/min/lb. Therefore, for the college student illustrated below who has a body weight of 124 lbs. the caloric expenditure while sitting quietly for 285 minutes in class is:

[.010 Cal/min/lb] [285 min] [124 lbs] = 353 Cal

An illustration of this process for a complete 24-hour period is seen below (Example B). It should be noted that the individual in this illustration is assumed to be under RMR conditions while sleeping. For this individual, her RMR equals 59.04 Cal/hr. Converting the 420 minutes she slept into hours:

[59.04 Cal/hr] [7 hrs of sleep] = 413 Cal

Example B. Sample Computation of 24-Hour Energy Expenditure of 23-Year Old Female College Student (Height = 66 inches; weight = 124 lbs.)

Time	Activity	Duration	Cal/min/lb[a]	Net Cal[b]
6:15 AM	Rise, dress, prepare for day	65 min.	.027	218
7:20	Eat breakfast	10 min.	.010	12
7:30	Drive to school	15 min.	.013	24
7:45	In-class including			
	sitting/writing	285 min.	.010	353
	standing	10 min.	.011	14
	walking	20 min.	.036	89
1:00 PM	Lunch	20 min.	.010	25
1:20	Walking	5 min.	.036	22
1:25	Study in library	125 min.	.010	155
3:30	Walking to gym	10 min.	.036	45
3:40	Change clothes	5 min.	.027	17
3:45	Aerobic exercise			
	warm up (light calisthenics)	10 min.	.036	45
	jog at 5.5 mph	30 min.	.067	249
	cool down	5 min.	.036	22
	shower & change	10 min.	.027	33

(Continued)

Time	Activity	Duration	Cal/min/lb[a]	Net Cal[b]
4:35	Walk to car	5 min.	.036	22
4:45	Drive to work	15 min.	.013	24
5:00	Work (check out counter)	120 min.	.027	402
7:00	Dinner break	30 min.	.010	37
7:30	Work (check out counter)	90 min.	.027	301
9:00	Drive home	15 min.	.013	24
9:15	Light activity at home	45 min.	.027	151
10:00	Study	60 min.	.010	74
11:00	Retire & prepare for bed	15 min.	.027	50
11:15	Sleep	420 min.	.008	413
	TOTAL	1440 min. (24 hrs)		2821 Cal

a From Appendix 6

b Numbers in this column are attained by multiplying *the duration* times *the rate of caloric expenditure/ minute/pound* times *the body weight in pounds.* E.g., for line 1:
[65 min.] [.027 Cal/min/lb] [124 lb] = 218 Cal

You will notice in Appendix 6 that the values for energy expenditure are dependent on body weight. In other words, the more you weigh, the greater the rate of energy expenditure, all else remaining the same. Although not always discernable from the numbers, the same is true when you work harder. For example, you will note that under running, the faster the pace, the greater the rate of energy expenditure. The same is true for virtually all other listed activities, even though this is not reflected in the table in each case. This is simply because information on the effect of different paces of playing soccer, for example, have not been determined. The value given in the table is merely an average value, assuming an average rate of energy expenditure in an average game by a player of average skill.

At times the objective of exercise is to do a given amount of work rather than to do something for a given amount of time.

For example, the gardener often decides to spade his flower bed in the spring and works until the job is completed and not when 30 minutes are up. Or a typical exerciser may decide on a sunny day to jog for 2 miles at a comfortable pace. If you were to determine the total caloric cost of running the 2 miles at a very fast pace and compare it to the caloric cost of jogging at a slower pace, the answers would be very similar. This is because, while the faster pace uses more energy per minute, the total duration of the run is shorter. Keeping this in mind, if one of your exercise goals is to maximize your energy expenditure, you may be more successful if you keep your pace at a relatively low to moderate level rather than trying to work intensively. By working at or near your maximum, you will probably fatigue quickly, which will shorten the overall length of your exercise bout. You may even make exercising unpleasant for yourself and be less likely to stay with it.

A Comprehensive Program for Weight Loss

If you find yourself wishing to lose excess weight because you have too much fat, what approach should you use? Will you be able to permanently maintain any loss you achieve? Unfortunately, the vast majority of people who undertake a weight loss program are not successful at keeping the weight off. Reasons explaining why this occurs will be presented later in the chapter, but before we address the reasons, a comprehensive program for weight loss will be presented. This program is designed to ensure permanent changes in body composition.

Rules for Losing Weight (Losing Fat)

The American College of Sports Medicine recently issued a position stand on proper and improper weight loss programs and included the recommendations listed below.

1. Weight loss should occur gradually and should not exceed 1–2 pounds of weight loss per week.
2. Weight loss should occur from a combination of a moderate diet and a regular aerobic exercise program.
3. Foods eaten while on this diet should be balanced with respect to nutritional requirements and should be compatible with personal tastes. Caloric intake should be at least 1200 calories/day.
4. Aerobic exercise should consist of gentle, rhythmic exercise using large muscle groups which is done a minimum of 3 days/week, for at least 20–30 minutes/day, at a minimum intensity of 60% of maximum heart rate reserve. At least 300 calories/session should be expended.
5. Behavior modification techniques should be employed to identify and eliminate dietary habits that lead to improper nutrition; these techniques will enable the individual to maintain the weight loss indefinitely.

The rationale for these guidelines is as follows:

1. Most nutrition experts have long recommended that the maximum rate of weight loss you should attempt is 1–2 pounds/week. One important reason for this is the simple fact that modest changes are more easily transformed into permanent habits that can be maintained throughout your life. What type of change will enable you to lose 1–2 pounds/week? Because one pound of fat contains 3500 calories of energy, a negative caloric balance of 500–1000 calories/day will help you accomplish this.

Consider an example. The daily caloric requirements for the average American female and male are 2000 calories/day and 2700 calories/day, respectively. In order to lose 1 pound/week, an average woman would have to consume 1500 calories while still expending 2000 calories daily (2000 − 500 = 1500 calories). (The recommended 1500 calories is considerably higher than the number of calories that the typical female consumes if she is on a diet.) Equivalent values for an average male to lose 1 pound/ week are: 2700 − 500 = 2200 calories/day.

Note that the above example assumes that the individuals have elected to go on a diet only, rather than also adding moderate aerobic exercise into their programs. Since most Americans, and especially those in need of weight loss, do not already engage in regular aerobic exercise, this diet-only approach does not take advantage of the long-term weight control benefits that can be obtained through regular exercise in a weight loss program. Dieting as an approach to weight loss and the numerous benefits of regular exercise for weight loss and weight control are discussed in the next two sections of this chapter.

A comment should be made regarding the nature of weight losses at different stages in a fat-loss program. Early in a program, pounds are lost more quickly because water is excreted along with fat losses. This means that initially you will be able to lose weight with less than the deficit of 3500 calories/lb that is needed when all the weight loss comes from fat. This is why it appears to become more difficult to lose weight after the first week or two.

2. Weight loss programs should involve a combination of a modest diet and regular aerobic exercise because you get the benefits of both approaches with fewer liabilities of either when you do them in combination. Example C below illustrates such a program. As you can see, the caloric cutback is modest and is not likely to cause great feelings of deprivation or craving. Further, because the diet is moderate and is accompanied by a moderate aerobic exercise program, it is not likely to cause a reduction in BMR, which may arise from more severe caloric restriction alone. A lowered BMR is a major drawback to a weight loss program because it virtually assures that you will regain weight once you terminate your program. More is explained about this problem in the following section on dieting.

Another advantage of including exercise in your weight loss program is that it causes a greater proportion of the weight loss to come from fat stores. Whenever you lose weight, just as when you gain weight, some of the loss (or gain) comes from fat stores, but importantly, some also comes from loss (or gain) of fat-free tissues. Research has shown that incorporating exercise into a weight loss program helps reduce the loss of fat-free tissues and forces more to be lost from fat stores.

3. It is recommended that at least 1200 calories be consumed even during a weight loss program in order to assure a nutritionally sound diet at all times. Crash diets that provide fewer calories than 1200 restrict not only calories but also numerous other nutrients that are needed for proper health and function. (Chapters 8 and 9 describe nutritional requirements and guidelines in great detail.) The only exception to this rule of consuming no fewer than 1200 calories should be if you are on a medically supervised diet. Unfortunately, many individuals, including athletes who are excessively concerned with body composition, teens, and children who are still growing, put themselves on diets that are considerably more restrictive than a 1200 calorie diet. Growing persons, especially, need a healthy diet to assure proper development of bodily tissues, and the use of crash diets puts their health status in jeopardy. Additionally, as noted above, severe caloric restriction causes a reduced BMR. It also causes a significant loss of fat-free weight in addition to fat weight.

4. Research into aerobic exercise programs indicates that when exercise is done 3 or more days/week, 20–30 minutes/day or longer, and at a minimum of 60% of heart rate reserve, individuals tend to lose fat. This has therefore become the basis for recommending how much exercise to do during a weight loss program. As mentioned later in the chapter, however, lower intensity exercise uses fat as a fuel to a greater extent than does higher intensity exercise. By keeping the intensity down, perhaps even below the level of 60% heart rate reserve, you will also be able to extend the duration of your exercise; and by maximizing duration, not only will fat utilization progressively increase, but total caloric expenditure will increase as well.

Example C. Example of a weight loss program following recommmended guidelines.

Name: Mildred Waitconscious   Weight: 150 pounds
                                      Height: 63 inches
                                      BMI: 27

Goal: Lose 1 pound/week

Program: If Mildred were to add slow running at 11:30 minutes/mile, 5 days/week to her normal activities, her total added energy expenditure from the exercise would be as follows:

Rate of energy expenditure (from Appendix 6): .061 Cal/min/lb
Body Weight: 150 lbs.
Duration: 30 minutes
Frequency: 5 days/week

Weekly caloric expenditure:

(.061 Cal/min/lb) (150 lbs) (30 min) (5) = 1372.5 calories

Subtracting the energy expenditure for the activity she would have been doing (seated office work) during the same time period each day had she not exercised:

(.010 Cal/min/lb) (150 lbs) (30 min) (5) = 225 calories

Net extra calories spent each week due to added exercise:

1372.5 − 225 = 1147.5 calories

Therefore, to lose 1 pound/week (remembering that 3500 calories = 1 lb of fat), she would have to reduce her caloric intake by:

3500 − 1147.5 = 2352.5 calories

On a daily basis, this means:

$$\frac{2352.5}{7} = 336 \text{ calories/day}$$

So by jogging slowly for 30 minutes/day, 5 days/week and restricting her diet by 336 calories/day, Mildred will lose fat at a rate of 1 pound/week. When she achieves her target weight, she can increase her caloric intake to normal and perhaps even allow herself to consume extra calories. She will not regain the lost weight, provided she continues with her exercise program indefinitely.

While 300 calories/session is the recommended minimum number of calories to be expended if body composition is to improve from an exercise program, this figure should be qualified: The majority of evidence on the topic of exercise and weight loss comes from research on men who, because of their greater size, spend more calories per minute than women. Were there just as much evidence on women, a reasonable guess is that the minimum number of calories required per exercise session for a woman would be slightly lower than that required for a man, perhaps around 250 calories per session.

Though we have thus far emphasized the use of aerobic exercise, this is not the only form of exercise that has an effect on body composition. Traditional forms of weight training using procedures designed to increase strength and muscular endurance have been shown to reduce body fat and increase fat-free weight. Circuit weight training has been shown to have similar effects in previously sedentary persons. The mechanisms explaining such changes are not clear but perhaps relate to the effects of such exercise on raising fat-free weight and hence BMR.

Exercise can alter fluid balance in a short period of time through sweat losses, particularly if the climate is hot and humid. This dehydrating effect of exercise has given rise to a number of fraudulent gimmicks for rapid weight loss including steam rooms, saunas, rubber suits, and other similar garments. Use of such practices for weight loss is strongly discouraged.

5. Behavior modification techniques that identify and change poor nutritional habits and/or identify ways in which food is being used inappropriately (for example, as a pacifier for stress, as a source of pleasure when nervous, and so on), will improve the likelihood of maintaining the weight loss permanently. Also, behavior modification techniques can and should be applied to the task of developing lifelong exercise habits to ensure successful and permanent weight control once weight-loss goals are met.

Dieting as a Method of Weight Loss

Effect on the Energy Balance Equation

Dieting (or restricting your caloric intake) so that stored fat is used for energy is one approach to weight loss that can be effective, provided basic nutritional principles are followed. Unfortunately, many people who diet are interested in rapid results that can be accomplished only through severe dieting and, using such methods, they create a number of problems which serve to defeat their objectives. For example, one consequence of severe caloric restriction already mentioned is that your BMR is lowered. It is almost as if your body doesn't know whether the dietary regime is likely to be long, arduous, and life-threatening (as in a famine) or whether it is just a temporary period of caloric restriction. Thus, your body reacts to severe caloric restriction in such a way as to defend against any possibility: it *conserves* the amount of energy that is expended. As a result, your BMR is lowered, and the consequences of a decline in BMR are twofold. First, your rate of fat loss will be slowed because your total energy expenditure per 24-hour cycle is reduced. Therefore, to continue achieving a weight loss you will have to restrict your caloric intake even further, which only continues the cycle. Second, if and when you attain your target weight and body composition, you will not be able to eat as much to maintain your weight at the new level because of your lower BMR. Thus the chances of achieving weight control at the new level are sabotaged and what occurs is the "see-saw" effect that so many Americans experience, namely the recurring cycle of weight loss followed by weight gain, followed by another diet and resultant weight loss, and so on. The net effect is that no real progress is made.

It should be noted that the decline in BMR is particularly significant if your caloric restriction is severe. Recent evidence suggests that such a decline may not occur if you go on a very modest diet.

Effect on Body Composition

Another important effect of severe or long-term dieting is that it results in significant loss of fat-free tissue along with loss of fat. As mentioned earlier, whenever you lose weight some of that weight loss is due to loss of proteins, water, minerals, electrolytes, and energy stores. All of these elements are needed for proper health and function, and the significant losses caused by fasting and severe caloric restriction can be medically dangerous.

Meeting Nutritional Requirements

Every time you enter a bookstore you are faced with endless diet books that claim new breakthroughs or some attractive gimmick that makes them sound plausible. It is not surprising that many people choose to try one of the many "fad" diets, many of which are unhealthy at best and dangerous at worst according to nutritional evidence. In reality, if you were to stand all such diets side by side and compare them fairly, equating them on the basis of total caloric intake, they would probably be very similar to one another. The only reason one might be more effective than another relates to the proportion of fat intake recommended by the diet. Recent evidence has demonstrated that dietary fat is converted into fat stores more efficiently than is dietary carbohydrate or protein, which means that any diet that restricts fat intake is likely to be more effective than a diet that does not, calorie for calorie.

Fad diets often recommend a severe restriction of a particular type of food, such as carbohydrates, or suggest that you eat all you wish of a certain type of food such as grapefruit. In such cases your intake of nutrients, vitamins, minerals, and fiber will be altered from desired levels, creating a dangerous or unhealthy nutritional deficiency. Since a well-balanced diet will be just as effective as a fad diet, given equivalent caloric restrictions, the most sensible approach is to choose the former. Chapters 8 and 9 discuss more fully the basic nutritional concepts behind a well-balanced diet, and practical suggestions are given. The same nutrition guidelines apply equally whether you are dieting or not; the only difference should be a reduction in the total number of calories by 500–1000 calories/day at most.

Exercise and Weight Control

There are a number of reasons why regular exercise is of great benefit to long-term weight control. These include the effect of exercise on body composition, caloric expenditure, fuel utilization, and appetite. Each of these factors is discussed more fully below.

Exercise and Body Composition

One important connection between regular exercise and weight control relates to its effect on the composition of the body. It is not uncommon for an individual to begin an exercise program only to discover that although fitness improves, body weight does not change much. This is particularly true if the individual is not overfat to begin with, or if his/her caloric intake increases to some degree after beginning the program. In reality, however, *body composition* changes. If the individual has been evaluated for body composition prior to beginning the program and is then remeasured at a later date, results will typically indicate that there has been a loss of body fat coupled with a similar gain in fat-free weight, thereby rendering the total body weight unchanged.

Of course, these predicted results are a generalization. Individual results will vary greatly due to differences in body makeup and as a result of the type, duration, and intensity of the exercise program. For example, if you choose a weight lifting program as your fitness activity, you will probably experience a greater gain in fat-free weight than if you spend the same amount of time doing an aerobics class. (This is true for both males and females.) On the other hand, if you are not regular in attending either to your weightlifting or to your aerobics, your changes in body composition will likely be much smaller, if any changes result at all. Generalizations about the benefits and results of an exercise program, then, must be qualified: people differ in ways that are as yet poorly understood and your results will depend partly upon factors that are unique to you.

One thing that does appear true, however, is that fat-free tissue expends more energy than does fat tissue. Fat-free tissue is said to be *metabolically active*, particularly if this tissue happens to be in the form of added muscle. If through regular exercise you build up your fat-free tissue, then hour-by-hour and day-by-day you will be expending more energy than if you had a larger proportion of fat and a relatively smaller porportion of fat-free tissue. Such an increase in daily energy expenditure will help tip the caloric balance equation in the desired direction and allow you to achieve weight control more easily.

Spot reducing refers to attempts to reduce localized fat stores by exercising the specific body part where the fat is located. Unfortunately, research on this topic indicates that this technique does not work. Exercise stimulates the mobilization of fat from deposits located throughout the body and not just from the fat cells located over the exercising muscle. The only benefits likely to be obtained from such exercises are improvements in flexibility, strength, and/or muscle endurance in the local body parts and related improvements in muscle tone. Such improvements can result in a loss of girth size, however.

Exercise and Caloric Expenditure

Another beneficial effect of regular exercise is that when you exercise you expend additional calories, which permits you to eat more food without the fear of gaining weight. It should be recognized also that the calories you expend during exercise are not the only additional calories spent. Following exercise for as long a period as 1–2 hours, depending on the nature and extent of the exercise and on the climatic conditions, your body continues to recover and continues to expend additional calories. The total caloric expenditure during this recovery period is not large, but it is nonetheless a part of your overall caloric expenditure.

Using exercise by itself as a means of weight loss, without any diet modification, is a relatively difficult method to choose. In fact, some experts suggest that the number of calories spent in exercise is so small that the effort may not be worth the trouble. To illustrate how the calorie expenditure is determined, sample calculations taken from one of the activities listed in Appendix 6 (easy running at 11 min 30 sec/mile) are provided in Example D below. By adding 2 miles/day, 3 days/week of such jogging into a previously sedentary routine, it would take 7 weeks for a 150 pound person to lose one pound of fat, a rate of fat loss which most Americans are likely to feel is too slow. However, while the immediate effects of the exercise are slow, if continued indefinitely the caloric effects can be considerable, simply because the caloric effects are cumulative. Over one year, 7.4 pounds of fat will be lost, all else remaining the same. Over 10 years this amounts to 74 pounds; over 20 years, 148 pounds. Thus, over a long time frame, the effects of regular exercise can be a powerful tool for losing fat and then for keeping fat levels under control. Between the ages of 20 and 40, the average individual gains 20–30 pounds of fat. If the majority of 40-year-olds had maintained a regular exercise program (with emphasis on regular!) during the previous 20 years, in all probability they would not have gained the extra fat.

Example D. Caloric effects of regular exercise.

If a 148 lb person were to jog on the horizontal at a pace of 11 min 30 sec/mile, the rate or energy expenditure in Appendix 6 is: 9.03 cal/min. Therefore, for 1 mile:

(9.03 Cal/min) (11.5 min/mi) = 103.8 Cal/mile

While sitting quietly this same person expends 1.48 Cal/min. Therefore, during the same time period, the person would have expended:

(1.48 Cal/min) (11.5 min) = 17.0 Cal

The net extra cost of jogging 1 mile is therefore:

(103.8 − 17.0) = 86.8 Cal/mi

Since 1 lb of fat = 3500 Cal, this means that

$$\frac{3500\ \text{Cal/lb}}{86.8\ \text{Cal/mi}} = 40.3 \text{ miles/lb of fat loss}$$

If this person jogged 2 miles/day for 3 days/wk = 6 mi/wk

Therefore: $\dfrac{40.3 \text{ miles/lb of fat}}{6 \text{ miles/wk}} = 6.7$ wks/lb

which is equivalent to: $\dfrac{52 \text{ wks/yr}}{6.7 \text{ wks/lb}} = 7.76$ lbs/yr

Over 10 years: (7.76 lbs/yr) (10 yrs) = 77.6 lbs

Over 20 years: (7.76 lbs/yr) (20 yrs) = 155.2 lbs

While no definite large survey data is available for documentation, some have suggested that, beginning in early adulthood, the typical American adds roughly 1–1.5 pounds per year of excess fat through a combination of slow fat-gain and slow loss of fat-free tissue. Since these two changes occur simultaneously, and since body weight may thus remain relatively unchanged, the fat accumulation is masked. Control of fat-weight gain through exercise is therefore to be recommended for all adults, even if an overall weight problem is not apparent.

Fuel Utilization in Exercise

The term "fuel" is used to refer to the foodstuffs used by the muscles during various types of exercise. There are three types of foodstuffs that contain energy: proteins, carbohydrates, and fats. For most circumstances, a simple generalization can be made, namely that proteins are not used at all as fuels for muscular exercise. Recent evidence has demonstrated that in prolonged exercise (such as marathon running), a small amount of the total energy production (<10%) comes from the breakdown of proteins. However, in all other types of exercise, the fuels that are used by the exercising muscles come from a mixture of fats and carbohydrates. Before describing the factors that influence the proportion of fat and carbohydrate used as fuel, it will be useful to describe in more detail the differences between aerobic and anaerobic exercise.

Aerobic exercises are ones which rely on oxygen in the production of energy. Oxygen does not supply the energy; it is simply needed to complete the last step in a large number of biochemical reactions required to break down food and release the energy that is contained within it. This process occurs within all cells in microscopically small structures called mitochondria.

Anaerobic exercises are ones which do not rely on oxygen for energy production (hence the term "anaerobic"). Instead they rely on immediate sources of energy found within the muscles or on the production of energy from the partial breakdown of carbohydrate. The immediate sources of energy are in short supply and are thought to be able to sustain the energy requirements of the muscles doing heavy exercise for only 5–10 seconds. The anaerobic breakdown of carbohydrate results in the production of a by-product called *lactic acid*, which is strongly implicated as a partial cause of muscle fatigue. For example, the weakness you experience when lifting a weight 15–20 times to the point of failure is thought to be partly due to the buildup of lactic acid in your exercising muscles.

Anaerobic exercises tend to be ones which last for short periods of time, usually less than 2–3 minutes. Whenever you complete a task within 2–3 minutes, particularly if it is vigorous (e.g., running up a flight of stairs, carrying a heavy suitcase in from the car, or running to catch up with a friend), you will rely primarily on anaerobic energy production. Depending on how long and how hard you push yourself, the fatigue you experience will vary accordingly.

Aerobic exercises are ones which last longer than 2–3 minutes. Since they are sustained for longer periods of time, such exercises tend to be done at a more gentle pace and as a result they are not as fatiguing as anaerobic exercises. For example, going for a walk, preparing a meal, working in the garden, are all examples of aerobic activities. So also are jogging, cycling, and swimming—the types of activities described in Chapter 5 as suitable for cardiorespiratory training. The latter activities tend to be more vigorous than the earlier examples and if you do them for long periods of time, they also tend to be fatiguing, particularly if you are not fit.

The needs of an exercising person depend on a number of factors, including the following.

1. *Diet:* If your diet is high in fat content, you will use fat to a greater extent as a fuel, all else remaining the same. The opposite is true if you eat a diet that is higher in carbohydrate content. This should certainly not be interpreted as a recommendation to increase your fat intake, as a number of health risks are associated with a high intake of dietary fat. More will be said on this matter in Chapters 8 and 9.

2. *Intensity of exercise:* In aerobic activities, both fats and carbohydrates contribute to the fuel requirements of the exercising muscles. Fats constitute the primary source of fuel used by the muscles in submaximal exercise, including activities during which you are at or nearly at rest. This fat comes from intracellular stores of fat within the muscles as well as from fat stores within fatty tissue. The greater the intensity of aerobic exercise, the more carbohydrates contribute to the fuel needs of the muscles and the less fats contribute.

Any anaerobic exercise relies exclusively on carbohydrates as a fuel once the immediate forms of stored energy are used up, which as mentioned earlier occurs after 5–10 seconds of heavy exercise. Thereafter, carbohydrates are the only form of fuel that can be relied on for anaerobic energy production.

3. *Duration of exercise:* When aerobic exercise is continued at a given pace, fats contribute increasingly to the fuel needs as duration of exercise increases. Thus, if you are to be able to keep up a jogging pace for 45 minutes, the relative contribution of fats will increase and be much greater toward the end of the workout than it was toward the beginning, all else remaining the same.

4. *Fitness status:* The more aerobically fit you are, the more you will be able to use fat in place of carbohydrate at a given level of exercise, all else remaining the same. This means that if you were to compare yourself under standardized conditions before and after 6 months of aerobic training, not only would a given level of exercise be much easier for you to perform because of your increased exercise capacity, but minute by minute you would also be using more fat and less carbohydrate to meet the energy demands of your muscles. This would be true at other times of the day as well, as for example while doing the tasks that make up your work day, or while driving to and from work. This is useful for at least two reasons. First, the fat stores in the body are many times greater than the stores of carbohydrate, even if you are relatively lean. Being able to rely on fat to a greater degree spares the more limited supply of carbohydrate for use only when it is absolutely required. Second, by being able to use fat as a fuel to a greater degree under all conditions, the total amount of fat stores tend to be lower, which is a pleasant outcome if you are concerned with weight control.

Exercise and Appetite

Contrary to what is commonly believed, adding regular exercise into your daily routine will not necessarily cause you to eat more. In fact, evidence suggests that the effects of moderate amounts of regular exercise will not increase your appetite at all; it may even lessen your appetite slightly, particularly if you exercise before a meal. In addition, recent evidence using lean persons suggests that when a meal is eaten in close proximity to an exercise session, more energy is expended than if the meal and exercise session are done separately. This adds further support to the argument favoring exercise in a weight loss program.

We should note, however, that this same accelerated energy expenditure due to the combination of meal and exercise has not been found to occur in obese persons. In fact, the energy expenditure that normally increases during and after a meal was instead reduced in the obese. This suggests that some people may be more prone to obesity than others due to this blunting of the normal increase in energy production as a result of a meal. The reasons for such differences remain unknown at present.

Liabilities of Exercise

The case favoring exercise is not so lopsided as to have no arguments against its use. There are many reasons why people do not turn to exercise, even when they are aware they should. First, exercise requires a commitment of time and often money (for clothing, equipment, gym fees, lessons, and so on), which are precious commodities in contemporary American society. In addition, many people dislike the fact that exercise leaves them tired and sweaty. There are risks involved as well: not only do you put yourself on display in many typical forms of exercise (that is, you risk exposure to others' observations), but there are also real risks of injury that many are unwilling to take. The problem is complicated further by the fact that our competitive, capitalistic marketplace offers hundreds of options from which to choose regarding agencies, instructors, books, testing facilities, and equipment, shoe, and clothing manufacturers. While this diversity may allow you to find the combination that best fits your needs (provided you take the time and energy to investigate the various options), it also puts you at risk of being taken in by fraudulent claims and offers. The only insurance against such practices is to be as informed as possible as a consumer.

Gaining Weight

For some people, the issue is not one of losing excess fat but rather one of gaining weight. Of course, most of any increase in weight should ideally come from an increase in fat-free weight, although for anyone whose percent fat is below the recommended level of essential fat (see earlier discussion), gaining extra fat is definitely a good idea and one which is compatible with an improved health status.

Gaining weight requires creating a positive caloric balance. Typically this is done by eating more calories than you expend. To assure that much of the weight-gain will be in the form of fat-free tissue, heavy resistance exercise (for example, weight training, calisthenics, circuit weight training) should be done as well. Protein supplementation may also be helpful to provide additional sources of complete protein for building muscle. If you elect to add extra protein, preferably it should not come in a form that also contains excessive fat (particularly saturated fat as in beef or pork) because of the risk such fats create for cardiovascular disease. Foods that are high in protein but lower in fat content, such as low-fat milk, egg white, and so on, would be better choices.

Summary

Some 15–20 percent of American adults are estimated to suffer from obesity, and countless others suffer from excessive fat even though they are not classified as obese. In addition to its negative social stigma, obesity is associated with numerous health problems, including higher risk for heart disease, cancer, and a higher overall death rate.

Determining your body composition is most accurately accomplished through hydrostatic weighing; however, skinfold measurement techniques that have been developed are easier to use and provide a general estimate of your percent fat. Such techniques are particularly useful if employed repeatedly over time. Experts are not in complete agreement regarding optimum levels of body weight and percent body fat.

Weight control is a function of energy balance, which is defined as the relationship between caloric intake and caloric expenditure. Recommended procedures for weight loss include a moderate diet in which no fewer than 1200 calories are consumed per day in conjunction with regular physical activity. Weight loss should not exceed 1–2 pounds/week. Activity should consist of moderate intensity aerobic exercise for 20–30 minutes or more per day, 3–5 days per week. As a method of weight loss, dieting by itself can be effective, but it may result in a decline in BMR, particularly if severe. If your dieting is severe you may also fail to take in a sufficient amount of daily nutrients to meet your nutritional requirements. Adding exercise to your routine may offset the loss in BMR that results from dieting, and it does not increase your appetite if done in moderation. In addition, exercise will force most of the weight loss to come from fat and not from loss of other tissues. Other benefits of regular exercise for long term weight control include a greater ability to use fat as a fuel (from aerobic training), overall improvement in body composition, and increased caloric expenditure, which assists in achieving long term caloric balance.

Gaining weight is best accomplished by eating more calories than you expend and by adding a supplemental heavy resistance exercise program to build lean tissue.

References

American College of Sports Medicine. Position stand on proper and improper weight loss programs. (1983). *Medicine and Science in Sports and Exercise* 15: ix–x.

Andres, R., Elahi, D., Tobin, J. D., Muller, D. C., and Bryant, L. 1985. Impact of age on weight goals. *Annals of Internal Medicine* 103(6), part 2:1030–1033.

Barrett-Connor, E. L. 1985. Obesity, atherosclerosis and coronary artery disease. *Annals of Internal Medicine* 103(6), part 2:1010–1019.

Bjorntorp, P. 1985. Regional patterns of fat distribution. *Annals of Internal Medicine* 103(6), part 2:994–995.

Bray, G. A. 1979. To treat or not to treat—That is the question. *Recent Advances in Obesity Research* II, ed. G. A. Bray. Westport, CT: Technomic.

Brehm, B. A. and Gutin, B. 1986. Recovery energy expenditure for steady state exercise in runners and non-exercisers. *Medicine and Science in Sports and Exercise* 18:205–210.

Brooks, G. A. and Fahey, T. D. 1984. *Exercise physiology.* New York: John Wiley and Sons.

Caspersen, C., Powell, K. E., and Christenson, G. M. 1985. Physical activity, exercise and physical fitness: Definitions and distinctions for health-related research. *Public Health Reports* 100(2):126–131.

Costill, D. C. 1985. Carbohydrate nutrition before, during and after exercise. *Fed. Proc.* 44:364–368.

Dohn, G. L., Kasperek, G. J., Tapscott, E. B., and Barakat, H. A. 1985. Protein metabolism during endurance exercise. *Fed. Proc.* 44: 348–352.

Frankel, H. M. 1986. Determination of body mass index. *JAMA* 255, No 10 (March 14).

Gollnick, P. D. 1985. Metabolism of substrates: energy substrate metabolism during exercise and as modified by training. *Fed. Proc.* 44: 353–357.

Health implications of obesity: National Institutes of Health consensus development conference statement. 1985. *Annals of Internal Medicine* 103(6), part 2:981–982.

Holloszy, J. O. 1982. Muscle metabolism during exercise. *Arch. Phys. Med. Rehabil.*, 63, 231–234.

Horton, E. S. 1985. Metabolic aspects of exercise and weight reduction. *Medicine and Science in Sports and Exercise* 18:10–18.

Is fat more fattening? 1987. *Tufts University Diet and Nutrition Letter* 4, No 12.

Jacobson, B. 1985. Anorexia nervosa and bulimia: Two severe eating disorders, *Public Affairs Committee, Inc.* Pamphlet No. 632.

Katch, F. I., Clarkson, P. M., Kroll, W., McBride, T., and Wilcox, A. 1984. The effects of sit up exercise training on adipose cell size and adiposity. *Research Quarterly for Exercise and Sport* 55:242–247.

Katch, F. I., and McArdle, W. D., 1983. *Nutrition, weight control, and exercise.* 2d ed. Philadelphia: Lea and Febiger.

Lohman, T. G., 1984. Research progress in validation of laboratory methods of assessing body composition. *Medicine and Science in Sports and Exercise* 16: 596–603.

McArdle, W. D., Katch, F. I., and Katch, V. L. *Exercise physiology.* 2d ed. Philadelphia: Lea and Febiger. 1986.

Metropolitan Life Insurance Co. 1984. 1983 Metropolitan height and weight tables. *Statistical Bulletin Metropolitan Life Insurance* 64:2–9.

New weight standards for men and women. 1959. *Statistical Bulletin Metropolitan Life Insurance* 40:1–4.

Oscai, L. B., 1973. The role of exercise in weight control. *Exercise and Sports Science Review* 1:103–124.

Oscai, L. B. 1981. Exercise and lipid metabolism. *Nutrition in the 1980's: Constraints on our knowledge.* New York: Alan R. Liss, 383–390.

Pollock, M. L. and Jackson, A. S. 1984. Research progress in validation of clinical methods of assessing body composition. *Medicine and Science in Sports and Exercise* 16:606–613.

Pollock, M. L., Wilmore, J. H., and Fox, III, S. M. 1984. *Exercise in health and disease.* Philadelphia: W. B. Saunders.

Ravussin, E., Lillioja, S., Anderson, T. E., Christin, L. and Bogardus, C. 1986. Determinants of 24-hour energy expenditure in man. *Journal of Clinical Investigation* 78:1568–1578.

Schlesier-Stropp, B. 1984. Bulimia: A review of the literature. *Psychological Bulletin* 95: 247–257.

Segal, K. R., Gutin, B., Nyman, A. M., and Pi-Sunyer, F. X. 1985. Thermic effect of food at rest, during exercise, and after exercise in lean and obese men of similar body weight. *Journal of Clinical Investigation* 76:1107–1112.

Thompson, J. K., Jarvie, G. J., Lahey, B. B., and Cureton, K. J. 1982. Exercise and obesity: Etiology, physiology, and intervention. *Psychological Bulletin* 91:55–79.

Webb, P. 1985. Direct calorimetry and the energetics of exercise and weight loss. *Medicine and Science in Sports and Exercise* 18:3–5.

Wilmore, J. H. 1983. Appetite and body composition consequent to physical activity. *Research Quarterly for Exercise and Sport* 54:415–425.

8

The Daily Dilemma: What's "Good" To Eat?

What nutrients do you need to be healthy?

How much of these nutrients should you be eating—and does it matter that much if you don't meet these requirements?

Most Americans are eating too much protein and fat and not enough carbohydrates; are you?

Can your diet affect your risk of contracting such diseases as cancer, heart disease, diabetes, osteoporosis, or even the common cold?

Is herb tea better for you than coffee? Wine better than beer? Mineral water better than soft drinks?

Introduction

Good nutrition is a rather demanding concept. It entails giving your body what it needs, when it needs it, and in the right amount to allow you to function in top form. This is no simple task because the body requires quite a variety of things to function at its best. In addition to energy, the body needs building blocks, transport carriers, regulators, facilitators, cleansers, and lots of water. To meet these needs, you have to eat over 45 different nutrients each day. Fortunately, you don't have to eat that many different foods to obtain these nutrients. Some foods, such as meat, milk, apples, oranges, and bread, contain many nutrients. Other foods, such as beer, soda pop, and pretzels, have almost none. The important point is that no one food or even a combination of several foods can provide all of the nutrients you need. There isn't any pill or capsule that can do the job either. Only by consuming a variety of foods with certain qualities and in specific amounts can you meet the body's needs. Thus *variety, quality, and quantity are the key determinants of good nutrition*. What foods have these qualities? How much of them do you need to eat and how often? Furthermore, how much does it really matter if you don't pay attention to these issues? These are the questions addressed in the first part of this chapter.

The nutrients the body needs to be supplied with daily are called *essential nutrients* because the body can't function properly without them and it has no way to get them unless you eat them. The six main categories of essential nutrients are protein, carbohydrate, fat (also called lipid), vitamins, minerals, and water. The essential nutrients in each of these categories are listed in Table 8.A. Of these, only protein, carbohydrates, and fat provide energy or fuel for the body. The amount of energy supplied by these nutrients is measured in calories (used in this book to mean kilocalories).*

Table 8.A   Essential Nutrients.

VITAMINS	MINERALS	PROTEIN	FAT	CARBOHYDRATE	WATER
Fat Soluble	Calcium	Amino Acids	Linoleic acid	Glucose	
A	Phosphorus	Leucine			
D	Sodium	Isoleucine			
E	Potassium	Lysine			
K	Sulfur	Methionine			
Water Soluble	Chlorine	Phenylalanine			
Thiamin	Magnesium	Threonine			
Riboflavin	Iron	Tryptophan			
Niacin	Selenium	Valine			
Biotin	Zinc	Histidine			
Folacin	Manganese				
Pyridoxine					
Vitamin B_{12}					
Pantothenic acid					
Ascorbic acid					

*Food energy is actually measured in kilocalories or Calories. A calorie (spelled with a small "c") is only 1/1000th of a kilocalorie or Calorie, but most Americans and even nutritionists simply use the term *calorie* to mean kilocalorie.

Although it is a potential energy source, the main role of protein is to provide the structural components or building blocks for body tissues. Vitamins and minerals function primarily as regulators and facilitators or catalysts of the millions of chemical reactions within cells that keep the body functioning. Water forms the major part of every body tissue (you are more than 70% water). It also provides the medium by which materials are transported to and away from cells and in which almost all body processes take place. The function(s) of each nutrient group are summarized in Table 8.B.

The ultimate purpose of this chapter is to help you make informed choices about what you eat each day. Toward this goal, the special characteristics/qualities of each of these essential nutrients will be discussed, and the best food sources of each identified.

Table 8.B   Basic functions of major nutrient groups.

	FUNCTIONS		
	ENERGY SOURCE	GROWTH, MAINTENANCE AND REPAIR OF BODY TISSUES	REGULATION OF BODY PROCESSES
Nutrient Groups	Carbohydrates		
	Fats		
	Proteins	Protein	Protein
	(Minerals)*	(Minerals)*	Minerals
	(Vitamins)*	(Vitamins)*	Vitamins

*Indirectly involved as catalysts for biochemical reactions

Protein

One of the most critical of the essential nutrients is protein. Its name was intended to connote its importance; *protein* means "in first place" after the Greek word *protos*. There are hundreds of different kinds of proteins in the body, all with very specialized functions. Typically only muscle is thought of as being protein, and the majority of protein is in muscle. However, protein is also a major structural component of *every cell* in the body. Table 8.C shows the distribution of protein among various body tissues. Protein is also used to make the antibodies in our blood and many of our hormones. It is used to transport nutrients to and from cells, and the protein *hemoglobin*, which contains iron, carries oxygen. A very special function of proteins is to catalyze or facilitate the chemical reactions in cells that keep the body functioning; these proteins are called *enzymes*.

Protein is made of nitrogen-containing components called *amino acids*. When you eat protein, the body digests it or breaks it down into these amino acids units. These

Table 8.C   Distribution of protein in the body.*

TISSUE	% OF BODY PROTEIN (APPROX.)
Blood proteins (albumin and hemoglobin)	10
Fat cells of adipose tissues	3–4
Body skin	9–9.5
Bones	18–19
Muscles	46–47

*The values have been obtained from different investigators and are presented in ranges to emphasize their variability in human bodies.

Reprinted with permission of the present publisher, Jones & Bartlett Publishers, Inc. From Y. H. Hui, *Principles and Issues in Nutrition,* Wadsworth Health Sciences, 1985, p.35.

are then absorbed into the bloodstream and carried to the cells where various of these amino acids are linked together to make the different proteins the body needs. There are some 22 different amino acids. Nine of these are called *essential amino acids* because the body cannot make them; they must be eaten. The other 13 amino acids can be made in the body as needed even if not specifically consumed. The 9 essential amino acids were listed in Table 8.A. Eight of these are considered essential for adults; the remaining one, histidine, is also essential for infants.

Any protein containing all 9 of these essential amino acids in sufficient quantity for the body to use is called a *complete protein*; all other proteins are called *incomplete*. They contain insufficient amounts of one or more of the essential amino acids. Consequently, the body will be able to use the amino acids supplied for building proteins only in relation to the amount of the *"limiting"* or *insufficient* amino acid(s). The situation is analogous to trying to make cookies when you have only one egg and the recipe calls for two. You can make only half the recipe. And if you are about to leave on a three month vacation and can't store the rest of the ingredients of which you have plenty, you will just have to use them in another way or throw them out. Similarly, the body has no way to store amino acids. Those that can't be used to make protein are stripped of their nitrogen and used for fuel, or stored as fat if other sources of fuel (carbohydrate and fat) are sufficiently abundant. The nitrogen is eliminated through the urine.

The only way to ensure that the body can make all the protein it needs, when it needs it, is to supply it with complete proteins periodically throughout the day. However, even when you eat enough protein, if the body receives insufficient calories for energy from its other fuel sources (carbohydrates and fats) protein will be used for energy instead of for building and repair, hormones, antibodies, and so on. It would be as if you weren't eating enough protein. In this sense, carbohydrates and fat are called "protein sparers."

Sources of Protein

All animals and animal products, except gelatin, provide complete proteins. This includes meat, fish, poultry, eggs, and dairy products. Vegetables and grains also provide proteins, but in general, these proteins are incomplete. Legumes are somewhat the exception: they are the richest sources of vegetable proteins and provide protein almost as complete as animal foods. Examples of legumes include lentils, peanuts, black-eyed peas, soy beans, chick peas, lima beans, kidney beans, pinto beans, black beans, and other types of dried peas and beans. Of these, soy beans and soy bean products most closely resemble animal protein. Seeds and nuts are excellent vegetable proteins, too, but they also contain so much fat — that is, calories — that their use as a major protein source is limited. All other vegetable and grain proteins are notably incomplete.

By eating certain combinations of vegetables and grains or by eating them with a source of complete protein like milk, it is possible to get complete protein without actually eating meat, poultry, or fish. Such protein combinations are called *complimentary proteins* and provide the basis for the vegetarian diet. Figure 8.1 shows how this works. Each of the 9 essential amino acids and the relative amount needed by the body is represented by a white bar graph. Superimposed over the bar graph in a dark shade is the amount of each essential amino acid in milk, soybeans, wheat, corn, and rice. You can see that by having milk with your cereal or toast, or by eating a combination of beans and rice, to use two examples, you can obtain a complete protein. On the other hand, toast and coffee (even whole wheat toast!), just won't fill the complete protein bill. Should you decide to have some milk or yogurt a bit later, within two hours or so, you could probably still complement your toast into "completeness," but the best advice seems to be to eat them together.

The limiting amino acid(s) for various categories of vegetable and grain proteins are listed in Table 8.D. Combining legumes with grains and seeds seems to be the best overall recommendation for obtaining complete protein without eating animal products. Other combinations will accomplish this also, but a full discussion of vegetarianism is beyond the scope of this book. The point is that getting the protein the body needs requires some knowledge and planning, and even more so if you choose not to eat any animal products.

Some other conditions affect the body's ability to use the protein you eat. These include the amino acid pattern of the protein, its digestibility, the availability of the vitamins and minerals needed to process it, and a sufficient intake of the "protein sparers," fat and carbohydrate, to prevent the protein from being used for energy. Vitamin and mineral needs will be discussed later in this chapter and the protein sparing effect of fats and carbohydrates has already been mentioned. The amino acid pattern and digestibility of proteins, however, deserve some explanation here. In brief, the more closely the amounts of essential amino acids in a protein you eat resemble the amounts in human protein, the more completely the protein can be used. This is referred to as the *biological value of protein*. In this respect, egg is the best protein source with a biological value of 100. It is followed by fish and dairy products, meats and soybeans, grains and nuts, in that order. However, you can't use what you don't digest and absorb, and the ability of the body to digest protein from different sources varies. Basically, the most easily digested proteins come from animal products, followed by soybeans and then other vegetables and grains.

In order to make protein, the human body needs eight or nine amino acids that must be supplied by the protein in food. And the body needs those essential amino acids in a certain proportion. If a food is low in one or more of the amino acids, the quality of its protein isn't as high as in a food that supplies all of them in the proper quantities.

We've superimposed the pattern for high-quality protein on the protein patterns (in blue) for five foods. Cows' milk and soybeans meet the pattern (as do meat, fish, and eggs); wheat, corn, and rice fall short. If you ate only one of those three grains, the quality of its protein would not improve, no matter how much you ate.

But by combining foods, the protein patterns can be improved. The extra lysine in milk, say, fills in the lysine missing in rice. That's protein complementation.

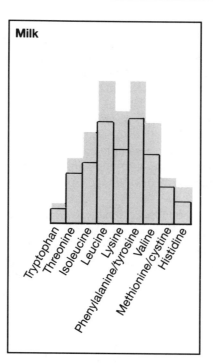
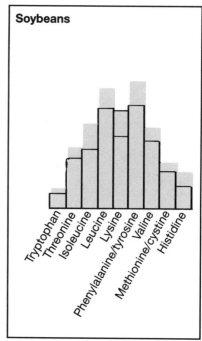
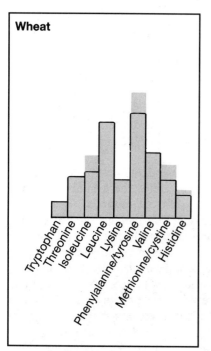
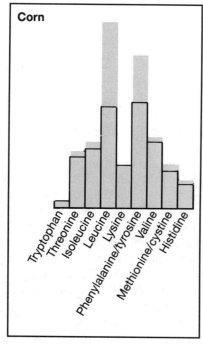
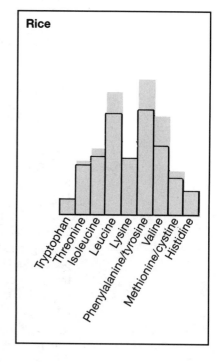

FIGURE 8.1   Protein qualities for different foods.

Table 8.D   Limiting amino acids in vegetable proteins.

VEGETABLE PROTEINS	LIMITING AMINO ACIDS			
	LYSINE	METHIONINE	THREONINE	TRYPTOPHAN
Most grains	√		√	sometimes (e.g., corn)
Most legumes		√		√
Nuts & seeds	√			
Green leafy vegetables		√		

Adapted from Hui, Y. H. *Principles & Issues In Nutrition*, Belmont, CA: Wadsworth, 1985.

The Body's Protein Requirements

Now that the quality of protein needed by the body has been defined, the final question is "how much protein do you need to eat?" Your size and age help to determine the answer. Look again at Table 8.C, which shows the distribution of protein among various body tissues. Almost 90% of our protein is located in lean or fat-free tissues. Obviously a large-sized person, someone with big bones and muscles, would need more protein to maintain these tissues than would a smaller person. Also, during those times in life when these tissues are being rapidly built, such as during pregnancy, infancy, and childhood, a higher intake would be needed compared to that needed just to maintain existing tissue.

Thus the amount of protein you need to eat is based on the amount of lean body tissue you have and/or are developing. For easier calculation, the reference standard used is average body weight or the midpoint of the weight range for medium-frame people according to height. You can determine this value for yourself from the height/ weight tables provided in Chapter 7. You can use the midpoint value for small or large-frame people if you think you fit better in one of these categories *or* use your own body weight if it is within the given range. The important point is not to over- or underestimate your protein needs should you weigh more or less than recommended.

It is estimated that the average adult needs only .45 grams of protein per kilogram (2.2 lbs.) of body weight. However, to allow for variation in individual need as well as in the quality of protein consumed, the official recommended intake for protein is .8 grams/kg., quite a generous allowance. This translates to .36 g/pound of body weight for adults 19 years of age and over. The recommended protein intake for various age groups is given in Table 8.E, per pound and per kilogram. You simply multiply your body weight (or the "average" body weight for your height) in pounds or kilograms times the unit given for your age to find the amount of protein recommended for you to eat. For the average 55 kg. (120 lbs.) female, this amounts to 44 grams of protein/day. For the average 70 kg. (155 lb.) male, the recommended amount is 56 grams of protein/day. However, given the generous safety margin built into this recommended intake, it is estimated that 80% of the population could actually be quite

Table 8.E   Recommended dietary allowance for protein.

AGE IN YEARS	GRAMS OF PROTEIN (PER POUND OR KILOGRAM OF IDEAL BODY WEIGHT)	
	G / POUNDS	G / KILOGRAMS
Infants		
0–0.5	1.0	2.2
0.5–1	.9	2.0
Children		
1– 3	.81	1.8
4– 6	.68	1.5
7–10	.55	1.2
11–14	.45	1.0
15–18	.39	.8
Adults		
19 and over	.36	.8
Pregnant women	.62	1.3
Nursing women	.53	1.17

Sources: (1) Food & Nutrition Board, *Recommended Dietary Allowances,* 9th Ed. Washington, D.C., 1980. National Academy of Sciences–National Research Council. (2) Jane Brody. *Jane Brody's Nutrition Book.* New York: Bantam, 1981.

healthy if they consumed only two-thirds this amount! It should be noted however, that this recommendation applies to people who are basically healthy. Illness, prolonged bed rest, and injury can increase the body's need for protein.

How much do you have to eat to get 44 grams or 56 grams of protein? The answer is far less than the average American thinks! As you can see in Figure 8.2, a breakfast of one egg and one piece of toast would provide 9 grams of protein. A peanut butter sandwich for lunch would add about 13 grams of protein. Should you choose to have a *small*, 6 oz. steak (6 oz. would be the petite cut in most American restaurants) on the same day, you would be consuming an additional 42 grams of protein. Just these foods alone total 64 grams of protein, 8 grams more than the average male needs and 20 grams more than the average female needs! And this total doesn't even consider the protein in the foods that accompany the entree such as fruit, vegetables, snacks, and dessert. Indeed, it's not difficult for the average American to consume 100 grams of protein a day, about twice the recommended amount. The average protein intake of Americans as reported by two national nutrition surveys is shown in Figure 8.3. As you can see, Americans from childhood through old age are overconsuming protein.

Overconsumption of protein presents several problems. Too much protein generally means not enough room for something else you need. In general it is thought that protein should comprise no more than 10–15% of our total calories; fat, no more than 30%, and carbhohydrate 55–60%. For a woman consuming about 2000 calories/day that translates to 200–300 calories from protein. Should she eat 100 grams of protein that contains 4 calories/gram, she would consume 400 calories or 20% of her calories

Example I			Example II		
		Protein (g.)			Protein (g.)
BREAKFAST	1 orange	1		1 banana	1
	1 poached egg	6		1 cup oatmeal	5
	1 slice whole			1 slice white	
	wheat toast	3		toast	2
	coffee			1 cup milk	8
		10 grams			16 grams
LUNCH	2 slices whole			Quarter Pounder	
	wheat bread	6		with cheese	30
	2 Tbsp. peanut-			Regular Fries	3
	butter	7		Milk Shake	9
	1 cup milk	8			42 grams
		21 grams			
SNACK	1/4 cup			1 cup	
	sunflower seeds	9 grams		popcorn	1 gram
DINNER	6 oz. steak	42		3 oz. broiled fish	17
	1/2 cup mashed			1/2 cup brown	
	potatoes	2		rice	3
	1/2 cup spinach	3		1/2 cup green	
	1 cup ice cream	5		beans	2
		52 grams		1 brownie	1
					23 grams
Total Protein = 92 grams			**Total Protein = 82 grams**		

FIGURE 8.2
Examples of daily
protein intake.

for the day in protein. If like most Americans she eats primarily animal products to obtain her protein, then her intake of fat is also likely to be higher than recommended. Many animal sources of protein actually contain more fat calories than protein calories. Vegetable sources of protein, on the other hand, generally contain very little if any fat, but rather have large amounts of carbohydrate. The percent of calories from fat, protein, and carbohydrates for various sources of protein is shown in Table 8.F.

Americans typically get 42% of their daily calories in fat rather than the recommended 30%. One of the main reasons for this high fat intake is high consumption of animal protein, especially popular foods like steak, hamburgers, hot dogs, bacon, eggs, cheese, and milkshakes. Even if the amount of protein consumed does not exceed recommended intake, eating a lot of foods like these can result in excessive fat intake, in particular saturated fats and cholesterol.

Crowded out of this picture are carbohydrates, found in fruits, vegetables, and grains. On the average Americans consume 46% or less of total daily calories in carbohydrates compared to the recommended 55–60%. Because fat contains 9 calories/gram compared to 4 calories/gram for carbohydrate, this high protein, high fat, low

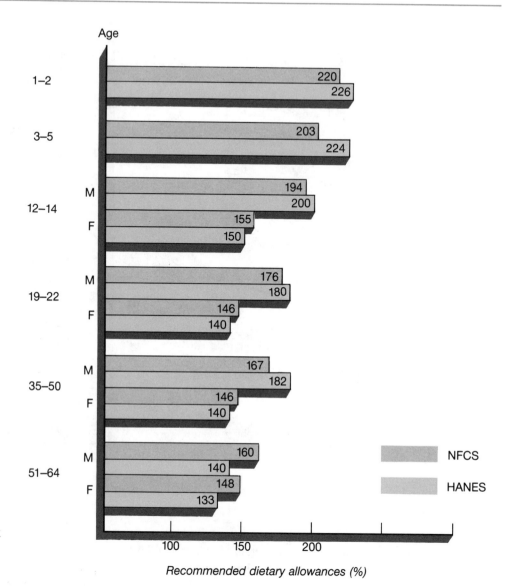

FIGURE 8.3
Mean protein intake of various age and sex groups in relation to recommended dietary allowances. Based on results of HANES I (1970–74) and Nationwide Food Consumption Survey (1977–78).

Reproduced by permission from Helen Guthrie, *Introductory Nutrition,* 5th Ed. St. Louis, 1983, The C. V. Mosby Co./Times Mirror/Mosby College Publishing.

carbohydrate diet can also be a high calorie diet. This is exactly the kind of diet associated with obesity, CVD, and cancer. High protein and high fat intakes also increase excretion of calcium, which can enhance the development of osteoporosis over time.

The bottom line for protein consumption seems to be to keep it in first place when it comes to quality and last place when it comes to quantity (percent of calories). To do this means selecting complete and/or complementary proteins to eat and emphasizing low fat sources such as fish, poultry, vegetables, and grains.

Table 8.F   Percent of calories from protein, fat, and carbohydrates for selected sources of protein.

FOODS	TOTAL CALORIES	% PROTEIN	% FAT	% CHO
Almonds, 1/4 cup whole shelled	212	10	79	11
Prime Rib with fat, 3 oz	375	19	80	—
Sirloin with fat, 3 oz	330	24	74	—
Sirloin, fat trimmed, 3 oz	175	63	35	—
Cheddar cheese, 1 oz	115	25	74	trace
Egg, hard boiled	80	30	67	3
Whole milk, 1 cup	150	21	48	31
Skim milk, 1 cup	85	40	trace	59
Hot dog, 8 per lb	170	16	80	2
Tuna, oil packed, 3 oz	170	57	40	trace
Tuna, water packed, 3 oz	117	90	6	trace
Chicken breast, with skin, 2.8 oz	160	65	30	3
Turkey, white meat (2 slices, no skin)	150	78	20	—
Kidney beans, 1 cup	230	25	4	71
Whole wheat bread, 1 slice	65	15	5	80
Peanut butter, 1 tbsp	95	17	70	13
Spaghetti, 1 cup	190	15	3	82

Note: All percentages are approximate.

Fats

Fat has such a bad reputation today that it may be hard to think of it as an *essential* nutrient. Most people know this about fat: (1) They're not supposed to be eating as much as they do; (2) they're not supposed to be "wearing" as much as they do; and (3) they're supposed to be "watching" their cholesterol. These perceptions are basically correct, but you must eat *some* fat and have some body fat in order to function normally. The fact that many Americans typically exceed these needs accounts for our perceptions of fat as harmful; such excesses are indeed linked to major health problems and premature death. Such types of fat as saturated fat and cholesterol are particular culprits in this regard. However, recent research suggests that there may be other types of fat that actually help to prevent or minimize these problems.

Dietary fat provides you with a concentrated source of energy and thus helps conserve protein for growth, maintenance, and repair. As previously noted, a gram of fat contains 9 calories as compared to 4 calories/gram for carbohydrate or protein. In essence, you obtain more than twice as much energy from the same size package. Without some fat in your diet you can not absorb vitamins A, E, D, and K since they are soluble only in fat. In addition, fat increases the texture, aroma, and flavor of foods, making them more inviting to eat. Fat is said to have a high *satiety value* because you feel more satisfied when you've eaten a food with some fat content, as compared to lettuce or celery for example. Since fat is digested rather slowly, it remains in the stomach longer and you feel fuller longer.

As a part of the body itself, fat provides padding to protect vital organs from injury. Fat beneath the skin serves as insulation against cold temperatures, and oils on the skin and hair give them a healthy sheen as opposed to a dried-out appearance. Fat is a constituent of hormones such as testosterone and estrogen. In fact, without sufficient body fat, women may lose reproductive function; that is, they may stop menstruating. And, of course, body fat stands as a ready fuel reserve whenever insufficient calories are consumed. It's your reserve fuel tank.

Types of Fat

Ninety-five percent of the fat you eat is called *triglyceride* to describe its chemical make-up. It consists of three ("tri") fatty acids attached to a glycerol molecule, like branches to a tree trunk. Our digestive process breaks this structure apart into individual fatty acids that can be absorbed into the blood.

There are three different types of fatty acids: saturated, monounsaturated, and polyunsaturated. These terms basically describe the chemical structures of the fatty acids. As shown in Figure 8.4, fatty acids consist of chains of carbon atoms with hydrogen atoms attached to them. When all of the possible attachment sites on each carbon atom are occupied by hydrogen atoms, the fatty acid is called *saturated*. If all the attachment sites are not occupied, the fatty acids are called *unsaturated*. *Polyunsaturated* fatty acids have many hydrogens missing (at least four) and *monounsaturated* fatty acids have two hydrogens missing (it is chemically impossible for only one hydrogen atom to be missing). In form, saturated fats are solid at room temperature and unsaturated fats are liquid.

Saturated Fatty Acid

Mono-Unsaturated Fatty Acid (one double bond)

Polyunsaturated Fatty Acid (two or more double bonds)

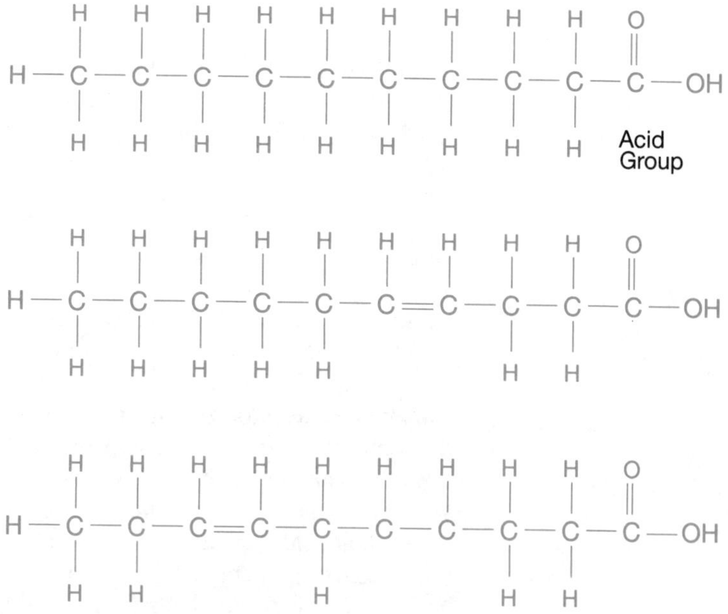

FIGURE 8.4 The chemical structure of fatty acids.

The importance of being aware of these different forms of fatty acids is related to their link with heart disease. Diets containing a lot of saturated fat increase the risk of cardiovascular disease whereas diets emphasizing polyunsaturated fats seem to provide some protection against cardiovascular disease. Recent research indicates that monounsaturated fats may be even more protective. While most foods actually contain mixtures of all three types of fatty acids, saturated fats predominate in animal products and mono- and polyunsaturated fats in vegetables and grains and fruits such as the avocado (most fruits have little or no fat at all).

Palm and coconut oils are natural exceptions to this general rule; they contain large amounts of saturated fats. There is also an unnatural exception: hydrogenated or partially hydrogenated vegetable oils. If you use margarine instead of butter because it is a polyunsaturated fat, you may have been surprised to read in the previous paragraph that unsaturated fats are liquid at room temperature. Whether you buy margarine in cubes or in tubs, it is definitely not a liquid. The reason for this more solid, saturated appearance is that manufacturers have *hydrogenated* the vegetable oil to make it look and behave more like butter and to increase its shelf-life. (Polyunsaturated fats spoil more quickly than saturated fats and hydrogenation retards this deterioration.) The reason hydrogenation makes vegetable oils appear and behave more like saturated fat is that it transforms polyunsaturated fat into saturated fat! Hydrogenation means "to add hydrogens." Thus, when the package label says the product contains hydrogenated vegetable oil, it really means saturated fat.

The term *partially hydrogenated* means that the vegetable oil is not fully saturated, but it certainly is much less polyunsaturated than a pure vegetable oil. It also contains a new type of fatty acid, a trans-fatty acid created during the partial hydrogenation process. These trans-fatty acids do not occur naturally in the body and there is concern that they may promote certain types of cancer. The evidence supporting this suspicion is not conclusive, but minimizing intake of trans-fatty acids seems wise at this point. Buying margarines listing liquid vegetable oil rather than partially hydrogenated oil as the first ingredient on the label is one way to minimize exposure to trans-fatty acids. Mixing soft butter with the same amount of safflower oil will produce a spread with the same degree of polyunsaturation as margarine, but with no trans-fatty acids at all.

In addition to triglycerides, there are other types of fat in our food, namely *phospholipids* and *sterols*. You may have heard of a substance called *lecithin*, a natural emulsifier, that is supposed to dissolve the fat in your arteries. Lecithin is a phospholipid and it does help to keep fats in solution in the blood as well as being an important cell membrane constituent. However, the lecithin the body needs can be made by the liver; you don't need to eat it. The lecithin you eat gets digested like other forms of fat before it can ever get into the blood stream. For this reason, buying lecithin supplements to prevent atherosclerosis will benefit the health food store proprietor more than the consumer.

Cholesterol, the most recognized form of sterols, is best known for its prominence in the fatty deposits that accumulate on blood vessel walls. Cholesterol is, however, sufficiently necessary to body functioning that the liver makes about 1000 mg. of cholesterol everyday. The liver can make cholesterol from either saturated fatty acid or glucose. Thus, it is not necessary to eat *any* cholesterol at all; nonetheless, average intake is 600 mg./day. The liver uses some of this cholesterol to make *bile*, which helps in the digestion of fats. Some cholesterol is used to make hormones. The rest is transported through the blood to cells, and some accumulates on blood vessel walls before reaching its destination. The cholesterol reaching the cells is used in many metabolic reactions and in parts of the cells' structure. The cholesterol that is not used is sent back to the liver.

As you will recall from Chapter 3, fats are transported through the blood by lipoproteins. The lipoproteins made by the liver to send to cells are called VLDLs and LDLs (very low density lipoproteins and low density lipoproteins, respectively). Of these, the LDLs are the prominent carriers of cholesterol; thus, a high level of LDLs in the blood is considered a risk factor for development of fatty deposits on blood vessel walls. Diets high in saturated fats and cholesterol seem to promote high levels of LDLs. Some people, however, seem to have inherited a propensity toward high LDLs in the blood.

Cholesterol being transported from the cells back to the liver travels in the form of HDLs, high density lipoproteins. People with high levels of HDLs in their blood seem less prone to developing fatty deposits on their blood vessels, and it even seems that increasing HDLs in the blood may result in some decrease in fatty deposits already formed. Regular vigorous exercise is the best way known to increase HDLs, although diets low in total fat, but higher in polyunsaturated fats than saturated, may also help. Women seem to have naturally higher levels of HDLs than do men.

Polyunsaturated fats from fish, especially a kind called omega-3, have recently been found to be particularly effective in reducing both cholesterol and triglyceride levels in the blood. In fact, Dr. William Castelli, director of the Framingham Heart Study in Framingham, Mass., has flatly stated that eating fish two times per week could cut the incidence of heart disease in half. Even shellfish, once considered loaded with cholesterol, are now being recommended as "protective fare." Newer methods of measuring cholesterol in food have shown the cholesterol level of most shellfish to be lower than that of canned tuna or broiled chicken breast. Even shrimp and lobster, which have the highest cholesterol content of the shellfish, are only slightly higher than lean beef or lamb in cholesterol. The cholesterol content of various types of fish is compared with chicken, pork, lamb, and beef in Table 8.G. Cholesterol is found only in animal products. Of these, the very lowest sources are clams, fresh fish, oysters, and scallops. These are also very low-calorie sources of protein. By far the highest sources of cholesterol are eggs and organ meats such as liver and kidney.

The types of fish with the highest omega-3 oil content are listed in Table 8.H. In this case, the fatter, higher-calorie fish are the best sources; for example, salmon and tuna. The fat and calorie content in these fish is still low when compared to most meats, however.

The Body's Fat Requirements

As previously mentioned, Americans currently eat about 42% of their daily calories in fat compared to a recommended intake of no more than 30%. It is also recommended that this 30% be evenly distributed among polyunsaturated, monounsaturated, and saturated fats, 10% of total calories for each. As shown in Figure 8.5, Americans currently consume more saturated and monounsaturated fat and less polyunsaturated fat than recommended.

The recommended intake of fat far exceeds actual need. The body needs only a small amount, 1–2% of total calories, of the polyunsaturated fat called *linoleic acid*. Linoleic acid is called an essential fatty acid because the body cannot synthesize it; you must eat it. One to two tablespoons of vegetable oil, especially safflower, wheat germ, corn, or soybean oil, will generally sypply the amount you need each day. The linoleic acid content of various oils is given in Table 8.I. Note the very small amount of linoleic acid in palm, olive, and coconut oils compared to other types.

Table 8.G   Cholesterol content of various meats, poultry, fish, and eggs.

FOOD	PORTION	MG. OF CHOLESTEROL
Clams	6 large	36
Fresh Fish	3 oz	42
Oysters	3 oz	45
Scallops	3 oz	45
Canned Tuna	3 oz	55
Crab	½ cup	62
Fresh Pork	3 oz	70
Chicken, White Meat, Skinned	3 oz	76
Lean Beef	3 oz	77
Lean Veal	3 oz	84
Lean Lamb	3 oz	85
Lobster	½ cup	90
Shrimp	½ cup	96
Egg	1 whole	256*
Beef Liver	3 oz	372
Chicken Liver	3 oz	480
Beef Kidney	3 oz	690

*All of the cholesterol is in the egg yolk.

Sources: *Wellness Newsletter,* Vol. 2, #3 (Dec. 1985). Berkeley: University of California. (2) Whitney, E. and Hamilton, E. *Understanding Nutrition,* 3d Ed. Minneapolis: West, 1984.

Table 8.H   Omega–3 oil content of species of fish.

SPECIES	OMEGA–3 OIL CONTENT IN 4 OUNCE-SERVING
Chinook Salmon	3.6 grams
Sockeye Salmon	2.3 grams
Albacore Tuna	2.6 grams
Mackerel	1.8–2.6 grams
Herring	1.2–2.7 grams
Rainbow Trout	1.0 grams
Whiting	0.9 grams
King Crab	0.6 grams
Shrimp	0.5 grams
Cod	0.3 grams

Adapted from data from *The Oregonian,* November 29, 1985.

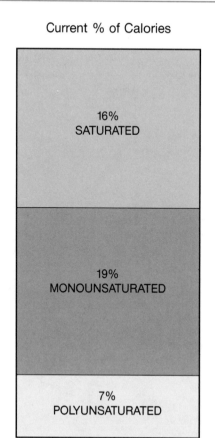

Current % of Calories

Recommended % of Calories

16%
SATURATED

19%
MONOUNSATURATED

7%
POLYUNSATURATED

10%
SATURATED

10%
MONOUNSATURATED

10%
POLYUNSATURATED

TOTAL = 42%

TOTAL = 30%

FIGURE 8.5
Current and recommended intake of types of fat.

The large difference between the recommended and needed amounts of fat reflects an attempt by scientists/nutritionists to be practical as well as safe. A diet in which fat accounts for only 10% of total calories has been proposed for years as a powerful combatant against atherosclerosis. However, the Pritikin diet, as it is called, has not been popular with Americans because it isn't very palatable; it just doesn't taste as good or feel very satisfying. We have grown accustomed to much higher amounts of fat in our diets and the level of satiety that accompanies that. Therefore, even though current research suggests that consuming a lot less than 30% of daily calories in fat would be healthier, it doesn't seem likely that many Americans would follow that recommendation at this time. However, a 25% decrease from the current 42% intake of fat is considered a strong step in the right direction. The current recommendation to consume 30% of calories in fat reflects this cutback.

It is likely that the recommended intake of fat will be reduced even more in the future because of the connection between high fat diets, heart disease, and cancer. As already noted, minimizing saturated fats in the diet seems particularly important to avoiding or minimizing atherosclerosis. Reducing cholesterol intake from 600 to 300 mg. per day is also being recommended. The primary intent of these measures is to reduce blood levels of cholesterol, especially in the form of LDLs.

Table 8.1 Linoleic acid content in various oils.

TYPE OF OIL	% LINOLEIC ACID
Safflower	74.5%
Sunflower	65.0%
Corn	58.7%
Soybean	58.0%
Cottonseed	51.9%
Sesame	41.7%
Peanut	32.0%
Palm	9.3%
Olive	8.4%
Coconut	1.8%

Adapted from Guthrie, H. *Introductory Nutrition,* 6th Ed. New York: Times Mirror/Mosby, 1986.

Using a new tool called the CSI, you can actually estimate the combined influence of the cholesterol and saturated fat in any given food on blood cholesterol levels. This procedure is shown in Box 1, below.

Diets high in fat, either saturated or polyunsaturated, also seem to increase the risk of cancers of the colon, breast, prostate, and endometrium. It is possible that the high fat content somehow encourages development of carcinogens in the intestinal tract. High fat diets are generally low in fiber, a non-digestible substance that helps move food through the intestines. This could result in a longer than usual passage time

---

BOX 1

A new way to estimate the cholesterol-raising effect of food is to calculate the Cholesterol-Saturated Fat Index (CSI). Because this formula considers *both* of the dietary fats known to increase blood cholesterol, it offers a more precise evaluation of your diet as a risk for Cardiovascular Disease.

To compute the CSI, you simply multiply the grams of saturated fat in food by 1.01 and the milligrams of cholesterol by .05 and add the two products together. The larger the result, the more risky the food!

For example:

A. 3 oz. regular hamburger has 6.9 g. saturated fat, 76 mg. cholesterol

   CSI = 6.9g. (1.01) + 76 mg. (.05)
   = **10.77**

B. 3 oz. water packed tuna fish has 0.3 g. saturated fat, 48 mg. cholesterol

   CSI = .3g. (1.01) + 48 mg. (.05)
   = **2.7**

The CSI for the average American's daily diet ranges from 51–60 for women and children and 69–82 for men and teenagers. A more healthy diet for your heart would yield a CSI of 16–19 for most women and children and 23–26 for men and teenagers.

through the intestines and more opportunity for carcinogens to build up. Whatever the mechanism(s), eating a low fat diet seems advisable in trying to avoid these types of cancer.

Choosing a low fat, low cholesterol diet means emphasizing consumption of vegetables, grains, and fruits. These have no cholesterol and are generally low in fat. Avocado, nuts and seeds are the exceptions. These foods are high in fat content and should be eaten infrequently and in small amounts if a low fat diet is your goal. Sources of animal products that are lower in fat, saturated fat, and cholesterol include fish, skim milk, and other low percent fat dairy products. Limiting intake of meats such as beef, pork, and lamb as well as butter and eggs will certainly help your cause.

The long term controversy about eating eggs warrants some additional attention. The cholesterol in an egg is very high, almost 260 mg. This is almost all of the 300 mg. to which you are advised to limit yourself per day. However, thus far research has not been able to firmly demonstrate that eating eggs, even every day, raises blood cholesterol levels. Some studies have supported the contention that eggs increase blood cholesterol; others have not. Since eggs are such an excellent and economical source of protein it seems premature to ban them from our diets. Until the evidence for or against eggs is clear, the best advice might be to limit consumption to two or three eggs per week.

Carbohydrate

With 40% of Americans overweight, it may seem absurd that nutritionists are urging you to eat more carbohydrate foods like potatoes, bread, and pasta. In fact, it may seem strange to hear about anything you are supposed to eat more of, especially something that sounds so fattening. So what is carbohydrate and why are you being encouraged to eat it?

Types of Carbohydrate

The term *carbohydrate* refers to molecules of sugar linked together in complexes, in pairs, or existing singly. Carbon, hydrogen, and oxygen are the elements that compose these molecules; hence the name carbohydrate. Single sugars and those in pairs are called *simple sugars*. Glucose, fructose, and galactose are the three forms of single sugar molecules, also called *monosaccharides*. Glucose and fructose are found alone or in combination in all fruits, vegetables, grains and milk; galactose is found only in milk. Paired combinations of these sugars are called *disaccharides*. The three forms of disaccharides are sucrose, a combination of glucose and fructose; maltose, a combination of two glucose molecules; and lactose, a combination of glucose and galactose. Sucrose is common table sugar and its cousins, powdered sugar and brown sugar. Lactose is milk sugar; milk is the only non-plant source of carbohydrates. Maltose is the sugar that seeds contain to fuel germination. Plants generally use it all themselves while growing, but we can get some maltose from the malt in beer.

Complex carbohydrates or *polysaccharides* are the names used for combinations of dozens of glucose molecules. Starch and undigestible fibers are complex carbohydrates. Of these, only starch provides nutrient; in fact, starch is the most abundant energy source in grain — such as wheat, rice, corn, rye, millet, barley, and oats — which is the basic food staple around the world. Beans and peas, especially dried beans, are also important sources of starch, as are tubers such as potatoes and yams. When carbohydrates are eaten, the body digests them into the basic units glucose, fructose, and galactose. The liver then converts fructose and galactose into glucose, the body's basic fuel source. Consequently, glucose is also called *blood sugar*.

Cellulose, hemicellulose, gums, pectin, and lignin are the types of complex carbohydrate that provide no nutrients for humans because we don't have the enzymes to digest them. Thus, fiber can't be called an essential nutrient, but few who understand its role in preventing constipation would say it's not important. In fact, as you will read later, fiber seems to be important in reducing the risk of several diseases including cardiovascular disease and cancer. Whole grains, vegetables, and fruits all are sources of fiber.

The Body's Need for Carbohydrate

There are several important reasons why you are being advised to eat more carbohydrate. First, consumption of carbohydrate is *not* associated with increased risk of cardiovascular disease and cancer. In fact, the incidence of these diseases is lower among people whose diets are high in carbohydrates. There is evidence that the fiber and certain vitamins and minerals in carbohydrate foods may even help to prevent these health problems. In fact, as the only source of fiber in our diets, carbohydrates are especially important.

Eating foods high in carbohydrates helps with weight control. As previously noted, carbohydrates provide as many calories as protein, 4 per gram, but foods high in carbohydrate are much lower in fat than many sources of protein. Also, because the fiber in carbohydrate foods adds bulk but no calories to the food, you will tend to eat less *and* will get fewer calories. For example, a dish of gourmet ice cream is high in fat and might have 360 calories. You would have to eat 3 or 4 apples or bananas or almost 5 slices of bread, both primary sources of carbohydrate, to equal those calories. While you might gladly eat a bowl of ice cream after dinner, you probably wouldn't consider eating that much fruit or bread. Therefore, choosing an apple or banana will save more than 200 calories while providing about the same amount of food. An added bonus will be decreased intake of fat.

Most foods high in carbohydrates also contain large amounts of vitamins and minerals, especially if the foods are eaten raw or in their natural state. However, sucrose or table sugar (and its various forms, brown sugar, powdered sugar, and raw sugar) is an excellent example of an "empty" carbohydrate. When the fructose and glucose of which it is composed were extracted from the sugar beets and/or sugar cane, none of the vitamins and minerals in those vegetables came with it. A teaspoon of sugar is 5 grams of carbohydrate or about 20 calories and that's it. You get nothing else from it. This also applies to any other type of processed sweetener such as corn syrup, honey, maple syrup, and fructose. Molasses, the exception, does contain useful amounts of calcium, iron, potassium, and B vitamins. Honey has minute quantities of these nutrients, but nothing significant. (If you need extra calories in your diet because of a rigorous activity level, however, refined sugars and syrups can certainly provide them for you.) The latest fad, refined or granulated fructose, has no more nutritional value than table sugar. It is sweeter, however, and *if* you use less of it you will save a few calories. If on the other hand you consume fructose by eating fruit, a good natural source of both fructose and sucrose, you will be taking in substantial vitamins and minerals plus additional carbohydrate in the form of fiber.

Refined white flour is another example of a calorie resource deprived of nutrients in the manufacturing process. In this case, the calories provided aren't totally empty, but they certainly don't offer the nutritional quality of the original grain. Even when white flour has been "enriched" by having vitamins and minerals added to it, it doesn't begin to have the nutrients contained in whole wheat flour, especially stoneground whole wheat. *Stoneground* refers to the milling process that does the least damage to the nutrient content of the grain. In essence, when you eat foods with lots of refined sugar and/or flour in them, you are taking in a lot of empty calories.

You can see, then, that pies, cakes, cookies, and donuts contain many empty calories. You should also realize that many canned vegetables, fruits, and other products—even peanut butters—have added sugar, and that many cereals on the market are loaded with it. The refined sugar content of numerous cereals and other foods is listed in Table 8.J for your examination.

From the body's standpoint, carbohydrate provides the ideal fuel. You will recall that the body can also use fat and protein for fuel, but this is not the desired use for

Table 8.J Refined sugar content in selected foods.

FOOD	PORTION	TEASPOONS OF SUGAR
Peanut butter	1 tbsp	1
Strawberry jam	1 tbsp	4
Honey	1 tbsp	3*
Applesauce, sweetened	½ cup	2
Orange juice	½ cup	2
Grape juice	½ cup	3⅖
Canned peaches	2 halves & 1 tbsp syrup	3½
Hotdog or hamburger bun	1	3
Doughnut	1	3
Doughnut, glazed	1	6
Brownie, unfrosted	1	3
Fig newton	1	5
Oatmeal cookie	1	2
Ice cream, regular	3½ oz	3½
Chocolate milk	1 cup	6
Sherbet	½ cup	9
Yogurt, sweetened fruit	1 cup	9
Custard pie	1 slice	10
Pumpkin pie	1 slice	5
Apple pie	1 slice	7
Hershey bar	1½ oz	2½
Fudge	1 oz	4½
Hard candy	4 oz	20
Seven-up	12 oz	9
Cola drinks	12 oz	9
Orange soda	12 oz	11½
Root beer	10 oz	4½

(Continued)

CEREALS	% OF CEREAL WEIGHT IN SUGAR
Shredded wheat, large biscuit	1.0
Cheerios	2.2
Special K	4.4
Wheaties	4.4
Corn flakes, Kroger	5.1
Grape Nuts	6.6
Corn flakes, Kellogg	7.8
Total	8.1
Rice Krispies, Kellogg	10.0
Raisin Bran, Kellogg	10.6
Life	14.5
Granola with dates or raisins	14.5
40% Bran flakes, Post	15.8
40% Bran flakes, Kellogg	16.2
Quaker 100% Natural with brown sugar and honey	18.2
100% Bran	18.4
All Bran	20
Nature Valley Granola with cinnamon and raisins	24
Quaker 100% Natural with raisins and dates	25
Country Morning	25.8
Nature Valley Granola with fruit and nuts	28
Sugar Frosted Flakes	29
Captain Crunch	43
Froot Loops	48.8
Lucky Charms	50.4
Apple Jacks	55
Sugar Smacks	61.3

*Actual sugar content, none added

Source: Whitney, E. & Hamilton, E. *Understanding Nutrition,* 3rd Ed. Minneapolis: West, 1984.

protein. Eating sufficient amounts of carbohydrate for fuel helps save protein for use in growth and maintenance of body tissue. Like fat, it is a protein-sparer.

Without a sufficient amount of carbohydrate in the diet, the body cannot properly utilize fat. When carbohydrate intake is inadequate, a toxic by-product of fat metabolism called *ketones* increases in the blood. The kidney's job is to get rid of this substance, but if this process goes on too long and the quantities of ketones become too great, the blood becomes "poisoned" with this substance. This conditon, called ketosis, is accompanied by feelings of fatigue, apathy, and nausea plus loss of weight in the form of protein and water. At its extreme, ketosis can result in coma, brain and kidney damage, and even death.

If you have diabetes or know someone who does, you may recognize the process just described as the physiological problem diabetics face. Their problem is severe because no matter how much carbohydrate they eat, their body doesn't metabolize it properly. For all intents and purposes, they are not eating enough, and the consequences are serious. A non-diabetic person who consumes a low carbohydrate diet (one of the popular approaches to weight reduction) for any length of time faces the same physiological problems as the diabetic, although the situation is certainly easier to remedy. This is also the process that occurs during starvation. In effect, a low carbohydrate diet sets up a "starvation syndrome" that has potentially dangerous consequences.

What is the least amount of carbohydrate you can eat before becoming a victim of the low carbohydrate, starvation syndrome just described? How much carbohydrate do you have to eat in order to get the protection from cardiovascular disease and cancer a high carbohydrate diet seems to offer? Does it matter what kind of foods you eat to get your carbohydrate? These are critical questions, and although not all of the answers are completely clear, there is sufficient information to provide the following guidelines.

Populations around the world who are less plagued by cardiovascular disease than Americans generally consume 60–80% of their daily calories in carbohydrates.* The incidence of various forms of cancer is also lower among people with high carbohydrate intakes. Consequently, nutrition experts are recommending that Americans try to eat at least 55–60% of their daily calories in carboydrates.

For the average American male weighing 154 lbs. (70 kg.) who eats about 2700 calories/day, a 60% carbohydrate diet would mean consuming at least 400 g. of carbohydrate or 1600 calories worth. The average woman who weighs 120 lbs. (55 kg.) and eats 2000 calories/day would have to eat at least 300 g. or 1200 calories of carbohydrate. At the present time, the average American eats only 46% of daily calories in carbohydrate; that's about 230 g. for women and 310 g. for men. As you will recall, the average American also eats about 12% more fat calories than is recommended. In essence, Americans are shorting the "nutrient account" that seems to provide some protection from cardiovascular disease and cancer to invest more in the one most highly associated with both diseases, fat!

Replacing fats in your diet is not the only way carbohydrate seems to reduce risk from cardiovascular disease and cancer. Eating certain types of fiber can decrease blood cholesterol and triglyceride levels. *Pectin,* found in most fruits and many vegetables, *lignin,* found in vegetables and grains, and *gums,* found in beans and oats, are especially effective in this regard. Bran, the food most of us think of when we think of fiber, does not affect blood fat levels. The cellulose and hemicellulose fibers contained in bran, cereals, whole grains, and vegetables, exert their influence by keeping waste moving smoothly and quickly through the intestines. This is thought to decrease risk of colorectal cancer. Fiber also tends to slow absorption of food from the gut, which is helpful to diabetics, who can handle small amounts of sugar over time much better than large quantities all at once. This slow absorption factor can be helpful in controlling weight, too, because fiber tends to make you feel full longer and on fewer calories.

The American Cancer Society is recommending that Americans increase their intake of fiber from a current level of 10–20 g. to 25–30 g./day. Some experts think 40 or more grams/day would be best. (Some vegetarians eat up to 60 g. of fiber/day.) However, fiber can decrease absorption of some important minerals such as calcium, iron, and zinc. It can also cause gas, bloating, and diarrhea in some people. If you think it wise to increase your fiber intake given the previous information, increasing your intake gradually will help minimize gas and bloating, and not going overboard in your end goal will help curtail excessive mineral loss. Food sources for and functions of the various types of fiber are listed in Table 8.K.

Besides providing fiber, carbohydrates are excellent sources of Vitamins A and C, which current evidence suggests may provide some protection against cancers of the larynx, esophagus, lung, and stomach. This evidence is sufficiently strong that the

---

*The exception is the Eskimos, whose diets are extremely high in fat and low in carbohydrates. The fat they eat, however, comes almost entirely from fish and contains very high amounts of the polyunsaturated fatty acid, omega-3, which as explained earlier seems to offer some protection against cardiovascular disease.

Table 8.K   The five kinds of fiber and where they are found.

	CELLULOSE	HEMICELLULOSES	GUMS	PECTIN	LIGNIN
Food Sources	Whole-Wheat Flour Bran Cabbage Young Peas Green Beans Wax Beans Broccoli Brussels Sprouts Cucumber Skins Peppers Apples Carrots	Bran Cereals Whole Grains Brussels Sprouts Mustard Greens Beet Root	Oatmeal & Other Rolled-Oat Products Dried Beans	Squash Apples Citrus Fruits Cauliflower Green Beans Cabbage Dried Peas Carrots Strawberries Potatoes	Breakfast Cereals Bran Older Vegetables Strawberries Eggplant Pears Green Beans Radishes
Function	Mechanically smooths function of large bowel: Absorbs water, increasing stool and decreasing transit time. Helps prevent constipation, and may protect against diverticulosis, colon cancer, hemorrhoids and varicose veins.		Influences absorption in stomach and small bowel: Binds with bile acids, thereby decreasing fat absorption and lowering cholesterol levels. Coats gut and delays glucose absorption, smoothing sugar surges for diabetics.		Influences other kinds of fiber: Binds with bile acids to lower cholesterol. Reduces digestibility of other fibers: Helps speed food through gut.

From Susan Lang, "Beyond Bran," *American Health* 3, No. 3 (May 1984):64.

American Cancer Society is urging greater consumption of dark yellow and green vegetables and deep yellow-orange fruit. These colors are guides to good sources of A and C in fruits and vegetables. Cruciferous vegetables such as broccoli, kale, brussel sprouts (all dark green too), cauliflower, and cabbage are also being recommended, not only because they provide Vitamins A and/or C, but also because they contain compounds called *indoles*, which in animal experiments seem to have reduced stomach and respiratory cancers. There is some evidence that Vitamin E and the mineral, selenium, may also help to minimize development of some cancers, but at this time the evidence is not considered sufficient by the American Cancer Society to officially acknowledge these substances as protective.

There are animal sources of Vitamin A; milk, cheese, butter, eggs, and meat are examples. A serving of liver can provide six times the amount of Vitamin A recommended for one day. The problem is the fat in these sources, and in particular, the cholesterol in liver. Since the strongest association of all between diet and cancer is a high fat diet, the best sources of Vitamins A and C would seem to be carbohydrates.

The Role of Refined Sugar in Meeting Carbohydrate Requirements

The recommendation to increase carbohydrate intake from 46% to 55–60% of daily calories also stipulates eating no more than 10% of calories in refined sugars. In essence, you should eat 45–50% of calories in complex carbohydrates. Currently

Americans eat 18% of their calories in refined sugar and 6% in natural sugars (from fruits, vegetables, and grains), leaving 22% for complex carbohydrates. A visual presentation of the differences between the recommended carbohydrate intake and current intake is shown in Figure 8.6.

Nutritionists are emphasizing complex carbohydrates because they are the sources of fiber in the diet; refined sugars have none. Complex carbohydrates also contain many vitamins and minerals; refined sugars have none or insignificant amounts of these. In fact, as discussed previously, refined sugar offers only "empty" calories.

Although the average American consumes a little more than one-third lb. of sweeteners every day or about 143 lbs. per year (an all time high!), it has so far not been possible to demonstrate a link between such a high refined sugar intake and the development of any major disease or health problem. In a major study of diet and heart disease conducted in 37 countries under the sponsorship of the World Health Association, no link with refined sugars was found; fat, especially saturated fat, was the culprit. Sugar intake has not been linked to cancer either, but high fat diets surely have.

It is also a misconception that sugar causes diabetes; there is no proof of this. Diabetics cannot metabolize sugar properly and struggle against the physiological consequences of this, but what *causes* this problem remains unknown. Overweight, however, is an important risk factor for diabetes, and overweight often reflects a high calorie, high fat diet. We do know that diabetics must be careful about eating any carbohydrate food that produces a large increase in blood sugar or glucose. While it used to be thought that only refined sugars did this, it is now clear that the situation

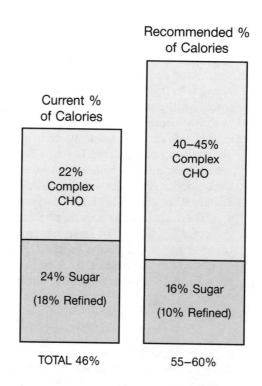

FIGURE 8.6
Current and recommended intake of carbohydrate and sugar.

is not that simple. For example, complex carbohydrates such as potatoes and carrots seem to increase blood sugar more than rice, fructose,* and dried beans. On the other hand, ice cream does not seem to increase blood sugar adversely in some diabetics. In sum, even for diabetics sugar does not seem so bad as was once thought.

Eating refined sugar is not problem free, however. Carbohydrates containing sucrose are major culprits in tooth decay, especially sources of these that have a sticky texture. Most dentists advise limiting refined sugar intake. A diet high in sugar also may cause episodes of reactive hypoglycemia, which means having too little sugar in the blood. This occurs when a sudden and large increase in blood sugar (which follows ingestion of high sugar foods) triggers release of more insulin than necessary. The excessive insulin drives too much glucose from the blood into the cells, resulting in a blood sugar level too low for proper brain/nerve function. If this happens to you, you will likely feel weak, dizzy, and anxious, and you may experience lack of neuromotor coordination. A small percentage of people are hypoglycemic due to chronic overproduction of insulin, but most who experience this situation have probably overdone the sweets and/or waited too long in between meals.

Three last issues involving sugar intake warrant comment. The connection between hyperactivity in children and high sugar intake remains unsubstantiated at this time. The biggest reason for minimizing refined sugar in your child's diet, and yours too for that matter, is to avoid empty calories and exposure to high fat and/or high calorie foods.

There may be a connection between consumption of lactose—the simple sugar natural to milk—and abdominal gas, pain, and diarrhea. Some adults, especially Black and Oriental people, lack the enzyme to digest this sugar. Fortunately this problem can be minimized if these people eat only small amounts of dairy products at one time and focus on those products containing yeast or added enzymes capable of rendering lactose digestible. Examples of such foods are yogurt and acidophilous milk.

To avoid calories, many Americans consume food with artificial sweeteners. Aspartame (marketed under the brand name *Nutrasweet*) and Saccharin are the predominant ones currently in use. Saccharin has been around for a long time, over 40 years, and is still in use despite some legitimate concern that large intakes might lead to bladder cancer. However, its popularity has waned significantly. Aspartame, a combination of two naturally occurring amino acids, phenylalanine and aspartic acid, is now the most popular artificial sweetener. So far there is no evidence to suggest it is harmful in any way except for people with phenylketonuria, a disorder characterized by inability to metabolize phenylalanine. (By this time you may be a little wary of things that are declared "harmless" one day and dangerous the next, however!)

If calories are a problem for you, aspartame can be of some help to you. Although it contains the same number of calories as sugar, it is 180 times sweeter. One teaspoon of sugar has about 18 calories; the same sweetening power can be obtained from .1 calorie of aspartame. Because aspartame loses some of its sweetening power when heated or baked, its use is somewhat restricted, however. It is currently used primarily in cereals, soft drinks, puddings, gums, mints, and as crystals for table use. The best advice seems to be to use it if you want or think you need to, but do not overdo it. With refined sugars, you fill up on empty calories; with aspartame you just fill up on

Caution: Fructose is converted by the liver into glucose which then must be metabolized, and the metabolism of glucose *is* the essential problem for diabetics. Studies indicate that indiscriminate use of fructose by diabetics could lead to a diabetic crisis.

fewer empty calories. Either way you may miss out on important nutrients you need. Also, if the future brings other than good news about aspartame's impact on our health, moderate or minimal intake might be considered more than just good choice.

Carbohydrates and Dieting

Since artificial sweeteners are so frequently used to allow consumers pleasure from sugary foods without weight gain, and since so many starchy foods like potatoes and bread are erroneously viewed as fattening, some comment is needed about carbohydrates and dieting. The facts are these: you will gain weight if you eat more calories than you need from carbohydrate foods. It doesn't matter whether you eat foods like potatoes, rice, pasta, and pancakes or foods like apples, oranges, tomatoes, and broccoli. The same can be said for protein foods of any kind and for all foods high in fat. In essence, too many calories from any type of food can end up as extra pounds.

Carbohydrates have gotten such a bad name largely because of the fat we consume in conjunction with them. For example, the gravy or sour cream plus bacon bits and cheese often added to potatoes may contain twice or more the calories of the potato itself. The same can be said for the butter on bread or pancakes. Nevertheless, many people equate carbohydrates with weight gain and think it quite logical that low carbohydrate diets will lead to weight loss. Since fat has so many more calories than carbohydrate or protein, it would of course be more logical to cut back on fat rather than carbohydrates in order to lose weight. It would also be safer and more effective since insufficient carbohydrate intake causes the body to fall into the starvation syndrome described earlier. Weight can certainly be lost by cutting out carbohydrates, but much of it will be in the form of protein and water rather than fat, which is hardly what the dieter desires.

To prevent the body from behaving as if it is starving you must eat carbohydrate, a minimum of 60 g./day. To allow for individual differences, it is recommended that you try to eat no less than 100 to 125 g. of carbohydrate per day to ensure proper metabolic functioning. And as discussed earlier, Americans are actually being encouraged to eat 3 to 4 times that much to decrease risk of chronic disease. As it turns out, carbohydrate is essential for everyone, even dieters.

Vitamins and Minerals

The essential nutrients called vitamins and minerals are substances that the body needs to function properly and/or to grow, but which provide no calories for energy. Most vitamins and minerals have been identified when their absence in the body has resulted in a function abnormality referred to as *deficiency syndrome* or disease.

The amounts needed to prevent deficiency problems are extremely small. The units of measurement are milligrams (mg.) or micrograms (ug.). A milligram is 1/1000th of a gram; a microgram is 1/1000th of a milligram. The recommended daily intake for Vitamins B_{12}, for example, is 5 ug. At 28 g./oz., an ounce of Vitamin B_{12} would be enough for 4,724,921 people!

Even with the technological advancements that have been made over the years, it is still not clear how much of some of these substances people actually need, what they do in the body, nor even if all of them have been identified yet. Such gaps in knowledge create much conjecture and controversy. Most nutrition and health authorities believe that if you eat a well-balanced diet containing a variety of foods you will get all of these substances you need. This belief is based largely upon the rarity of deficiency diseases in this country today. Others believe that the vitamin and mineral amounts needed to prevent deficiency aren't necessarily the same as the amounts needed for optimal health and well being, or for preventing or minimizing susceptibility to diseases of all sorts, or for retarding the aging process. Consequently you may feel bombarded with contradictory advice regarding vitamin and mineral supplements.

Some of this advice/conjecture about vitamins and minerals is based on legitimate, but as yet inconclusive, research. Some is based on nothing more than personal experience. Undoubtedly you've heard such testimonials: "I take this or that and it works for me." Unfortunately such observations fall far short of scientific evidence. Conjecture is also stimulated simply by the desire to make money by selling dietary supplements. Caught in the middle of all this are millions of people who do not want to spend money needlessly, but who do want to protect themselves from illness and aging as much as possible. Until scientists can provide the answers to these controversies, the decision about what to take is yours to make. The following information about the vitamins and minerals for which need has been established should help you with these decisions. First, however here are some general guidelines for checking the validity of claims about vitamins and minerals. These are summarized in Table 8.L.

1. *Learn about vitamins/minerals, what they can and can't do, and how much we seem to need.* Basic information is provided in this text. Additional reliable sources of information include the U.S. Department of Agriculture (U.S.D.A.), the Food and Drug Administration (F.D.A.), the American Dietetic Association (A.D.A.), and the

---

Table 8.L   Guidelines for determining the validity of claims for vitamins and minerals.

---

1. *Learn about vitamins and minerals.*

   Reliable sources include:

   U.S. Department of Agriculture

   FDA

   American Dietetic Association

   American Medical Association

   Certified physicians, nutritionists and dieticians at your public health department, hospital, Heart Association, and university

2. *Challenge health claims for scientific evidence.*

   a. Any evidence beyond personal anecdotes?

   b. Effects of the vitamin/mineral compared with other treatments.

   c. Use of the vitamin or mineral as claimed safe? If risk, how great?

3. *Investigate health experts and organizations making claims.*

   a. What degrees do they hold?

   b. What experience do they have?

   c. Who funds them?

4. *Find out if you are deficient or at risk.*

   Dietary analysis by trained personnel

   Blood/urine tests

   Physical exam

From Andresky, J. *The A.B.Cs of Vitamins.* Consumers Digest, July/August 1981.

American Medical Association (A.M.A.). Look in your phone book for the local numbers of these national organizations or government units. You can also get free information and consultation from the nutritionists (Registered Dietitians) or nutrition education units at your local public health department, American Heart Association unit, and hospital. You can also read about vitamins and minerals in general nutrition textbooks obtainable at your local public or university library.

2. *Challenge the validity of claims about vitamins and minerals.* Is there evidence for the claim beyond personal observations and experiences? If so, did researchers compare the effectiveness of the vitamin/mineral with a control treatment or substance (for example, a pill or placebo)? Is the dosage claimed to be effective actually safe? If there's risk, how high is that compared to the potential benefit? If there are no answers to these questions or if the answers are *no*, suspicion and caution are in order.

3. *Investigate the "health expert."* In this country you are free to say just about anything about everything. You do not have to have a degree in nutrition in order to give advice about it. The initials Ph.D. after someone's name simply means the person has a doctorate or graduate degree in some field; it could be any area of study. One very popular writer of diet books has a Ph.D. in Radio Communications! Find out what degrees or training an advocate for a certain supplement has before "buying" his/her claim. Institutes, foundations, and other organizations you haven't heard of should be checked out, too. The Institute for Vitamin Experimentation and Cancer Prevention (to the authors' knowledge, a fabrication) could well be funded by the vitamin industry and may not even perform actual research.

4. *Find out if you are deficient or at risk of low level intake of the vitamin or mineral.* Blood and urine tests are one set of reasonably reliable indicators. Diet analyses can be helpful, too, if carefully done and analyzed by trained persons. These tests should be accompanied by a general physical exam. Self analysis should be used only as a rough estimate of your dietary intake. The same goes for computerized analysis. In fact, a computerized analysis can be purposefully programmed for higher than recommended vitamin/mineral needs and may indicate deficiencies that do not actually exist. You should inquire about the source(s) of the standard used by the computer to rate your diet. The most accepted standard today would be the Recommended Dietary Allowances (RDAs). Other techniques such as hair analysis simply aren't valid for predicting vitamin/mineral adequacy.

Vitamins

Vitamins are organic substances—that is, derived from plant and animal life—that perform a myriad of functions in the body. Acting primarily as *coenzymes* (assistants to enzymes), they help in the processing of other nutrients and in the formation of various substances and structures needed for proper functioning, such as hormones, blood cells, bone, membranes, and so on.

Currently 13 organic substances are known to be required by the body and must be consumed. These are the fat soluble vitamins A, D, E and K, and the water soluble B and C vitamins. The B vitamins include thiamin (B_1), riboflavin (B_2), niacin (B_3), pantothenic acid, pyridoxine (B_6), cobalamin (B_{12}), folic acid (folacin), and biotin. There are other substances, such as choline, inositol, and PABA (para-amino-benzoic acid), that some people proclaim as vitamins, but to date no deficiency syndrome has been related to these and no dietary needs established.

The fat soluble vitamins are carried into the body with the aid of fat in the diet and are stored in fat in the body. Because they can be stored, it is not absolutely critical to eat them each day unless you are eating only small amounts of them compared to the daily recommended intake. For example, you can get enough Vitamin A in a week by eating one cooked carrot every other day. On the other hand, because they can be stored, fat soluble vitamins can accumulate to toxic levels in the body if consumed in excess.

Water soluble vitamins are not stored in the body to any great extent, although small resources are maintained. In general these vitamins need to be eaten daily to maintain adequate fluid concentrations since they are constantly being metabolized and lost in urine and sweat. Consuming large quantities of these vitamins in excess of body needs generally just results in vitamin rich urine. However, recent research has indicated that megadoses, ten times or more the amount needed by the body, can produce some undesirable and even harmful side effects in some people.

The 13 fat and water soluble vitamins are listed in Table 8.M along with their respective recommended daily intakes, basic functions in the body, and food sources. Space doesn't permit a discussion of each of these, but some additional information is provided about Vitamins A, C, and E due to their controversial association with cancer, heart disease, colds, aging, and so on.

Vitamin A

As previously stated, the American Cancer Society has recently suggested that you eat more foods containing Vitamin A because diets high in this vitamin are associated with lower levels of cancer of the lung, larynx, and bladder. Specifically you are urged to eat more dark green and yellow-orange vegetables because these provide the best sources of *retinoids*, in particular beta-carotene, which are precursors of Vitamin A (that is, substances converted to Vitamin A in the body). It is primarily the presence of these substances in food, and not Vitamin A itself, that has been associated with lower levels of cancer. Almost all *preformed* Vitamin A is found in animal products (or in vitamin capsules).

At this point in time, there is no indication that people gain any benefit from consuming large amounts of Vitamin A. In fact, because Vitamin A is a fat soluble vitamin, consuming megadoses may be dangerous. Headaches, drowsiness, nausea, loss of hair, dry skin, and diarrhea can occur. More seriously, menstruation can cease in women and bone substance can be lost in adults in general.

The amount of Vitamin A you need to eat has traditionally been given in International Units (I.U.) rather than milligrams. This has been necessary because the different forms (precursors) of Vitamin A don't all produce the same level of biological activity inside the body. Today, however, *retinol equivalents* (R.E.) are the preferred unit of measure because they provide greater precision in estimating this biological activity. This new system of measurement has not yet totally replaced the old and you may see either or both of these unit measures listed for Vitamin A. The recommended daily intake for men is 5000 I.U. or 1000 R.E. For women, it is 4000 I.U. or 800 R.E.

Almost 30% of Americans have intakes below 70% of the recommended intake for Vitamin A. Given the important functions of this vitamin and its possible influence over cancer, it would seem prudent to assess the adequacy of your own intake and to make sure that you are eating some of those recommended dark green and yellow vegetables at least every other day. However, daily ingestion of more than 25,000 I.U. or 7500 R.E. of Vitamin A may be toxic over time, so avoid excessive doses of this vitamin.

Table 8.M Vitamins: A fact sheet.

VITAMIN	ADULT RDA*	SOURCES	WHAT IT DOES
A	800–1,000 mcg (micrograms)	Liver, eggs, fortified milk, carrots, tomatoes, apricots, cantaloupe, fish	Promotes good vision; helps form and maintain healthy skin and mucous membranes; may protect against some cancers
C	50–60 mg (milligrams)	Citrus fruits, strawberries, tomatoes	Promotes healthy gums, capillaries, and teeth; aids iron absorption; may block production of nitrosamines; maintains normal connective tissue; aids in healing wounds
D	5–10 mcg (200–400 IU)	Fortified milk, fish; also produced by the body in response to sunlight	Promotes strong bones and teeth; necessary for absorption of calcium
E	8–10 mg	Nuts, vegetable oils, whole grains, olives, asparagus, spinach	Protects tissue against oxidation; important in formation of red blood cells; helps body use vitamin K
K	70–140 mcg**	Body produces about half of daily needs; cauliflower, broccoli, cabbage, spinach, cereals, soybeans, beef liver	Aids in clotting of blood
B_1 Thiamine)	1–1.5 mg	Whole grains, dried beans, lean meats (especially pork), fish	Helps release energy from carbohydrates; necessary for healthy brain and nerve cells and for functioning of heart
B_2 (Riboflavin)	1.2–1.7 mg	Nuts, dairy products, liver	Aids in release of energy from foods; interacts with other B vitamins
B_3 (Niacin)	13–19 mg	Nuts, dairy products, liver	Aids in release of energy from foods; involved in synthesis of DNA; maintains normal functioning of skin, nerves, and digestive system
B_5 (Pantothenic acid)	4–7 mg**	Whole grains, dried beans, eggs, nuts	Aids in release of energy from foods; essential for synthesis of numerous body materials
B_6 (Pyridoxine)	1.8–2.2 mg	Whole grains, dried beans, eggs, nuts	Important in chemical reactions of proteins and amino acids; involved in normal functioning of brain and formation of red blood cells
B_{12}	3 mcg	Liver, beef, eggs, milk, shellfish	Necessary for development of red blood cells; maintains normal functioning of nervous system
Folacin	400 mcg	Liver, wheat bran, leafy green vegetables, beans, grains	Important in the synthesis of DNA; acts together with B_{12} in the production of hemoglobin

(Continued)

VITAMIN	ADULT RDA*	SOURCES	WHAT IT DOES
Biotin	100–200 mcg**	Yeast, eggs, liver, milk	Important in formation of fatty acids; helps metabolize amino acids and carbohydrates

*These figures are not applicable to pregnant women, who need additional vitamins.
**Although there is no RDA for this vitamin, the Food and Nutrition Board recommends this range of intakes.

Adapted from "Vitamins: Fact and Fancy," *University of California, Berkeley, Wellness Letter,* Vol. 2, Issue 1 (Oct. 1985) P.O. Box 10922, Des Moines, IA, 50340. © Health Letter Associates, 1985-1986.

Vitamin C

Vitamin C has also been linked with reduced risk of cancer, stomach and esophagal cancers in particular. The evidence seems to support Vitamin C as a *preventive* measure; that is, diets high in Vitamin C may *reduce the risk* of cancer. There is no evidence that Vitamin C can cure cancer.

Not so widely known is the importance of Vitamin C to the integrity of body tissues, both bone and soft tissue. For example, Vitamin C is necessary for the proper formation of the connective tissue called *collagen*, which forms that part of the bony structure in which calcium and other minerals are deposited. Collagen plays a critical role in the maintenance and repair of body tissues in general; thus, so does Vitamin C. In fact, extra Vitamin C is often prescribed before and after surgery to facilitate healing of tissues. Vitamin C also enhances the absorption of calcium when the two are consumed together. All of this evidence emphasizes the importance of an adequate intake of Vitamin C to minimize the degradation of bone and other tissues that occurs with age. However, there is no evidence that large doses of Vitamin C offer any additional benefits in this regard.

Claims that Vitamin C reduces blood cholesterol have not been substantiated by research efforts thus far, but there is some evidence that Vitamin C can minimize the symptoms of a cold. At the doses required, however, the risks might outweigh the benefits, especially since colds generally go away by themselves whether or not they are treated. In contrast to the recommended daily intake of 60 mg. of Vitamin C, many proponents of Vitamin C's cold-fighting capabilities would recommend intake of a *minimum* of 1000–2000 mg. or 1–2 g. The thinking is that if this is more than you actually need, it will simply wash out of the body in urine. With Vitamin C, however, this is not necessarily the case. Megadoses of C can interfere with copper metabolism, cause premature bleeding in pregnant women, cause kidney stones and, over time, increase the amount of Vitamin C required to prevent scurvy, its primary deficiency disorder. In addition, some Black people, Orientals, and Sephardic Jews lack an enzyme needed to handle large doses of Vitamin C and may develop a form of anemia by megadosing.

Any decision to take supplements of Vitamin C has to be weighed against the potential hazards just described. A safer way to get more than the recommended intake is to include lots of fruits and vegetables in your diet. An 8 oz. glass of orange juice, for example, provides almost twice the recommended daily intake. If you smoke, drink lots of caffeine-containing beverages such as coffee, tea, and colas, or take large quantities of aspirin, you may want to increase your intake of Vitamin C since all of these practices diminish Vitamin C supplies in the body.

Vitamin E

Vitamin E is popularly acclaimed for its power to slow the aging process, increase sexual potency, and prevent heart disease. All of these claims are gross misrepresentations of what little is actually understood about this vitamin. It is known that Vitamin E is an antioxidant, as are Vitamins A and C, and that antioxidants curtail the incidence of oxidative reactions that degrade and destroy normal tissue. Some gerontologists believe, in fact, that these oxidative reactions are primarily responsible for the loss of cells that underlies the aging process. While there have been reports of increased longevity in cell cultures and in mice fed antioxidants, no data of this sort exist regarding humans.

The amount of Vitamin E you need is not really known because the only deficiency syndrome identified in humans thus far is a type of anemia generally observed only in premature infants and adults unable to absorb fat properly. Consequently, average intake has basically become the recommended intake: 10 mg./day for men and 8 mg./day for women. Whether these amounts optimize healthy functioning is just not known.

With health food stores and other vitamin proponents recommending intakes up to 1000 mg./day based on proposed benefits that are largely unsupported by available evidence, it becomes important to know if there is danger in consuming such quantities. For the most part, however, the answer is not clear. There have been reports that intakes of 600 mg./day increase levels of fat in the blood, in particular triglycerides, in women, especially those taking oral contraceptives, and decrease levels of thyroxine, the major regulator of metabolic rate, in both men and women. Increased fat in the blood and a decrease in the rate of overall body functioning (and thus a decrease in caloric expenditure) are not desirable conditions for most people. Neither are nausea and diarrhea, which have also been observed in some studies. Vitamin E is stored in body fat and thus, like Vitamin A, has a potential toxicity level even though that level remains to be defined. For now the important thing to remember is that claimed benefits for megadoses of Vitamin E are unsubstantiated.

Minerals

Unlike vitamins, minerals are inorganic substances. They are not derived from living things, but are inert elements that have been part of the earth since its beginnings. Twenty-one minerals are known to be essential to body functioning. These fall into two categories, macrominerals and microminerals. *Macrominerals* are needed in quantities of 100 mg. or more. Calcium, phosphorous, sulfur, sodium, potassium, chlorine, and magnesium are macrominerals. *Microminerals* are needed in extremely small amounts, a few milligrams or less per day. For this reason they are sometimes also called "trace" minerals or elements. Included in this category are iron, copper, zinc, fluorine, iodine, chromium, selenium, manganese, molybdenum. It is thought that other minerals like cobalt, tin, nickel, vanadium, and silicon may be essential, too, because they are contained in the body. However, deficiency syndromes have not yet been identified for these minerals.

Some minerals act as co-factors with enzymes like vitamins do. Others are involved in regulating body fluids, blood clotting, transmission of nerve impulses, maintenance of acid levels, muscle contraction, absorption of nutrients, oxygen transport, and so on. The list of functions is quite lengthy. Many minerals are also constituents of major body structures like bone.

It may appear that quite a lot is known about these minerals, but actually that is not the case. So far, recommendations for daily intake have been made for only six minerals; for another nine, only "estimated safe and adequate" amounts have been stipulated. This situation is potentially very dangerous for someone taking mineral supplements because minerals tend to be toxic at much lower levels than vitamins and for many minerals toxicity levels haven't been clearly established. In addition, excess amounts of one mineral can create deficiency in another. For example, too much zinc decreases the body's supply of copper; too much iron decreases zinc supplies. If this seems complicated and confusing, you are right. Researchers are only beginning to learn how minerals interact with each other. This makes experimentation with mineral supplements very risky business. Even being well informed doesn't ensure safety since so little is known at present. The fifteen minerals about which there is at least some information are listed in Table 8.N. Estimated or recommended intake, food sources, and functions are included.

Calcium and iron are two minerals most often found lacking in the American diet. Others like sodium and chloride (the combination of these yields table salt) are so abundant in our diets that deficiencies are unheard of. Instead, the problem seems to be too much salt. Because of the health consequences and public attention associated with calcium, iron, and salt, some additional information about each of these might be helpful.

Calcium

Calcium has attracted a great deal of attention in the last few years primarily because of a growing concern about osteoporosis. This problem was described earlier in Chapter 3. In hopes of minimizing the net loss of bone, physicians and nutritionists are now encouraging an increase in calcium intake from the previously recommended 800 mg./day to 1000–1200 mg./day. For women after menopause, the recommendation is 1500 mg./day. Since the current average calcium intake for women is closer to 600 mg. or less/day, these new recommendations for calcium will mean quite an increase in calories unless a supplement is used. Since men generally consume more calcium than women, increasing their intake to 1000–1200 mg. can be achieved simply by drinking one more glass of milk at 90 to 150 calories, depending on the fat content. A woman will probably need three additional glasses, which means an increase of 270 to 450 calories every day. The average calcium intake for males and females is shown in Figure 8.7; as you can see, women have thus far done a poor job of getting the calcium they need.

Additional pressure to increase calcium intake stems from recent studies that show high blood pressure to be more prevalent in adults consuming low amounts of calcium in comparison with those eating the recommended amounts. Blood pressure levels have dropped "beneficially" in some people when calcium supplements were taken.

Calcium will command even more attention if reports linking increased calcium intake with prevention of colon cancer in high risk families prove true. Researchers have observed a return to normal of precancerous colon cells after 8 weeks of calcium supplementation in subjects from families with a high incidence of colon cancer.

How to get more calcium safely is a controversial issue. Again, as with all the minerals, information to guide you is limited. The best advice for the moment includes the following recommendations and precautions:

1. Try to get more calcium from the foods you eat. Good sources of calcium are listed in Table 8.O. The lactose in milk products enhances absorption of calcium,

Table 8.N   Minerals: A fact sheet.

MINERAL	ADULT RDA OR ESTIMATED INTAKE	FOOD SOURCES	WHAT IT DOES
Calcium	800 mg* (1,200–1,500 mg for older women, according to an NIH consensus report) 1 quart milk = 1,250 mg	Milk and milk products, sardines and salmon eaten with bones, dark green leafy vegetables, shellfish, hard water	Builds bones and teeth and maintains bone density and strength; helps prevent osteoporosis in older population; plays a role in regulating heartbeat, blood clotting, muscle contraction, and nerve conduction; may help prevent hypertension
Chloride	1,900–5,000 mg**	Table salt, fish, pickled and smoked foods	Maintains normal fluid shifts; balances pH of the blood; forms hydrochloric acid to aid digestion
Magnesium	300 mg (women), 350 mg (men)* 1 cup spinach = 160 mg	Wheat bran, whole grains, raw leafy green vegetables, nuts (especially almonds and cashews), soybeans bananas, apricots, hard water, spices	Aids in bone growth; aids function of nerves and muscles, including regulation of normal heart rhythm
Phosphorus	800 mg* 1 cup milk = 993 mg; 1 serving chicken = 231 mg	Meats, poultry, fish, cheese, egg yolks, dried peas and beans, milk and milk products, soft drinks, nuts; present in almost all foods	Aids bone growth and strengthening of teeth; important in energy metabolism
Potassium	1,500–6,000 mg** 1 cup raisins = 524 mg; 1 banana = 400 mg; 1 small potato = 400 mg	Oranges and orange juice, bananas, dried fruits, peanut butter, dried peas and beans, potatoes, coffee, tea, cocoa, yogurt, molasses, meat	Promotes regular heartbeat; active in muscle contraction; regulates transfer of nutrients to cells; controls water balance in body tissues and cells; contributes to regulation of blood pressure
Sodium	2,000–3,300 mg** 1 frozen pot pie = 1,600 mg	All from salt	Helps regulate water balance in body; plays a role in maintaining blood pressure
Chromium	.05–.20 mg**	Meat, cheese, whole grains, dried peas and beans, peanuts, brewer's yeast	Important for glucose metabolism; may be a cofactor for insulin
Copper	2.0–3.0 mg**	Shellfish (especially oysters), nuts, beef and pork liver, cocoa powder, chocolate, kidneys, dried beans, raisins, corn oil margarine	Formation of red blood cells; cofactor in absorbing iron into blood cells; assists in production of several enzymes involved in respiration; interacts with zinc
Fluorine (fluoride)	1.5–4.0 mg**	Fluoridated water, foods grown with or cooked in fluoridated water; fish, tea, gelatin	Contributes to solid bone and tooth formation; may help prevent osteoporosis in older people
Iodine	.15 mg*	Primarily from iodized salt, but also seafood, seaweed food products, vegetables grown in iodine-rich areas, vegetable oil	Necessary for normal function of the thyroid gland; essential for normal cell function; keeps skin, hair, and nails healthy; prevents goiter

(Continued)

MINERAL	ADULT RDA OR ESTIMATED INTAKE	FOOD SOURCES	WHAT IT DOES
Iron	10 mg (male), 18 mg (female, during childbearing years, expected to be lowered to 16 mg)* 4 oz calf's liver = 12 mg	Liver (especially pork liver), kidneys, red meats, egg yolks, peas, beans, nuts, dried fruits, green leafy vegetables, enriched grain products, blackstrap molasses	Essential to formation of hemoglobin, the oxygen-carrying factor in the blood; part of several enzymes and proteins in the body
Manganese	2.5–5.0 mg** ½ cup peanut butter = 2 mg	Nuts, whole grains, vegetables, fruits, instant coffee, tea, cocoa powder, beets, egg yolks	Required for normal bone growth and development, normal reproduction, and cell function
Molybdenum	.15–.50 mg**	Peas, beans, cereal grains, organ meats, some dark green vegetables	Important for normal cell function
Selenium	.05–.20 mg** 4 oz fish = .038 mg	Fish, shellfish, red meat, egg yolks, chicken, garlic, tuna, tomatoes	Complements vitamin E to fight cell damage by oxygen
Zinc	15 mg* 5 oysters = 160 mg; 2 slices whole wheat bread = 2 mg	Oysters, crabmeat, beef, liver, eggs, poultry, brewer's yeast, whole wheat bread	Maintains normal taste and smell acuity, growth, and sexual development; important for fetal growth and wound healing

*Amount adequate to meet the needs of practically all healthy persons except pregnant or lactating women. Established by the Food and Nutrition Board of the National Academy of Sciences.
**No RDA established. Estimated safe intake given.

Adapted from "Minerals: Fact and Fancy," *University of California, Berkeley, Wellness Letter*, Vol. 2, Issue 1 (Oct. 1985) P.O. Box 10922, Des Moines, IA, 50340. © Health Letter Associates, 1985-1986.

which makes them good sources. When Vitamin D is added to these products, they are even better because Vitamin D also increases calcium absorption. So does Vitamin C, so eating an orange with milk is a good choice. Avoid heavy consumption of soda pop, especially colas, and coffee; large amounts of phosphorous (in pop) and caffeine interfere with calcium absorption. Try to consume low fat or skim dairy products to minimize fat intake. High fat as well as high protein intakes interfere with calcium absorption and/or increase excretion of calcium from the body.

2. Take a supplement if you can't or won't get enough calcium from the foods you eat. However, don't count on a supplement to replace calcium-rich foods in your diet. Large doses of calcium supplements may actually interfere with the absorption of manganese, another mineral that may turn out to be as important as calcium to bone integrity. As the calcium in milk and milk products does not interfere with manganese, food remains your best source of calcium. If you do take a supplement, make sure it is just that! Some criteria to guide selection of a supplement are:

a. Of the various forms available, calcium carbonate is better absorbed. Some Vitamin D combined with it enhances absorption but care should be taken not to exceed 800–1000 mg. of Vitamin D per day, including what you eat. Excess Vitamin D can be toxic.

(List continued on page 238)

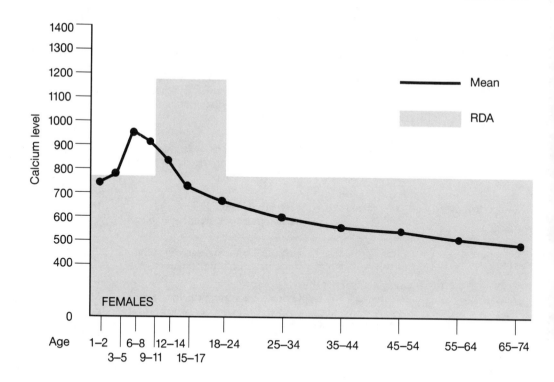

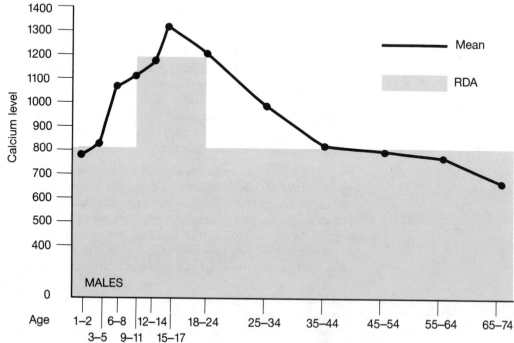

FIGURE 8.7
Daily calcium intake (mg) for females and males, U.S. population, 1976–80.

Data from M. Carroll, S. Abraham, and Dresser, C. Dietary Intake Source Data: United States 1976–1980. *Vital and Health Statistics* 11, #231, DHHS Pub. PHS-83-1681. National Center for Health Statistics, Government Publishing Office, Washington, D.C.

Table 8.O Calcium content per serving of selected foods.

MG. CALCIUM	DAIRY	FRUITS/VEGETABLES	LEGUMES/NUTS/SEEDS	GRAINS	MEAT/FISH/FOWL
LESS THAN 100 MG	1 egg – 28	1 banana – 7 1 apple – 10 1 baked potato with skin – 20 1 c cooked carrots – 48 1 orange – 54 1 c green beans – 61 1 c sauerkraut – 71 1 c mashed sweet potato – 77	1 tbsp peanut butter – 5 1 oz dry roasted cashews – 13 1 oz peanuts – 24 1 oz sunflower seeds – 33 1 c cooked lentils – 50 1 oz filberts – 53 1 oz almonds – 75 1 c chick peas (garbanzo beans) – 80 1 c pinto beans – 86 1 c navy beans – 95	1 c spaghetti noodles – 14 1 c oatmeal – 14 1 slice whole wheat bread – 20 1 c brown rice – 23 1 plain bagel – 29 1 slice white bread – 32 1 pancake – 36 1 pita bread – 49 1 buckwheat pancake – 59 1 bran muffin – 60 1 English muffin – 96	2 slices bacon – 2 2.8 oz lean beef roast – 4 2.5 oz pork chop – 4 1 hot dog (10/pkg) – 5 2.5 oz lean sirloin steak – 8 1/2 roast chicken breast – 13 3 oz light meat turkey – 16 3 oz broiled halibut – 14 3 oz water packed tuna – 17 3 oz baked salmon – 26 3 oz baked clams – 59 3 oz crabmeat – 61 3 oz shrimp – 96
100 + MG	1 c 2% cottage cheese – 155 1 c hard ice cream or ice milk – 176	1 c cooked dandelion greens – 147 1 c cooked chopped kale – 179	1 piece tofu – 108 (2½ × 2¾ × 1") 1 c refried beans – 141		3 oz canned salmon with bones – 167
200 + MG	1 oz cheddar cheese – 204 1 oz part skim mozzarella cheese – 207 1 oz provolone – 214 1 oz swiss cheese – 272 1 c whole milk – 291 1 c 2% milk – 297 1 c baked custard – 297	1 c cooked broccoli – 205 1 c cooked chopped turnip greens – 249 1 c cooked spinach – 277			1 c oysters – 226
300 + MG	1 c nonfat (skim) milk – 302 8 oz lowfat fruit flavored yogurt – 343 8 oz lowfat plain yogurt – 415	1 c cooked rhubarb – 341 1 c cooked chopped collard greens – 357			3 oz canned sardines with bones – 372

b. Supplements with the words "dolomite," "bone meal" or "oyster shell" on the label may contain lead contaminants. Using these could lead to lead poisoning.

c. The amount of calcium actually available to you from a tablet is called "elemental calcium" and should be listed on the product label. It is possible for more calcium to be in a tablet than you can get out of it. For example, a tablet of the antacid TUMS contains 500 mg. of calcium, but only 200 mg. is elemental calcium.

Iron

Iron is so important to life that the body has no way of excreting it. It is needed to deliver oxygen to the cells, form muscle, produce antibodies, synthesize collagen, convert beta-carotene to Vitamin A, and detoxify drugs in the liver, among other things!

The amount of iron you need to eat each day depends upon how much you lose in urine, feces, perspiration, and desquamation (that is, loss of hair, skin cells, and nails). For children, adolescents, and pregnant women, new tissue growth also creates more need for iron. For the average adult man, iron loss totals about .9–1.2 mg./day. Menstruation increases the average iron loss for women to 1.4–2.2 mg./day. Because the body only absorbs about 10% of the iron you eat, the recommended intake is 10 mg./day for men and for post-menopausal women. Menstruating women need at least 18 mg. of iron each day.

National nutritional surveys in the late 1970s indicated that about 18% of women 19–64 years of age consumed the amount of iron recommended. Another 26% consumed 70% of the recommended amount; for the remaining 56% of women intake was below 70%! Men did a lot better. Eighty-eight percent of the men in this age group ate the recommended amount of iron. The fact that women need more iron than men during these years accounts for some of this difference, but not all. As you can see in Figure 8.8, even after age 65 men still eat more iron than women.

It is difficult for women to obtain needed iron since a diet adequate in most other nutrients provides only 6 mg. of iron per 1000 calories. Unless a woman eats 2500–3000 calories a day, she very likely won't get the iron she needs. An iron supplement may be needed; ferrous sulphate is probably the least expensive and most effective form. Whether or not you need such a supplement is best determined through blood test and discussion of the results with a physician.

Where to get iron and how to get the most iron out of what you eat are important questions, especially for women. The following information about sources of iron provides some answers.

Food sources of iron. Liver is the only really good source of iron, pork liver offering the most per serving. Unfortunately, liver also offers high levels of cholesterol. Perhaps more importantly, many Americans don't (won't!) eat liver very often. Other meats, cereals, vegetables, and beans provide most of the iron in American diets. Fruits are rather poor sources although the pulp of fruit has twice as much iron as fruit juice. Eggs seem to be a good source of iron on paper, but only 2% of the iron in egg can be absorbed. Milk and milk products contain very little iron. A non-food source of iron is iron pots and pans: foods cooked in them can pick up additional iron. The amount of iron in selected, frequently-consumed foods is listed in Table 8.P.

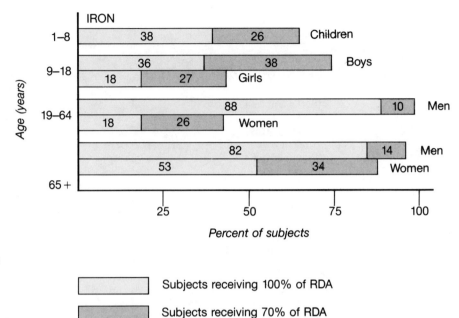

FIGURE 8.8
The inadequacy of iron intake in the North American population, according to the NFCS (U.S. government, 1977-78).

Reprinted by permission from Helen Guthrie, *Introductory Nutrition,* 6th Ed. St. Louis, 1983, The C. V. Mosby Co./Times Mirror/Mosby College Publishing.

Absorption of iron.

1. The iron in animal foods is better absorbed than that in vegetables and grains. However, consuming meat with vegetables and grains increases the absorption of iron from these sources two to three times.
2. Consuming a source of Vitamin C with sources of iron increases its absorption This is also true when taking a supplement; you will get more iron from a supplement taken with a glass of orange juice than with water.
3. Small amounts of iron are more easily absorbed. Eating small doses of iron three to four times throughout the day is better than consuming one big dose. The same applies to supplements. Also, you will get about twice the iron from your supplement if it is taken with a meal than if you take it before eating.
4. Drinking coffee or tea with a meal can decrease iron absorption between 40–95%. Tannins in tea and polyphenols in coffee are iron-binding substances.

Salt (Sodium Chloride)

The combination of two minerals, sodium and chlorine, is most commonly known as salt. It is given special attention here because diets high in salt are associated with high blood pressure, and American diets *are* high in salt. As previously noted, one in six Americans has high blood pressure.

Sodium appears to be the mineral responsible for the connection between salt and high blood pressure. However, sodium is not solely to blame for this health problem.

Table 8.P Iron content per serving of selected foods.

FOOD	SERVING SIZE	CALORIES	MG. IRON
Meat, Fish, Eggs, Poultry, Nuts & Legumes			
Egg, fried	1 large	83	0.9
Beef roast, lean	3 oz	165	3.1
Hamburger	3 oz	285	3.2
Chicken breast	3 oz	160	1.3
Tuna in water	3 oz	120	1.6
Peanut butter	2 tbsp	178	0.6
Bacon, lean	3 slices	89	2.8
Beef liver	3 oz	195	7.5
Shrimp	3 oz	100	2.5
Haddock, Perch, Salmon, etc.	3 oz	160	1.0
Raw clams	3 oz	65	5.2
Oysters (7–8 med.)	4 oz	80	6.0
Tofu (soybean curd)	4 oz	85	2.5
Chick peas	½ cup	145	2.9
Sunflower seeds (dry, hulled)	¼ cup	200	2.5
Pumpkin seeds (dry, hulled)	¼ cup	195	3.9
Peanuts (roasted in oil & salted)	¼ cup	210	.7
Filberts	¼ cup	182	1.0 scant
Cereals			
Cornflakes	1 cup	88	1.9
Shredded wheat	1 biscuit	83	1.1
Saltines (10 grams)	4 crackers	43	0.5
Rice	½ cup	112	0.9
White bread	1 slice	81	0.6
Whole-wheat bread	1 slice	73	0.5
Dairy Products			
Whole milk	8 oz	157	0.1
2% fat milk	8 oz	121	0.1
Skim milk	8 oz	90	0.1
Cheddar cheese	1 oz	114	0.2
Fruits			
Apple	1 med	81	0.4
Banana	1 med	105	0.9
Orange juice, frozen	4 oz	56	0.1
Peach	1 med	37	0.5
Vegetables			
Corn, canned	4 oz–½ cup	98	0.8
Green beans	4 oz–½ cup	52	0.7
Green peas	4 oz–½ cup	88	1.8
Lettuce (100 grams)	¼ head	13	0.5
Tomatoes	1 med	22	0.5
Potato, baked	1 med	93	0.7

As noted earlier, a low calcium intake, overweight, smoking, race, age, and family history are also risk factors. To further complicate the picture, not all people who eat salt develop high blood pressure, and reducing salt intake certainly doesn't guarantee a return to normal pressure once high blood pressure has developed.

While there is some confusion and controversy about salt and high blood pressure, one fact has emerged rather clearly: certain people have a genetic propensity to develop high blood pressure and/or are sodium sensitive. For these people, a high salt diet will, in time, probably contribute to high blood pressure. It is estimated that 20% or more of Americans may have this tendency, with Black Americans being at even greater risk. It is also possible that long term high salt intake is an important factor since almost three out of four people over age 65 have problems with high blood pressure. Recent research suggests, however, that the impact of high salt intake may be minimized if adequate amounts of potassium and calcium are consumed.

At this point in time there is no way to predict who can eat salt liberally without concern and who can not. This is unfortunate because desire for salt appears to be acquired through dietary practices, and not by a need for it. The body only needs about 220 mg. of sodium/day to regulate the balance of water and dissolved substances outside of cells (potassium does this inside cells). To allow for variation in individual need plus exercise and environmental conditions, nutritionists suggest that 1100–3300 mg. of sodium/day should be adequate. This amounts to 3 to 8 g. of salt per day or ½ to 1½ tsps. However, the average American adult eats 10–20 g. of salt/day, betweem 2–4 tsps.

Why do Americans like salt so much? The explanation may lie in reports from the Food and Drug Admnistration that American infants consume about the same amount of salt as adults, 18 g./day, and that toddlers get even more, about 25 g./day. How do they get so much salt? They get it from adults, of course, who prepare foods to their own tastes, often with salt. Adults also buy and serve prepared foods, also called processed foods, which supply about two-thirds of all the salt Americans consume.

The use of processed foods doesn't necessarily mean that parents are giving their children "junk food." It simply means that foods you buy in cans and packages very often contain a lot of added salt. For example, fresh peas contain only 2 mg. of sodium per 3½ oz. serving but canned peas contain 236 mgs. In comparison, an ounce of Planters Peanuts contains 132 mgs. and a one ounce bag of Lay's Potato Chips has 191 mgs. of sodium. A ten ounce serving of Campbell's Tomato soup has a whopping 1,050 mgs. The sodium content of these and other processed and fresh foods are listed in Table 8.Q. A more complex list is given in *The Sodium Content of Foods*, published by the U.S. Department of Agriculture.

With processed foods comprising 55% of the American diet, the difficulty of reducing an over-developed taste for salt should be apparent. Difficult or not, that is exactly what health experts are recommending. They believe that limiting salt intake to 5 g./ day, which is equivalent to 2000 mg. of sodium, will help curtail the incidence of high blood pressure. Should you want to reduce the salt in your diet, the following suggestions will help you:

1. Add little or no salt to food at the table, and certainly not until after you've tasted it.

2. Cut down on salt used in cooking and baking. First cut the amount in half. As you become accustomed to that, you can reduce it further.

3. Use sodium-free spices and flavorings in place of salt. Some of these are onion, garlic, curry, ginger, nutmeg, parsley, pepper, sage, thyme, mustard, sesame seeds, and vanilla, walnut, lemon, almond, and peppermint extracts. The American Heart Association can provide a more complete list of these plus low sodium recipes.

4. Use fresh meats, vegetables, and fruits as much as possible. Frozen vegetables are next best.

5. Reduce intake of canned soups and vegetables, cold cuts, canned meats, hot dogs, sausage, salted and smoked fish, processed cheese, boullion cubes, and sauces like worcestershire, soy, and barbeque.

6. Reduce intake of salty snacks like potato chips, pretzels, salted nuts, crackers, and popcorn.

7. Look for the word "sodium" on product labels even if it's part of another word like monosodium glutamate, sodium bicarbonate, sodium propionate, or sodium saccharin. Avoid as many of these as you can.

8. Pickled vegetables contain lots of salt. Limit your intake of these.

9. Avoid eating at fast-food restaurants. Many of the usual entrees like hamburgers and fried chicken are very high in sodium (see Table 8.Q).

10. Check with your local water district to find out if the sodium content of your drinking water is higher than 45 parts per million. If it is, buy a filter to attach to your tap; otherwise, simply drinking water could nullify your efforts to reduce sodium in your diet.

Water and Other Sources of Liquid

"Last, but not least" is certainly an appropriate description for the last nutrient to be discussed. In fact, you need more of this than any of the other nutrients and without it, you would probably die within a week. The magic nutrient is water. It supplies no calories for energy, but it provides the medium for *all* essential body functions. As such it is a solvent, growth promotor, lubricant, temperature regulator, catalyst, and source of trace elements. Indeed, the human body is composed largely of water: the average adult body contains about 40–50 quarts.

The average person loses about 2½ to 3 quarts of water daily in urine, perspiration, feces, and by evaporation in the lungs. In hot environments or with heavy exercise, water loss can approach 4 quarts. To maintain optimum functioning this fluid has to be replaced each day.

A guide to estimating the amount of water you need each day is 1 quart or 4 cups for every 1000 calories consumed. For most people, that would mean drinking between 8 and 16 cups of water every day. Fortunately, you don't actually have to drink this much water because the food you eat contains water. Fruits and vegetables have an especially high water content, most about 80%. Meats are about 50% water, breads 35%. Water is also created inside the body through various metabolic reactions. In all, these sources will probably provide almost half the water you need; the rest you have to drink.

It is generally recommended that you consume a minimum of 6 to 8 glasses of water per day. Some of this can be in the form of other beverages such as milk, which

Table 8.Q Sodium content of selected foods.

FOODS	PORTION	SODIUM (MG.)
Dairy:		
Milk	1 cup	130
Chocolate milk	1 cup	150
McDonald's chocolate shake	1	330
Ice cream, hard	1 cup	85
Ice cream, soft	1 cup	154
Cheddar cheese	1 oz	176
Cottage cheese	1 cup	910
Mozzarella cheese	1 oz	106
Swiss cheese	1 oz	74
Swiss, processed	1 oz	388
Homemade chocolate pudding	1 oz	146
Jello chocolate instant pudding	1 cup	820
Yogurt, fruit flavored	1 cup	135
Egg	1 whole	60
Egg white	1 white	50
Fats:		
Butter	1 pat	41
Margarine	1 pat	49
All oils	1 cup	0
French dressing	1 tbsp	219
Low calorie	1 tbsp	126
Italian dressing	1 tbsp	314
Low calorie	1 tbsp	118
Thousand Island	1 tbsp	112
Low calorie	1 tbsp	112
Meats:		
Canned tuna, Del Monte	3 oz	430
Canned shrimp	3 oz	1955
Fresh shrimp	3 oz	118
Salmon, broiled	3 oz	99
Pink salmon, canned	3 oz	443
Halibut, broiled	3 oz	114
Scallops, steamed	3 oz	225
Bacon	2 slices	250
Beef, pot roast	3 oz	46
Chipped beef	2½ oz	1188
Ground beef	3 oz	40
McDonald's Big Mac		1510
Burger King Whopper		909
Lamb Chop	3 oz	47
Ham	3 oz	560
Pork chop	2.7 oz	23
Canned lunchmeat	1 slice	720
Oscar Mayer beef franks	1	425
Oscar Mayer bologna	2 slices	450
Kentucky Fried Chicken, Original Recipe	3 pieces	2285
Broiled chicken	½ or 6 oz	116
Swanson turkey dinner	1	1735
Roast turkey, light	2 slices	70

(Continued)

Table 8.Q   Sodium content of selected foods. *(Continued)*

FOODS	PORTION	SODIUM (MG.)
Fruit:		
Apple, large	1 cup	2
Applesauce	1 cup	5
Banana	1	1
Grapefruit	½	2
Cantaloupe	½	57
Honeydew	1/10	27
Orange	1	1
Pear	1	3
Strawberries	1 cup	2
Grains:		
Bagel	1	320
Whole wheat bread	1 slice	132
Pumpernickel bread	1 slice	182
French bread	1 slice	203
White bread	1 slice	142
Shredded wheat	1 biscuit	1
Oatmeal, cooked	1 cup	1
Oatmeal, instant	1 cup	400
Kelloggs Corn Flakes	1 cup	320
Post Raisin Bran	1 cup	389
Pancakes, homemade buckwheat	3	345
Hungry Jack extra light pancakes, 4 inch	3	1150
Rice, cooked without salt	1 cup	1
Instant rice, cooked	1 cup	767
Vegetables		
Peas, fresh	½ cup	2
Peas, canned	½ cup	236
Green beans, fresh	1 cup	5
Green beans, canned	1 cup	319
Beets, fresh	1 cup	74
Beets, canned	1 cup	378
Tomatoes, cooked/fresh	1 cup	10
Tomatoes, canned	1 cup	390
Corn, fresh	1 cup	1
Corn, canned	1 cup	384
B & M Brick Oven baked beans	1 cup	810
Potatoes, baked	1	4
Hashbrowns, cooked from frozen	1 cup	446
Potato chips	10	215
Sauerkraut	1 cup	1554
Miscellaneous		
Jif peanut butter	2 tbsp	155
Campbell's tomato soup	10 oz	1050
Lipton Cup-A-Soup, vegetable	8 oz	1058
Heinz kosher dill	1 large	1137
Nabisco wheat thins	16 (1 oz)	260
Planter's peanuts	1 oz	132
Olives, green	10 large	926
Olives, ripe	10 extra large	385
A-1 barbeque sauce	1 tbsp	275
Soy sauce	1 tbsp	1029

is 87% water, and bottled waters.* Soft drinks are also a source of water, but they are loaded with sugar (only about 10% of the soft drinks sold are diet). It's estimated that 25% of the sugar we eat annually comes from soft drinks. For those needing only extra calories and more water in their diets, soft drinks are a good choice since in general the only nutrients they have are calories and water!

Colas, regular or diet, also give you a dose of caffeine fairly equivalent to that in a cup of coffee or tea, depending on how the latter are brewed. The caffeine in a 12 oz. cola drink ranges from 40–72 mg. A cup of instant tea has about 25 mg. of caffeine, but brewed tea has twice as much or more. Instant coffee has about 65 mg. of caffeine per cup, but perked coffee may contain as much as 140 mg., and drip coffee 155 mg. or more.

Caffeine acts as a stimulant to the heart and central nervous system and as a relaxant to the digestive system and kidneys. In small doses, as in one or two cups of coffee, caffeine can enhance the efficiency of the heart and other muscles and increase mental alertness and thought processes. Larger doses, however, can be trouble. Drinking 3 to 4 or more cups of coffee in succession can cause rapid and irregular heart rhythms, shakinesss, headache, diarrhea, and excessive urine output. All of these reactions are suitably unpleasant, and certainly not conducive to health. However, the major concern with caffeine is its possible long term effects. Numerous studies, primarily of coffee drinkers, have indicated a possible link between caffeine and increased risk of heart disease, cancer, fibrocystic breast disease, and birth defects. To date the evidence remains inconclusive. Until more information is available, it appears that the caffeine in several cups of coffee, tea, or soda pop should not be a problem for most people. Pregnant women and people with heartbeat irregularities, however, should check with their physicians about the safety of drinking these beverages. Consumers of caffeine in general might want to consider moderating the amounts they drink just in case the possible negative effects of caffeine are eventually confirmed. In all cases, users of caffeinated beverages risk loss of water soluble vitamins and minerals, especially iron and calcium, in their urine due to the diuretic effect of caffeine.

To avoid caffeine, some people have begun drinking decaffeinated coffee and herbal teas. A word of caution is needed in each case. Many decaffeinated coffees contain chemicals derived from the decaffeinating process that some researchers feel may be cancer causing. Evidence of this is inconclusive at this time. Coffee decaffeinated by a steam process developed in Switzerland does not contain these chemicals, and might be a safer choice for consumers. Look for water-processed decaffeinated coffee if you want to be extra cautious in this matter.

Herbal teas have become popular replacement beverages for coffee. Although most of them don't contain caffeine, some do, and in amounts equal to or greater than those in coffee. The product label should indicate this. Besides indicating caffeine content, if any, the label should indicate the plants used to make the tea. This information is especially important because many herbal teas come from plants that have historically been used as drugs. Some of these teas are actually poisonous in sufficient quantities. Teas made from sassafras, ginsing, or chamomile are examples. If you want to drink herbal teas, the best advice is to first learn about the plants they are made from and then to drink only very dilute preparations not too frequently. Herbal teas are not a very safe way to fulfill your water needs.

---

*Mineral water, seltzer, and club soda are especially popular drinks today. It should be noted, however, that the health benefits of these drinks beyond increased water intake have not been established. Some of these do offer extra minerals, but large amounts of these can be a hazard. As previously explained, too many minerals can upset the body's natural balance of these substances. Persons with heart disease or high blood pressure should examine labels closely to see if sodium is one of the minerals present, as in club soda.

Alcoholic beverages provide water, too, but they also contain the drug alcohol. Alcohol is a central nervous system depressant. Besides its sedating effect on the brain, it acts as a diuretic. Thus, when you drink alcoholic beverages you risk loss of water soluble vitamins and minerals. Heavy use of alcohol is also prominently associated with fatal accidents, liver disease, cancer, gastrointestinal problems, and birth defects.

Technically alcohol is a nutrient because it provides calories, 7 per gram. Some alcoholic beverages like wine contain small amounts of vitamins and minerals, but for the most part alcohol, like refined sugar, represents "empty calories." Because it provides essentially nothing but calories and its presence in the body is not in anyway needed, it is usually not considered a nutrient.

Since the mid 1970s several studies have indicated that people who consume moderate amounts of alcohol (one to two drinks per day) live longer than tee-totalers or heavy drinkers. In general, these moderate drinkers have lower rates of cardiovascular disease. It was thought that this lower rate was possibly due to alcohol's ability to increase the level of HDLs in the blood. However, it has recently been discovered that there are several types of HDLs; one type helps to minimize damage to blood vessel walls and another type doesn't seem especially useful at all. This "useless" form of HDL is the one increased in the blood by drinking alcohol. It will take further study to determine exactly why moderate drinking characterizes those who are living longer, but for now alcohol itself doesn't appear to be the reason.

As a beverage or as a nutrient, alcohol offers very little, especially in light of its association with numerous serious health problems. It is thought best to limit consumption to one or two drinks per day or less. If weight control is a problem, eliminating the empty calories you get from alcohol would be best; next best would be no more than one drink per day.

The RDAs, USRDAs, and U.S. Dietary Goals

For each of the nutrients discussed in this chapter, the amount the body needs for optimal functioning was indicated as well as a larger recommended intake that included a built-in safety margin. Recommendations were also made regarding the proportions of proteins, fats, and carbohydrates and the amounts of certain vitamins and minerals that seem most likely to minimize risk of major illness. The primary sources of these recommendations were the Recommended Dietary Allowances (RDAs) and the U.S. Dietary Goals.

The RDAs are established by the Food and Nutrition Board, a committee of the National Academy of Sciences National Research Council (NAS-NRC). They are reviewed and reissued about every five years. The board's goal is to recommend a daily intake for each essential nutrient that will be adequate to meet the needs of practically all healthy persons. To accommodate individual variations in need and usage of nutrients, the board's recommendations actually exceed the nutrient requirements for most people. The RDAs for 1980 are listed by sex and age group in Appendix 7. The 1985 version has been delayed to allow closer examination of new research findings.

Often confused with the RDAs are the U.S. Recommended Daily Allowances (USRDAs), the government's standards for nutritional information given on food product labels. The USRDAs are based on the RDAs, but use only the highest intake recommended for any age group (excluding pregnant and lactating women) as the standard that manufacturers must use to indicate the nutrient content of their products. Any food processor who adds any nutrient to food or who wishes to make any nutritional statements about a product must indicate on the package label the percentage of the USRDA his/her product contains in protein, iron, calcium, and the vitamins A, C, thiamin, riboflavin, and niacin. The number of calories and the amount of protein, carbohydrate, fat and sodium (required after July, 1986) must also be listed by weight for a stated serving size. The manufacturer can choose to provide data on twelve other nutrients, but is not required to do so. An example of a product label with required USRDA data is shown in Figure 8.9 and one with the optional data added is shown in Figure 8.10.

The U.S. Dietary Goals were developed in 1977 by the Senate Select Committee on Nutrition and Human Needs. They reflect the recommendations of the nation's foremost nutrition and health experts for reducing the incidence of disability and death due to chronic diseases like cardiovascular disease, cancer, and diabetes. Since that time, dietary goals and/or guidelines have also been issued by the National Academy of Sciences, the Surgeon General of the United States, the American Heart Association, and the U.S. Department of Agriculture. A comparison of all these guidelines is presented in Table 8.R. They are strikingly similar. Basically these guidelines suggest following nine steps to minimize the risk of chronic disease:

1. Maintain weight by balancing caloric intake with expenditure.
2. Increase carbohydrate intake to approximately 60% of total calories. Limit refined sugars to 10%.
3. Increase fiber intake.

FIGURE 8.9
Product label with mandatory nutrient information only.

```
Sugar-Free Hot Cocoa Mix

Nutrition Information Per Serving
Serving Size:   1 envelope (0.53 oz.)
Servings Per Container:        10

Calories  ......................... 50
Protein  .......................... 4 grams
Carbohydrate  ..................... 8 grams
Fat  ....................... less than 1 gram
Sodium  ......................... 160 mg.

Percentages of U.S. Recommended
Daily Allowances (% U.S. RDA):

Protein  .......................... 8%
Vitamin A  ........................ *
Vitamin C  ........................ *
Thiamine  ......................... 2%
Riboflavin  ....................... 10%
Niacin  ........................... *
Calcium  .......................... *
Iron  ............................. 4%

*Contains less than 2% of U.S. RDA
 of these nutrients.
```

4. Reduce total fat intake to 30% or less of total calories. Limit saturated fat to 10% or less.

5. Reduce cholesterol intake to 300 mg./day or less.

6. Reduce salt intake to 5 g./day or less.

7. Increase consumption of fruits, vegetables, and grains.

8. Use alcohol in moderation or not at all.

9. Eat a variety of foods.

Nutrition Information
Serving Size: 1.4 oz. (1 oz. bran flakes with 0.4 oz. raisins; about 3/4 cup)
Servings Per Package: 15

	Cereal and Raisins	With 1/2 C. Skim Milk	With 1/2 C. Whole Milk
Calories	110	150	180
Protein	3 g	7 g	7 g
Carbohydrate	31 g	37 g	37 g
Fat	1 g	1 g	5 g
+Cholesterol	0 mg	0 mg	15 mg
Sodium	210 mg	270 mg	270 mg
+Potassium	230 mg	430 mg	410 mg

Percentage of U.S. Recommended Daily Allowances (U.S. RDA)

Protein	4	15	15
Vitamin A	25	30	30
Vitamin C	*	2	2
Thiamin	25	30	30
Riboflavin	25	35	35
Niacin	25	25	25
Calcium	*	15	15
Iron	100	100	100
+Vitamin D	10	25	25
+Vitamin B_6	25	25	30
+Folic Acid	25	25	25
+Vitamin B_{12}	25	35	30
+Phosphorus	15	25	25
+Magnesium	15	20	20
+Zinc	25	30	30
+Copper	10	10	10

*Contains less than 2% U.S. R.D.A. of this nutrient

+Carbohydrate Information

	Cereal and Raisins	With Milk
Starch & related carbohydrates	15 g	15 g
Sucrose & other sugars	12 g	18 g
Dietary Fiber	4 g	4 g
Total Carbohydrates	31 g	37 g

+Optional Information

FIGURE 8.10
Product label with mandatory and optional nutrient information.

The Impact of Good Nutrition on Health

The dietary guidelines just presented leave no doubt that the health experts in this country believe that what we eat can increase or decrease our risk of developing serious degenerative disease, especially cardiovascular disease, cancer, and diabetes. In the years to come, researchers will continue to explore and clarify the relationship between nurtition and these conditions, but there is no doubt even today that nutrition does play a critical role.

The same can be said for the role of nutrition in the aging process. As explained in Chapter 3, the physical losses in function that occur with age seem to result primarily from two conditions: disuse and cell dysfunction and death. Since cells cannot function properly at any age without an adequate nutrient supply, the importance of good nutrition in maintaining maximum possible function and minimizing premature dysfunction is clear. Though we have only theories to explain what goes wrong with cells to ultimately cause dysfunction after 70–80 plus years, it is notable that nutrition is a factor in all of these theories. Research indicates that nutrition does indeed have the power to increase or decrease the speed of the aging process.

The impact of nutrition on health extends further than simply minimizing the development of diseases and aging changes. Good nutrition is critical to feeling and doing your best. The importance of adequate nutrients for proper physiological functioning has already been noted; you can't be in top physical condition without them. What you eat can also influence your emotional state. For example, you can't feel really well if your blood sugar is low. In fact, if it becomes too low you may feel not only weak, but anxious. A primarily carbohydrate breakfast such as a donut and an orange can leave you feeling rather sleepy for your morning duties whereas eating some protein with that same breakfast can make you feel "ready to go." More dramatically, nutrition has been linked with feelings of depression and, in later life, with symptoms that mimic senility.

If health can be described as being able to do the things you want and need to do and feeling like *now* is the best time to be alive, then good nutrition is essential to health.

Table 8.R Comparison of dietary advice to the public from various government and health groups.

	WEIGHT CONTROL	CARBOHYDRATE	FIBER	ANIMAL LIPID
Dietary Goals, USDA, 1978	To avoid overweight, decrease energy intake, and increase energy expenditure.	Increase complex carbohydrate to 48% of energy intake. Reduce refined sugar to 10% of calorie intake.		Reduce to 10% of calories
Healthy People, Surgeon General, 1979		Reduce simple carbohydrate; increase complex carbohydrate.		Reduce intake.
Diet and Cancer, National Academy of Sciences, 1982			Increase fiber intake.	Reduce intake.
American Heart Association, 1978		Increase carbohydrate intake to 55% of calories, mostly complex. Increasing to 65%.		Reduce to 10% of calories.
Dietary Guidelines, USDA, HHS, 1985	Maintain desirable weight	Avoid too much sugar.	Increase fiber intake.	Avoid eating too much.
Nutritional Guidelines for Health Education in Britain, 1983	Adjust food intake and exercise to maintain optimal weight for height.	Reduce sucrose to 10 kg/yr.	Increase from 20 to 30 g/day.	
Nutrition Recommendations for Canadians, 1979	Reduce excess consumption of calories and increase physical activity.			Include source of linoleic acid.
Dietary Guidelines for Japan, 1984	Eat to match your energy requirements.			

(Continued)

	VEGETABLE LIPID	TOTAL LIPID	CHOLESTEROL	SODIUM	OTHER ADVICE
Dietary Goals USDA, 1978	Increase to 10% of calories.	Reduce to 30% of calories.	Reduce to 300 mg/day.	Decrease use of salt and foods high in salt.	
Healthy People, Surgeon General, 1979		Reduce total fat intake.	Reduce intake.	Reduce intake.	Exercise and eat a variety of foods.
Diet and Cancer, National Academy of Sciences, 1982	Reduce intake.	Reduce to 30% of calories.			Increase the use of fruits, vegetables, and whole-grain cereals. Avoid smoked and salt-cured food. If alcohol is used, drink in moderation.
American Heart Association, 1978	10% of calories.	Reduce to 30% of calories, and then to 20%.	300 mg/day.		Protein should comprise 15% of caloric intake.
Dietary Guidlines, USDA, HHS, 1985		Avoid eating too much.	Decrease intake.	Decrease intake.	Eat a variety of foods.
Nutritional Guidelines for Health Education in Britain, 1983		30% of total energy intake.	None.	Decrease salt intake.	Decrease alcohol to 4% of total energy intake. Increase proportion of vegetable protein to other nutrients.
Nutrition Recommendations for Canadians, 1979		Reduce to 35% of calories.			Emphasize whole-grain products, fruits, and vegetables in the diet; minimize alcohol, salt, and refined sugar.
Dietary Guidelines for Japan, 1984		Avoid eating too much. Eat more vegetable than animal fat.		Eat no more than 10 g of salt/day.	Eat 30 different food-stuffs every day; enhance the pleasure of your table.

Reproduced with permission from Helen Guthrie, *Introductory Nutrition*, 6th Ed. © 1986 by Times Mirror/Mosby College Publishing, St. Louis.

Summary

Variety, quality, and quantity are the key determinants of good nutrition. In terms of quality, your diet needs to contain those nutrients the body cannot function properly without and cannot make on its own. There are six main categories of these essential nutrients: protein, carbohydrate, fat, vitamins, minerals, and water. Quantity standards are not yet definite for all nutrients. However, the U.S. Dietary Goals and the Recommended Dietary Allowances (the RDAs) are cited as the prevailing quantity guidelines at present.

One of the most critical essential nutrients is protein, which is composed of nitrogen-containing components called amino acids. Nine of these amino acids are called essential because the body cannot make them. Any protein containing all nine of these essential amino acids in sufficient quantity for the body to use is called a complete protein; all other proteins are incomplete. All animal products except gelatin provide complete proteins. With the exception of legumes, vegetable proteins are incomplete. By eating certain combinations of vegetables, grains, nuts, and seeds or by eating them with a source of complete protein like milk, it is possible to get complete protein without actually eating meat.

The recommended intake for protein is .8 g/kg of average body weight for a given height. This amounts to 44 g. of protein/day for the average woman and 56 g. for the average man. However, national nutrition studies indicate that the average American over-consumes protein from childhood through old age. Nutrition experts currently advise limiting protein to no more than 12% of total daily calories.

Americans are also eating more fat than the recommended 30% or less of daily calories. The average American consumes about 42% of his/her daily calories in fat. About 95% of the fat in the diet is composed basically of three kinds of fatty acids: saturated, monounsaturated, and polyunsaturated. While most foods actually contain mixtures of all three types, saturated fats predominate in animal products and mono- and polyunsaturated fats in vegetables and fruits such as the avocado (most fruits have little or no fat at all). Diets high in saturated fat increase the risk of cardiovascular disease whereas diets emphasizing mono- and polyunsaturated fats seem to provide protection from this problem. High fat diets, regardless of the type of fat, increase risk of several forms of cancer.

Cholesterol is another type of fat found in the diet of those who consume animal products. Americans eat about 600 mg. of cholesterol/day even though the liver can make all that the body needs, and despite the fact that high levels of cholesterol in the blood increase the risk of cardiovascular disease. Reducing cholesterol intake to 300 mg. or less is recommended.

All evidence indicates that choosing a low fat, low cholesterol diet is advisable for overall good health. This requires emphasizing consumption of vegetables, grains, and fruit and limiting intake of meats such as beef, pork, and lamb, as well as butter and eggs.

The incidence of cardiovascular disease and cancer is lower among people whose diets are high in carbohydrate. There is some evidence that the fiber and vitamins and minerals in carbohydrate foods may actually help prevent these problems in addition to supplying the body with essential nutrients. For these reasons, nutrition experts are recommending that Americans increase their carbohydrate intake from the current 46% of daily calories to 55-60%. This recommendation, however, stipulates eating no more than 10% of daily calories in the form of refined sugars. Refined sugars or simple carbohydrates contain none of the fiber or vitamins and minerals found in the complex carbohydrates—fruits, vegetables, and grains.

In terms of fuel for body functioning, protein and carbohydrate each provide the body with four calories of energy per gram. Fat is more energy-dense, providing nine calories per gram. Of these three nutrient groups, carbohydrate and fat are the body's preferred fuel sources. If these are in sufficient supply, protein can be "spared" for structural growth and repair, its primary role.

The essential nutrients called vitamins and minerals are substances the body seems to need to function properly and/or to grow, but which provide no calories for energy. Even with the technological advancements that have been made over the years, much remains unknown about these substances, including how much of them people actually need for good health. Consequently, controversy prevails regarding the quantities of certain vitamins and minerals that people should consume. Vitamins A, C, and E are prominent examples of this. It is important to check the validity of claims made for these and other nutrients before consuming large amounts; guidelines for doing this are suggested.

Currently 13 vitamins are known to be required by the body and must be consumed. These are the fat soluble vitamins, A, D, E, and K and the water soluble B complex (eight total) and C vitamins. The fat soluble vitamins are carried into the body with the aid of fat in the diet and are stored in fat in the body. Thus, it is not absolutely critical to eat them each day unless the amounts being consumed and in body stores are very low compared to recommended intake. In fact, fat soluble vitamins can accumulate to toxic levels if consumed in excess over a period of time. Water soluble vitamins are not stored in the body to any great extent, and thus need to be eaten daily. However, even these vitamins, when consumed in very high amounts, can cause undesirable and even harmful side effects. The controversial Vitamins A, C, and E are discussed in detail.

Twenty-one minerals are known to be essential to body functioning. Calcium, phosphorus, sodium, and potassium are examples of macrominerals, needed in quantities of 100 mg. or more per day. Iron, copper, and zinc are examples of microminerals, needed in amounts less than a few mg. per day.

Thus far, the body's daily need for minerals has been established for only six of the twenty-one minerals; for nine of these, the amounts suggested are described only as "estimated safe and adequate." This ignorance regarding minerals is potentially very dangerous since minerals tend to be toxic at much lower levels than vitamins. For many minerals, toxicity levels have not even been clearly established. Because calcium and iron are often found lacking in the American diet and because consumption of sodium and chloride (salt) is close to excessive, specific discussions are provided regarding these minerals.

Because the body loses 2½ to 3 quarts of water in urine, perspiration, and feces and by evaporation in the lungs, this fluid must be replaced each day. This requires consuming about 1 quart of water or 4 cups for every 1000 calories consumed. Fortunately, some of this water can be supplied by food, leaving 6–8 cups to be consumed in beverage form. The benefits and detriments of various sources of water such as coffee, tea, soda and mineral waters, soda pop, and alcohol are discussed.

In all, the information provided in this chapter makes one very clear statement: good nutrition is essential for health.

References

Altscul, A. & Grommet, J. 1980. Sodium intake and sodium sensitivity. *Nutrition Reviews* 38:393.

Are you sure you're getting enough iron? 1985. *Tuft's University Diet and Nutrition Letter* 3 (October):3.

Assessing changing food consumption patterns. 1981. Committee on Food Consumption Patterns, Food and Nutrition Board. Washington, D.C.: National Academy Press.

Beer or skittles? 1986. *The Harvard Medical School Health Letter* 11. (January).

Bishop, J. 1986. America's new hunger for calcium presents a nutritional dilemma. *The Wall Street Journal,* January 20.

Brody, J. 1981. *Jane Brody's nutrition book.* New York: Bantam Books.

Buying guide: sugar substitutes. 1986. *University of California Berkeley Wellness Letter* 2 (June):9.

Deciding on decaf. 1986. *University of California, Berkeley Wellness Letter* 2 (June):9.

Diet and behavior. 1985. *Dairy Council Digest* 56 (July/August):19.

Diet, nutrition and cancer prevention: A guide to food choices. 1984. Public Health Service. Department Health & Human Services. NIH publication #85-2711. Washington, D.C.: Government Printing Office.

Dietary goals for the United States 2d ed. 1977. Select Committee on Nutrition & Human Needs, U.S. Senate. Washington, D.C.: Government Printing Office.

Durbin, B. 1985. Researchers say benefits from eating more fish all positive. *The Oregonian,* November 29.

Fear of shellfish: An instant cure. 1985. *University of California Berkeley Wellness Newsletter* 2 (December):7.

Glomset, J. 1985. Fish, fatty acids, and human health. *New England Journal of Medicine* 312:1253.

Guthrie, H. 1986. *Introductory nutrition.* St. Louis, MO: C. V. Mosby Publishing.

Hui, Y. 1985. *Principles and issues in nutrition.* Monterery, CA: Wadsworth.

Hubbard, J., et al. 1985. Nathan Pritikin's heart. *The New England Journal of Medicine* 4:52.

Jukes, T. 1984. Diet and Cancer. *Physician and Patient,* April.

Kagan, D. 1985. Mind nutrients. *OMNI* 7:36.

Krombout, D. et al. 1985. The inverse relationship between fish consumption and 20-year mortality from coronary heart disease. *New England Journal of Medicine* 312:1205.

Lang, S. 1984. Beyond bran. *American Health* 3 (May).

Lecos, C. 1983. A compendium of fats. *FDA Consumer* 17 (March):4.

McCarran, D. 1982. Low serum concentrations of ionized calcium in patients with hypertension. *New England Journal of Medicine* 307:226.

Nestle, M. 1983. Dietary recommendations: What constitutes good nutrition and for whom. *Consultant* 23 (January):271.

Newell, G. 1984. Nutrition and cancer: The provocative role of diet in carcinogenesis. *Consultant* 24 (January):116.

Osteoporosis. 1984. National Institutes of Health Consensus Development Conference Statement 5, #3. Washington, D.C.: Government Printing Office.

Recommended Dietary Allowances. 9th ed. 1980. Committee on Dietary Allowances, Food & Nutrition Board, Washington, D.C.: National Academy of Science.

Swan, B. 1983. Food consumption by individuals in the U.S. *Annual Review of Nutrition* 3:413.

Taking warnings about coffee to heart. 1986. *Tuft's University Diet and Nutrition Letter* 3 (January):1.

The sodium content of your food. 1982. U.S. Department of Agriculture, Department Health & Human Services. Home & Garden Bulletin #233. Washington, D.C.: Government Printing Office.

Vegetarianism: Can you get by without meat? 1980. *Consumer Reports* 45 (June):357.

Whitney, E. & Hamilton, E. 1984. *Understanding Nutrition.* 3d ed. New York: West Publishing.

Why sugar continues to concern nutritionists 1985. *Tuft's University Diet and Nutrition Letter* 3 (May):3.

Wrap-Up: Minerals 1986. *University of California, Berkeley Wellness Letter* 2 (January):4.

9

Checking-Up
On Eating Well

How well are you eating? Do you really know?

What guidelines can you follow to choose a health-promoting diet for yourself?

Do you know how to shop for and prepare the most nutritious foods?

Should you be taking supplements or shouldn't you?

Introduction

According to the statistics reported in Chapter 8, Americans in general need to change many of their eating habits in order to enjoy optimum vitality and longevity. The problem is, even statistically supported evidence such as this doesn't seem to cause very many people to change their behavior. People all have a tendency to read such evidence, believe it, be concerned about it, and yet not *do* much about it. It's easy to think that statistics apply only to other people, but only a nutrition "check-up" will indicate whether that's true or not.

You may feel that, while your diet could certainly use some improvement, overall it is not that bad. Or, you may feel rather sure that your diet is poor. One way or another, checking-up on your diet—that is, comparing your diet to the recommendations—is the best way to find out what, if anything, you need to change or improve. The techniques and procedures to help you do this type of dietary analysis are provided in the first part of this chapter. The second part of the chapter offers practical guidelines you can use as needed to implement the recommendations made in Chapter 8. Eating patterns, supplement use, and the selection and preparation of food to help you eat well are the specific issues addressed.

Nutritional Assessment

Determining whether or not you are well nourished is quite an involved task. A complete nutritional assessment would include an in-depth personal history, anthropometric measurements, a physical examination, and biochemical and dietary analyses. The specific data that would be collected under each of these categories are indicated in Tables 9.A and 9.B. The services of trained professionals would obviously be required to analyze all of this material appropriately. Such an assessment would be not only time consuming but expensive. However, if you are in nutritional trouble, it could be worth it to both your quality and quantity of life.

Although diet analysis is just one small part of a thorough nutritional assessment, it does provide an inexpensive, do-it-yourself way of "guestimating" whether or not you are eating sufficiently well to provide the nutrients you need. Should the results suggest you are significantly over- or under-eating in terms of calories or specific nutrients, you might then wisely seek professional consultation to help you remedy the problem(s).

Of course, a diet analysis does not tell you if you are properly metabolizing and absorbing the food you eat, so periodic physical examinations and blood tests could prove beneficial even if your diet analysis shows no problems. This precaution could be especially important if one or more of the nutritional risk factors or deficiency symptoms listed in Tables 9.A and 9.B apply to you.

One of the more accurate techniques for analyzing your diet is the food diary. You simply record everything you eat and the amounts for a 24 hour period. If your dietary intake varies a lot from day to day, it would be best to do this for a minimum of three days and preferably for an entire week. Once you have recorded your food intake for at least one day, you will need to determine the nutrient content of what

Table 9.A Nutritional assessment data: Possible indicators of poor
nutrition status.

MEDICAL PROBLEMS
Recent major illness/surgery
Over or underweight
Anorexia/Bulimia
Diarrhea or vomiting
Heavy smoking
Alcoholism
Cancer
  Radiation or drug therapy
Cardiovascular Disease
  Hyperlipidemia
  Hypertension
Diabetes
Diseases of lung, liver or kidney
Neurologic Disorders
  Depression
  Other
Drug use, regular or long-term
  Legal: Prescription and
         nonprescription
  Illegal

DIET PRACTICES/PROBLEMS
Very low calorie intake
Fad diets
Fasting 10 days or more
Dental problems
  Chewing/swallowing difficulty

SOCIOECONOMIC CONDITIONS
Inadequate income
Inadequate knowledge
Inadequate food storage or preparation
Living/eating alone

ANTHROPOMETRIC MEASURES
Height
Weight
Skinfold or other body fat indicator

Adapted from Whitney, E. and Hamilton, E. *Understanding Nutrition.* Minneapolis:
West, 1984.

Table 9.B Nutritional assessment data: Possible laboratory tests and physical indicators of
vitamin and mineral deficiency/toxicity.

VITAMIN		SELECTED PHYSICAL SIGNS/SYMPTOMS OF DEFICIENCY (D)/TOXICITY (T) IN ADULTS	LAB TESTS
Vitamin A	(D)	Triangular gray spots on eye, dryness of eyes, night blindness, dry, scaly, "goosebump" skin	Serum Vit. A Serum Carotene
	(T)	Joint pain, bleeding, loss of appetite, loss of hair, menstrual cessation, jaundice	
Thiamin (B₁)	(D)	Muscle weakness, calf muscle pain, loss of ankle and knee jerk reflex, edema in lower limbs	Urinary thiamin Thiamin load test
Riboflavin (B₂)	(D)	Redness, scaling and cracking at corners of mouth, magenta-colored tongue, light sensitivity, mental confusion	Urinary Riboflavin Riboflavin load test
Niacin (B₃) (Nicotinic acid)	(D)	Enlarged, reddened & "smooth" tongue, irritability, bi-lateral skin irritation on backs of hands, forearms, legs, etc.	Urinary N-methyl-nicotinamide
	(T)	Skin burning, itching and flushing, nausea and diarrhea	
Pyridoxine (B₆)	(D)	Cracking at corners of mouth, enlarged, red tongue, irritation of sweat glands, weakness, nervousness	Urinary B₆ Tryptophan load test
	(T)	Nerve damage	

Continued

Table 9.B   Nutritional assessment data: Possible laboratory tests and physical indicators of vitamin and mineral deficiency/toxicity. *(Continued)*

VITAMIN	SELECTED PHYSICAL SIGNS/SYMPTOMS OF DEFICIENCY (D)/TOXICITY (T) IN ADULTS		LAB TESTS
Folacin (Folic acid)	(D)	Cracked and swollen tongue, diarrhea, anemia	Red cell folate
Cobalamin (B_{12})	(D)	Smooth, swollen tongue, numbness in fingers and toes, skin sensitivity, anemia, lemon-yellow color	Serum B_{12} Urinary methyl-malonic acid
Vitamin C	(D)	Bleeding spongy gums, pin-point hemorrhages into skin, weakness, poor wound healing	Urinary Vitamin C Serum Vitamin C Capillary fragility test
	(T)	Cramps, diarrhea, nausea	
Vitamin D	(D)	Bone softening and bending; muscle cramps and twitching	Serum 25-hydroxy-cholecalciferol Serum calcium and phosphorous
	(T)	Calcification in soft tissue, loss of appetite, thirst, nervousness	
Vitamin E	(D)	Rare: red blood cell fragility, possible edema and flaky dermatitis	Hydrogen peroxide hemolysis test Plasma tocopherol
	(T)	Not definitely known. Some reports of cramps, diarrhea, possible impaired clotting time, increased blood lipids in women using oral contraceptives, decreased serum thyroid hormone	

MINERAL			
Calcium	(D)	Osteoporosis, uncontrollable muscle contractions, seizures	Serum calcium
Potassium	(D)	Muscle weakness, hypotension, respiratory failure, arrhythmia	Serum potassium
	(T)	Abnormal heart function	
Magnesium	(D)	Uncontrollable muscle contractions, nervousness and tremors, nausea, lethargy, arrhythmias	Serum magnesium
Iron	(D)	Fatigue, weakness, pallor, headache, difficulty breathing upon exertion	Hemoglobin Hematocrit Serum ferritin
	(T)	Iron deposits in tissues, bronze-colored skin, blackened stools, arrhythmias, infections	
Iodine	(D)	Goiter, sluggishness and weight gain	Serum protein bound iodine Urinary iodine
Zinc	(D)	Impaired sense of taste and smell, poor appetite, slow wound healing, infections, impaired growth	Serum zinc Hair analysis?
	(T)	Nausea, exhaustion, anemia, diarrhea	

Sources: (1) Whitney, E. & Hamilton, E. *Introductory Nutrition.* Minneapolis: West, 1984. (2) Hui, Y. *Principles and Issues in Nutrition.* Belmont: Wadsworth, 1985. (3) Guthrie, H. *Introductory Nutrition.* New York: Mosby, 1986. (4) Brody, J. *Jane Brody's Nutrition Book.* New York: Bantam, 1981.

you've eaten. You can do this by consulting the Nutritive Value of Foods listed in Appendix 8. You can then compare the nutrient quality of the foods you have eaten with the Recommended Dietary Allowances (RDAs) and the U.S. Dietary Goals. These comparisons will provide at least an indicator of how well you are eating to optimize body functioning and to minimize risk of chronic disease.

You can also compare the total calories you consumed in a day with your caloric expenditure. This should provide some help in analyzing present weight control problems and/or in preventing future ones. Instructions for calculating your daily caloric expenditure were given in Chapter 7. It would be best, of course, to calculate your expenditure for the same day or days you recorded your food intake. If done carefully, this should provide the most accurate estimate of your caloric expenditure. You can, however, *estimate* your expenditure using the formula shown in Table 9.C or by using the values listed in the RDA table. The RDA table will be your least accurate estimate unless you are exactly the weight and activity level of the standard reference male or female.

Inaccuracy in recording the amounts of food you eat greatly diminishes the value of the food diary. Before beginning your food diary, you may need some practice in estimating amounts of food. It is fairly easy to say how many slices of bread or how many bananas you have eaten, although even with these, sizes vary. An extra thick slice of bread, for example, will have to be listed in your food diary as 1½ or 2 slices in order to accurately indicate the quantity of bread you ate. Thus, you will have to pay close attention to the size of the item you consume. Estimating the amount of roast beef you ate in ounces, the amount of milk your favorite mug holds, or the amount of rice on your plate requires more than just close attention. You will have to have some idea what standard serving sizes look like on your plate or in your glass.

Servings of meat are usually listed in 2 to 3 ounce portions in the Nutritive Value of Foods; however, the dimensions of these portions are also given. If you're not very good at envisioning written dimensions, you may want to study the portions of meat illustrated in Figure 9.1 to see how much a serving size actually is compared to what you usually eat.

Table 9.C Estimated daily caloric need.

ACTIVITY LEVEL	CALORIES PER POUND EXPENDED
1. Very sedentary — no activity; confined to house.	13
2. Sedentary — typical American with office job/light work.	14
3. Moderate — #2 plus weekend recreation	15
4. Very active — complies with American College of Sports Medicine standards of vigorous exercise 3 × /wk.	16
5. Competitive athlete — vigorous activity	17 +

Formula: Weight in pounds × Activity Level Expenditure

Example: 120 lb. female × Sedentary Activity Level
120 lb. × 14 = 1680 calories
Estimated daily caloric need = 1680 calories

Adapted from American Heart Association

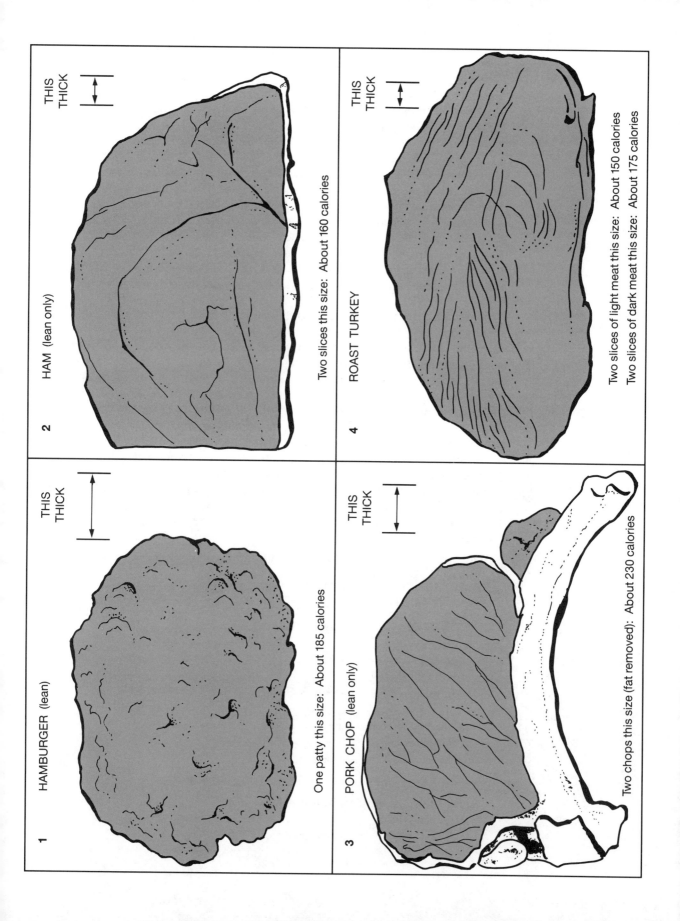

1

HAMBURGER (lean)

THIS
THICK

One patty this size: About 185 calories

2

HAM (lean only)

THIS
THICK

Two slices this size: About 160 calories

3

PORK CHOP (lean only)

THIS
THICK

Two chops this size (fat removed): About 230 calories

4

ROAST TURKEY

THIS
THICK

Two slices of light meat this size: About 150 calories
Two slices of dark meat this size: About 175 calories

Serving sizes for foods other than meats and individual items like apples and oranges are usually given in fluid ounces, cup portions, or tablespoons. You can increase your ability to estimate these portions accurately by actually measuring the amounts of food you eat for a day or two before doing your food diary. If this is too time-consuming or bothersome, at least allow yourself one practice session. In your practice session fill a measuring cup (8 oz.) with water and pour it into your favorite juice or milk glass to see how much it really holds. If you drink 3 glasses of milk a day from a 10 oz. glass which you assume to be only a cup or 8 oz., you will under-record your intake by 3/4 cup. If you drink whole milk, you will be under-estimating your intake of calories by 120 and of calcium by 215 mg.

To envision portions of cereal, rice, peas, and so on, fill a cup measure with these substances and pour it into a bowl or plate. Do the same with a 1/2 cup measure. To estimate quantities of such things as jam, salad dressing, and gravies, measure out a tablespoon of the substance (or of water if you wish) and pour it into a cup or dish until you have about the amount you might normally use. Note how many tablespoons you used and the total quantity in ounces or cup portions.

When you feel reasonably confident about estimating portions of food, you are ready to begin your food diary. It is important to eat just as you normally would on the day or days you record your intake. People have a tendency to eat less when they know they have to record the information; in fact, this is one of the techniques used to help people lose weight. For the purpose of analyzing your diet, however, it's important to avoid this tendency.

At the end of this chapter are samples of forms you can use to record your food intake and energy expenditure. Forms 1 and 2 are for that purpose. Forms 3 through 7 are provided to assist you in comparing the nutrient value of your diet with the RDAs and U.S. Dietary Goals. You will note that Form 3, for recording the nutrient content of the foods you have eaten, provides space only for the vitamins and minerals that were discussed in detail in the last chapter, plus three B vitamins: thiamin, riboflavin, and niacin. The reason for this is that diets providing adequate amounts of these key nutrients *generally* also contain the other essential nutrients you need.

When you have completed Form 3, you will have gathered all the nutrient data you need to analyze how well you are eating. Using Form 4, you can then determine if your calorie intake is in balance with your expenditure, and if not, what the impact of this imbalance would be on your weight over time if you ate and exerted yourself similarly every day. You can also calculate the number of pounds you might gain or lose in a year if you chose to modify your intake or expenditure patterns.

A note of caution is necessary at this point. If there is a large difference between your intake and expenditure and you are not gaining or losing weight, you have probably erred in recording or calculating your data. It is also possible that you did not eat or exercise as you normally do during the time you recorded your data. Either way, you might want to recheck your initial calculations or even repeat your data collection before proceeding further with the analysis, so you know you are working with accurate information. If you show a large deficit in caloric intake compared to expenditure and are reasonably certain your data are correct and representative of your eating habits, *but* you are not losing weight, your BMR may have fallen below normal as a result of your habitual very low calorie intake. In this case, the weight loss and gain calculations you make on Form 4 will not be accurate until you re-establish your normal BMR. The rest of your analysis, however, can be completed using the data you have. (*Note:* How to increase your BMR to normal levels was discussed in Chapter 7.)

FIGURE 9.1
Calories in portions of various meats, shown here actual size.

Reproduced from *Calories and Weight: USDA, A Pocket Guide*. 1970. U.S. Dept. of Agriculture. DHHS Home and Garden Bulletin #153. Washington, D.C.: Government Printing Office.

The next step in analyzing your diet is to determine if you are eating the proportions of protein, fat, and carbohydrate suggested in the U.S. Dietary Goals as important for minimizing the incidence of major chronic disease. Use Form 5 to calculate the percent of your total calories comprised by each of these major nutrients and to compare these proportions to the U.S. Dietary Goals. By determining your cholesterol-saturated fat index (CSI) on Form 6, you can check to see if the kind of fat you are eating minimizes or increases your risk of heart disease.

The last step is to determine if your diet provides the RDAs for eight key nutrients which, as previously explained, are general indicators of the overall quality of your diet in terms of essential nutrients. Use Form 7 to compare the amounts of the key nutrients you consumed with the RDAs for your sex and age groups. You might also want to identify the best source of each key nutrient in your diet as well as some additional foods you could eat that would contribute these nutrients. Space to do this is provided on the form. Making sure you get some of these foods every day could help maintain or improve the quality of your diet.

Choosing a Health-Promoting Diet

Just as diagnosing a disease doesn't cure it, neither does a dietary analysis automatically improve one's diet. In the first instance a prescription of some sort is generally given in hopes of restoring health. Prescriptions have also been written to help people select foods to eat that optimize healthy functioning and minimize risk of disease. The Basic Four Plan and the Dietary Guidelines for Americans are two of these. If you are one of the few people whose diet analysis indicated you are eating well in all categories of comparison, congratulations! The information in the rest of this chapter will simply help you to refine your already good nutritional habits. If your diet did not meet recommendations, the following dietary "prescriptions" could make a significant difference in your well being now and in the future.

The Modified Basic Four

The Four Food Groups Plan or the Basic Four was devised several decades ago to help people select foods to eat that would supply all the needed nutrients in appropriate amounts without your having to have a degree in nutrition to do it. The Basic Four plan, shown in Table 9.D, recommends eating two servings of meat or meat substitutes, two servings of milk products, four servings of fruits and vegetables, and four servings of whole or enriched grain products. The Basic Four is attractive because of its simplicity, but depending upon the choices you make in each food group, you may end up eating too many calories, too much fat, too much salt, and not enough of certain nutrients. The Center for Science in the Public Interest has prepared a modified version of the Basic Four that emphasizes food selections that minimize these problems. This modified version is presented in Table 9.E. Selecting foods according to this plan should provide you with the nutrients you need at an acceptable calorie intake to maintain weight. There are two exceptions to this. It is unlikely that the iron or calcium requirements of women will be met using this diet plan, or any other for that matter. As previously indicated, most women probably need to consume additional

Table 9.D   Servings in the four food group plan.

FOOD GROUP	SERVINGS (ADULT)	SERVING SIZE
Meat and meat substitutes	2	2–3 oz cooked meat, fish, or chicken; ¼ cup tuna; 2 eggs; 4 tbsp peanut butter; 1 cup cooked legumes; ½ cup nuts
Milk and milk products	2[a]	1 cup (8 oz) milk; 1 cup yogurt; 1½ cup cottage cheese; 2 cups ice cream ; 5 tbsp milk pudding; 1–2 oz cheese
Fruits and vegetables	4[b]	½ cup fruit, vegetable, or juice; 1 medium apple, orange, banana, or peach
Grains (bread and cereal products)	4[c]	1 slice bread; ½ cup cooked cereal or 1 cup (1 oz) ready-to-eat cereal; ½ hamburger or hot dog bun or English muffin; ½ cup cooked rice, grits, macaroni, or spaghetti; 2 tbsp flour; 6 saltines; 1 6-inch tortilla

[a]For children up to 9, 2–3 cups; for children 9 to 12, 3–4 cups; for teenagers and pregnant women, 3–4 cups; for nursing mothers, 4 cups or more.
[b]One should be rich in vitamin C; at least one every other day should be rich in vitamin A.
[c]Enriched or whole-grain products only.

Table 9.E   The modified basic four food groups: A planning guide.

ANYTIME	IN MODERATION	NOW AND THEN
	BEANS, GRAINS, AND NUTS *(4 or more servings per day)*	
Bread and rolls (whole grain)	Cornbread[8]	Croissant[4, 8]
Bulgur	Flour tortilla[8]	Doughnut[3 or 4, 5, 8]
Dried beans and peas	Granola cereals[1 or 2]	Presweetened cereals[5, 8]
Lentils	Hominy grits[8]	Sticky buns[1 or 2, 5, 8]
Oatmeal	Macaroni and cheese[1, (6), 8]	Stuffing (with butter)[4, (6), 8]
Pasta, whole-wheat	Matzoh[8]	
Rice, brown	Nuts[3]	
Sprouts	Pasta, refined[8]	
Whole-grain hot and cold cereals	Peanut butter[3]	
Whole-wheat matzoh	Pizza[6, 8]	
	Refined, unsweetened cereals[8]	
	Refried beans[1 or 2]	
	Seeds[3]	
	Soybeans[2]	
	Tofu[2]	
	Waffles or pancakes with syrup[5, (6),8]	
	White bread and rolls[8]	
	White rice[8]	

[1]Moderate fat, saturated.
[2]Moderate fat, unsaturated.
[3]High fat, unsaturated.
[4]High fat, saturated.
[5]High in added sugar.
[6]High in salt or sodium
[(6)]May be high in salt or sodium.
[7]High in cholesterol.
[8]Refined grains.

(Continued)

Table 9.E   The modified basic four food groups: A planning guide. *(Continued)*

ANYTIME	IN MODERATION	NOW AND THEN
	FRUITS AND VEGETABLES *(4 or more servings per day)*	
All fruits and vegetables except those at right Applesauce (unsweetened) Unsweetened fruit juices Unsalted vegetable juices Potatoes, white or sweet	Avocado[3] Cole slaw[3] Cranberry sauce[5] Dried fruit French fries[1 or 2] Fried eggplant[2] Fruits canned in syrup[5] Gazpacho[2,(6)] Glazed carrots[5,(6)] Guacamole[3] Potatoes au gratin[1,(6)] Salted vegetable juices[6] Sweetened fruit juices[5] Vegetables canned with salt[6]	Coconut[4] Pickles[6]
	MILK PRODUCTS *(3 to 4 servings per day for children, 2 for adults)*	
Buttermilk (from skim milk) Low-fat cottage cheese Low-fat milk (1%) Low-fat yogurt Nonfat dry milk Skim-milk cheeses Skim milk Skim-milk and banana shake	Cocoa with skim milk[5] Cottage cheese, regular[1] Frozen yogurt[5] Ice milk[5] Low-fat milk (2%)[1] Low-fat yogurt, sweetened[5] Mozzarella, part-skim[1,(6)]	Cheesecake[4,5] Cheese fondue[4,(6)] Cheese soufflé[4,(6),7] Eggnog[1,5,7] Hard cheeses: blue, brick, Camembert, cheddar, muenster, Swiss[4,(6)] Ice cream[4,5] Processed cheeses[4,6] Whole milk[4] Whole-milk yogurt[4]
	POULTRY, FISH, MEAT, AND EGGS *(2 servings per day; vegetarians should eat added servings from other groups)*	
Cod Flounder Gefilte fish[(6)] Haddock Halibut Perch Pollock Rockfish Shellfish, except shrimp Sole Tuna, water-packed[(6)] Egg whites Chicken or turkey, boiled, baked, or roasted (no skin)	Fried fish[1 or 2] Herring[3,6] Mackerel, canned[2,(6)] Salmon, canned[2,(6)] Sardines[2,(6)] Shrimp[7] Tuna, oil-packed[2,(6)] Chicken liver[7] Fried chicken in vegetable oil (homemade)[3] Chicken or turkey, boiled, baked, or roasted (with skin)[2] Flank steak[1] Leg or loin of lamb[1] Pork shoulder or loin, lean[1] Round steak or ground round[1] Rump roast[1] Sirloin steak, lean[1] Veal[1]	Fried chicken, commercial[4] Cheese omelet[4,7] Whole egg or yolk (limit to 3 a week)[3,7] Bacon[4,(6)] Beef liver, fried[1,7] Bologna[4,6] Corned beef[4,6] Ground beef[4] Ham, trimmed[1,6] Hot dogs[4,6] Liverwurst[4,6] Pig's feet[4] Salami[4,6] Sausage[4,6] Spareribs[4] Red meats, untrimmed[4]

Reprinted from *The New American Eating Guide,* which is available from the Center for Science in the Public Interest, 1501 16th St., N.W., Washington, D.C. 20036 for $3.95. © 1981.

foods rich in these minerals or consider taking a supplement in order to get the amounts recommended.

Dietary Guidelines for Americans

Since 1977, when the U.S. Dietary Goals were issued in the hope of reducing the incidence of chronic disease, recommendations have been developed to provide some guidance in reaching these goals. These recommendations, called *Dietary Guidelines for Americans*, are listed in Table 9.F. An easy way to follow most of these guidelines is simply to choose the majority of foods you eat from the "anytime" column of the

---

Table 9.F Dietary guidelines for Americans.

- Eat a variety of foods.
- Maintain ideal weight.
- Avoid a lot of fat, saturated fat, and cholesterol.
- Avoid a lot of sodium and salt.
- Avoid a lot of sugar.
- Eat foods with starch and fiber.
- Drink only moderate amounts of alcohol.

Nutrition and Your Health: Dietary Guidelines for Americans.
Home and Garden Bulletin #232, U.S. Dept. of Agriculture,
USDHHS, February 1980.

Modified Basic Four Plan in Table 9.E. More specific suggestions for adding starch and fiber to the diet and avoiding too much fat, cholesterol, sugar, alcohol, and salt were presented in Chapter 8. Combining these suggestions with the recommended food selections from the Modified Basic Four produces a diet plan that provides the RDAs you need and minimizes risk of major chronic diseases. This plan emphasizes consumption of fruits, vegetables, and grains accompanied by smaller amounts of lean meats and dairy products, and very limited quantities of high fat foods such as gravies, baked goods, dressings, and alcohol. A visual representation of this diet plan is presented in Figure 9.2.

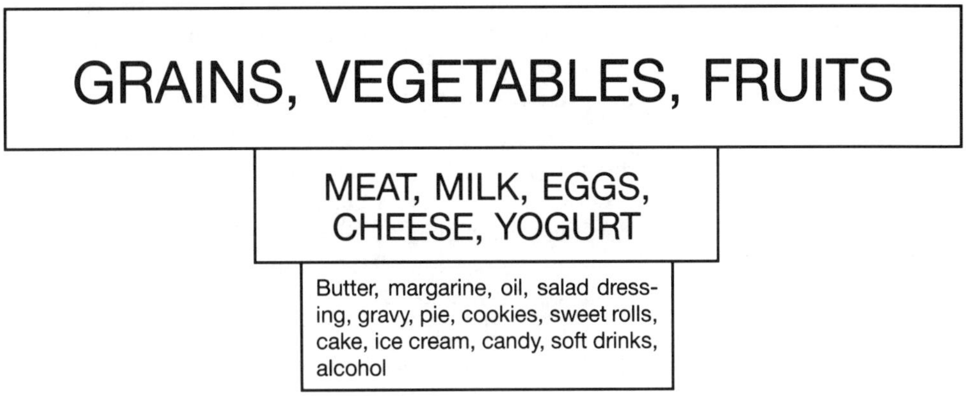

GRAINS, VEGETABLES, FRUITS

MEAT, MILK, EGGS, CHEESE, YOGURT

Butter, margarine, oil, salad dressing, gravy, pie, cookies, sweet rolls, cake, ice cream, candy, soft drinks, alcohol

FIGURE 9.2
Visual representation of a diet plan that supplies RDAs but minimizes chronic disease risk.

Getting the Most From Your Food

Deciding what foods are best to eat is only part of the diet planning job. How often you eat, what you buy at the store, and how you prepare it all influence the nutrients you get from food. The following information may help you with these choices.

Three Meals or More

If your food intake record indicated no intake until after 5:00 P.M., it's possible that you aren't as well nourished as your analysis indicates. The body simply doesn't handle large amounts of nutrients very well. For example, you may recall that the absorption rate for iron is very low when a large amount is supplied all at once, but is much higher when only small amounts are available. The recommendation is to eat small amounts of iron throughout the day. This recommendation also applies to consuming sources of complete protein. Small, frequent meals are recommended, too, as a means of controlling weight and body fat. In essence, the body makes best use of food when you provide it in small amounts, a minimum of 3 times per day or preferably four to six. Eating in relation to your activity pattern also seems to help the body use food better. If you are more active during the day, that's when to eat most of your food. "Breakfast like a king, lunch like a prince, and dinner like a pauper" seems to be the best advice though most people do not eat this way. If you can move just a little in that direction, you will be doing a better job of eating to enhance yourself.

Shopping, Health-Wise

Getting the most for your money is every consumer's goal. To do it, however, generally requires some knowledgeable shopping. In this regard, food shopping creates some heavy demands. When you walk into a supermarket, you are faced with 5,000 to 10,000 items from which to choose. Some general guidelines are offered here to help you make the most nutritious selections.

1. Start reading labels. Ingredients are listed in descending order according to the amount in the product. Decide if the first several ingredients are basically what you want to get from that product. If not, don't buy it or check another brand. It might have more of what you want.

Some descriptions you might find on a product label and what they mean include:

Low Calorie: Contains no more than 40 calories per serving.

Sugar Free: Contains no sucrose, but may have other sweeteners such as fructose, corn syrup, honey, sorbitol, mannitol, molasses, or artificial sweeteners.

Fortified: Supplemental vitamins and minerals have been added. (This does *not* mean you can get all 47 nutrients from this product.)

Enriched: Some, *but not all*, of the ingredients lost in processing have been added back into the product.

Very Low Sodium: Contains 35 mg. or less/serving.

Low Sodium: Contains 140 mg or less/serving.

Reduced Sodium: Normal sodium content reduced by 75%.

Crude Fiber: A measure of fiber content in food. "Dietary fiber" is a new and better measure of this. One gram of crude fiber equals two to three grams of dietary fiber.

2. When buying cereals, breads, and other grain products, choose those that list "whole grain" as the first ingredient rather than refined or bleached ingredients. You will get more vitamins and minerals. For the same reason, choose "enriched" over "unenriched," "stoneground" grain over any other form, and brown rice over white.

3. Choose fresh fruits and vegetables over canned. Frozen are your next best choice, and perhaps your best choice if you can't shop very often. Fresh produce can lose significant amounts of vitamins if stored in the refrigerator for several days. To minimize losses, refrigerate produce in moisture-proof bags, or at least in the vegetable crisper section. When buying fresh produce, select the fruits and vegetables that are darkest in their natural color. Dark greens and deep yellows, oranges, and reds offer the most vitamin A.

4. Buy fresh meats if you can, but frozen meats, fish, and poultry offer similar nutrient content *if* they have been wrapped well.

Cooking It Right For You

How food is cooked can also significantly influence the nutrients you get. The concern here is largely with loss of water soluble vitamins, but increasing nutrient content is also a possibility. For example, frying food will markedly increase its caloric content. And using iron pots and pans will add some iron to the foods you prepare in them.

To minimize loss of water soluble vitamins in cooking, try the following suggestions:

1. Minimize exposure of foods to water; the B and C vitamins dissolve in it.
   a. Don't soak vegetables to wash or store them.
   b. Use as little water as possible in cooking and cook for the shortest time possible.
   c. If cooking time is prolonged as in braising or stewing meat, try to use the broth in some way, e.g., for soup or in dressing.
   d. Cook vegetables whole if possible. The more you cut them up, the greater the vitamin loss.
2. The best cooking methods for preserving vitamins are pressure cooking, steaming, boiling, poaching, and stewing. Although significant vitamin loss occurs with the last three of these because of the water exposure, using the broths recaptures the vitamins.

   Microwave cooking, oven broiling, roasting, and frying do less damage to vitamins than braising or stewing (if you can't or won't reuse the broth), but frying so significantly adds fat and calories to the diet that it just can't be recommended.

   It is thought that charcoal broiling or barbecuing may add carcinogens to foods through the smoke and/or flames. Wrapping foods in foil or placing them in a pan to protect them from the smoke and flames can eliminate this problem, but may also reduce desired flavors. A compromise would be to raise the grill higher above the flames or coals and cook foods more slowly.

3. Over-cooking meats causes loss of the B Vitamin, thiamin, (unless the broth is eaten), and can decrease the availability of certain amino acids.

4. Prepare salads as close as possible to the time they'll be eaten. This will preserve Vitamin C.

Deciding About Supplements

At this point you may be thinking, "This is just too much to bother with! I'll just take a supplement to make sure I'm getting what I need." While it's possible you might need a supplement, there are several problems with assuming that supplements can be substitutes for food. The first problem is a practical one: there simply isn't a supplement on the market that contains all the nutrients you need. That creates the problem of trying to buy some or all of the nutrients you need individually and then combining them in the appropriate dosages so you're not getting too much of one or too little of another. Too much of one nutrient might interfere with absorption or utilization of another. Too little of another nutrient might make it worthless, or render another nutrient unusable, and so on! This description is meant to sound confusing and complex because that's the situation regarding supplements today. Not even the experts can tell you how to use supplements in place of a good diet because the information simply isn't available. Anyone who claims such knowledge is deliberately or unintentionally misrepresenting the "state of the art" in nutrition.

Experimentation is on-going, of course, not only in regard to what we need to function, but also in terms of possibly curing disease. In some research, the effects of megadoses of vitamins and minerals (ten or more times the known or assumed requirement) are being examined, but there is no hard evidence from which to derive safe recommendations at this time. In fact, these studies are generally indicating that all vitamins and minerals can be toxic in large enough doses. Anyone who chooses to take such large amounts sporadically or on a regular basis is taking a risk.

The truth is there is relatively little information about how much of the different nutrients the body needs, what combinations promote the greatest utilization of what is consumed, and exactly when the body needs what. It is clear, however, that all the nutrients the body requires are present in foods. It is also known which foods contain a lot of nutrients and which contain only a few. This is the knowledge base behind the recommendation to eat a variety of high quality foods in moderation throughout the day. With the help of diet planning guides like the Modified Basic Four Food Groups, eating becomes far easier and certainly a more pleasurable way to try to meet nutritional needs than relying on supplements. Thus, the important points regarding supplements are:

1. There is just no adequate replacement for food for obtaining the necessary vitamins and minerals; and

2. The word supplement means "added to," not "substituted for"!

There are those, however, who may need to supplement nutrients in their diets. Some of these people were identified in Chapter 8, during discussions of the individual nutrients. Also, a detailed list of conditions that might cause a person to require supplementation was given in Table 9.A. The more common of these conditions are summarized in Table 9.G, accompanied by suggestions of the vitamins or minerals probably needed. If you find yourself described in the list in Table 9.A or Table 9.G, you may need a supplement of vitamins and/or minerals. Your safest action would be to take a supplement that provides no more than the recommended amount of the nutrient(s) you need. If you think more than that would be better, take some time to find out what is known about the effects of large amounts of that vitamin or mineral before using yourself as a guinea pig. Some reliable sources to consult were listed in Table 8.L.

The seriousness of some of the conditions listed in Tables 9.A and 9.G warrants some additional comment. Excessive drinking, anorexia/bulimia, extreme fad diets (such as liquid protein formulas), and very low calorie diets or fasting are more than just nutritional problems; they are, in fact, potentially life-threatening. A vitamin/mineral supplement may help offset some of the negative effects of such nutritional problems, but it certainly won't solve the problem. The most important action you can take if you are experiencing one or more of these problems is to seek professional help. Contacting Alcoholics Anonymous, Eating Disorders Groups, Overeaters Anonymous, or Weight Watchers will make a good starting point. The people involved with these groups have all struggled with similar problems. They can provide support, information, and direction in locating additional sources of help as needed.

Table 9.G   Situations in which supplements are useful.

The following are common conditions in which vitamin supplements—or an increased consumption of vitamin-rich foods—are valuable.

1. *Pregnancy and breast-feeding* increase a woman's vitamin requirements. A multi-formula tablet with iron guarantees meeting these needs. In fact, all women of child-bearing age need extra iron, whether from foods or supplements.
2. *Oral contraceptives* lower bloodstream vitamin levels by disrupting the body's ability to utilize B vitamins (particularly niacin and B_6). Some physicians recommend a B-complex tablet to counter this.
3. *Smoking* depletes vitamin C supplies by as much as 30 percent, which can be harmful, depending upon dietary habits. A small supplement (100 mg.) will be enough to compensate.
4. *Dieting* reduces overall vitamin intake, at times dangerously, and this is especially true for the fad diets and very low calorie diets. Unless the diet is nutritionally balanced (an example is Weight Watchers), multi-vitamin tablets are needed.
5. *Alcohol* can disrupt diet. Multi-tablets (especially those high in B-complex vitamins, which absorb alcohol) may prevent serious physical damage.
6. *Caffeine,* taken in large quantities from coffee, tea, or cola drinks, causes the body to flush out the water-soluble vitamins more rapidly. Small daily supplements of the B-complex and C vitamins will replenish supplies.
7. *Vegetarians* who eat no animal products at all need a supplement of vitamin B_{12}.

Adapted from *Consumer Digest*, July/August 1981.

Summary

Nutritional studies indicate that the average American needs to change some of his/her eating habits in order to enjoy optimum vitality and longevity. Unfortunately, most people don't really know if they are eating better or worse or the same as the "average" person. You can, however, determine how well you are eating and if you should consider making changes by comparing your diet to nutritional recommendations. The techniques and procedures to help you do this type of dietary analysis are described in this chapter. The steps involved in conducting your personal dietary analysis include: (1) keeping a food diary of everything you eat, and the amounts, for at least a 24 hour period (three days or an entire week would provide greater accuracy); (2) recording all activities and calculating energy expenditure for the same day or days the food diary is kept; (3) determining if calories consumed balance with calories expended and, if not, the probable impact on your weight over time; and (4) comparing the nutrient content of the food you ate with the Recommended Dietary Allowances for your sex and age group and with the U.S. Dietary Goals for protein, fat, and carbohydrate intake.

Guidelines for eating well are offered to help those whose diet analyses were less than optimal and those wishing to refine good nutritional habits. A modified version of the Basic Four Food Group Plan and the Dietary Guidelines for Americans is recommended as a guide for selecting foods that provide the required nutrients while helping you avoid excessive fat, cholesterol, sugar, alcohol, and salt.

Since getting the most from the food you do select for your diet can depend upon when you eat it and your shopping and cooking skills, some guidelines are also offered regarding these practices. Eating smaller meals, three times or more a day, allows the body to make the best use of food. Eating in relation to your activity pattern is also helpful in this regard.

Shopping skills that promote a healthier diet include careful reading of labels for major ingredients and such added features as "fortified," "enriched," and "low sodium"; buying whole grain products; and choosing fresh vegetables, fruits, and meats whenever possible.

How you cook food can significantly influence its nutrient content. Frying markedly increases the caloric content of any food. Prolonged cooking in water generally causes major losses of C and B vitamins. Recommended cooking techniques include pressure cooking, steaming, baking, poaching, and stewing. The last three of these do cause significant vitamin losses, but these can be regained if the broth is used, as in a soup.

Regarding vitamin and mineral supplementation, remember that *there is no adequate replacement for food for obtaining all the vitamins and minerals you need.* Among those people who may *need* to supplement nutrients in their diets are those people who consume very low calorie diets, drink excessive amounts of alcohol, have been ill for a prolonged period, and/or take oral contraceptives. The safest choice is a supplement that provides no more than the recommended amount of the needed nutrient(s).

Probably the two most important dietary practices to begin following right away, if you currently don't, are (1) eat small amounts often, and (2) avoid fatty foods.

FORM 1.   CALORIC INTAKE RECORD

Directions: Keep a 24-hour diary of all foods and beverages consumed. Be specific as to type, method of preparation and quantity. For mixed dishes, estimate amount of each ingredient. Check package labels or *Nutritive Value of Foods* (Appendix 8) to assess calorie content. Include all butter, dressings, mayonnaise, etc.

FOOD ITEM	QUANTITY (tsp, cup, oz)	CALORIES	TOTALS

Breakfast
_____ _____ _____
_____ _____ _____
_____ _____ _____
_____ _____ _____
_____ _____ _____
_____ _____ _____

Breakfast Total: _____

Snack
_____ _____ _____
_____ _____ _____
_____ _____ _____

Snack Total: _____

Lunch
_____ _____ _____
_____ _____ _____
_____ _____ _____
_____ _____ _____
_____ _____ _____
_____ _____ _____

Lunch Total: _____

Snack
_____ _____ _____
_____ _____ _____
_____ _____ _____

Snack Total: _____

Dinner
_____ _____ _____
_____ _____ _____
_____ _____ _____
_____ _____ _____
_____ _____ _____
_____ _____ _____
_____ _____ _____
_____ _____ _____

Dinner Total: _____

Snack
_____ _____ _____
_____ _____ _____
_____ _____ _____

Snack Total: _____

DAILY TOTAL: _____

FORM 2. CALORIC EXPENDITURE RECORD

Directions: Keep a 24-hour diary of your activities. Be sure to include sleeping and sitting so that your records show the full 24 hours. Find calories expended per activity (Appendix 6). Add calorie column to find daily totals.

	ACTIVITY	LENGTH OF TIME	CALORIES EXPENDED
Morning			
Afternoon			
Evening			
Night			

TOTAL HRS = 24   Daily Calorie Total _____

FORM 3. NUTRIENT COMPONENTS OF FOODS

Make a nutritional evaluation of foods consumed during a 24-hour period. List food, precise amount and quantity of each component listed below.
Use *Nutritive Value of Foods* (Appendix 8) for nutrient quantities. Add columns to find daily totals.

(A) Food	(B) Approx. Measure or Weight	(D) Food Energy (Calories)	(E) Protein (gm)	(F) Fat (gm)	(J) Carbo- hydrate (gm)	(K) Calcium (mg)	(M) Iron (mg)	(O) Vitamin A (I.U.)	(P) Thiamin (mg)	(Q) Ribo- flavin (mg)	(R) Niacin (mg)	(S) Ascorbic Acid (Vit. C) (mg)
TOTALS												

FORM 4.   CALORIC BALANCE COMPUTATION SHEET

Directions: Refer to caloric intake record and caloric expenditure record for determining energy balance and body weight change.

A.   Total calories consumed in 24 hour period: _____ Cal.

B.   Total calories expended in 24 hour period: _____ Cal.

C.   Caloric balance (difference between A and B): _____ Cal.

D.   Indicate whether negative (expenditure greater than intake) or positive (intake greater than expenditure) caloric balance.

    Circle One: Negative   Positive

E.   Weight change should take place at a rate of 1 pound for every 3500 calories in excess or deficit. A negative balance produces weight loss while a positive balance yields weight gain. If this 24 hour calorie pattern would continue unchanged, the following body weight changes could be expected:

   1. Weekly weight change $\dfrac{\text{(Caloric Balance)} \times 7}{3500}$ = _____ lbs.

   2. Monthly weight change $\dfrac{\text{(Caloric Balance)} \times 30}{3500}$ = _____ lbs.

   3. Annual weight change $\dfrac{\text{(Caloric Balance)} \times 365}{3500}$ = _____ lbs.

F.   List two modifications you could make in your eating and activity patterns and project the effect of each on weight for a period of one year.

$$\text{lbs./year} = \frac{(\text{cal/wk} \times 52)}{3500}$$

  1. Eating Modifications:

Food	Calories	Servings/Wk	Cal/Wk		
_____	_____	_____	_____	=	_____ lbs/yr
_____	_____	_____	_____	=	_____ lbs/yr

  2. Activity Modifications:

Activity	Time	Calories	Periods/Wk	Cal/Wk		
_____	_____	_____	_____	_____	=	_____ lbs/yr
_____	_____	_____	_____	_____	=	_____ lbs/yr

FORM 5.   PERCENT OF CALORIES FROM PROTEIN, FAT AND CARBOHYDRATE

The contribution which protein, fat and carbohydrates make toward total caloric intake is an important health consideration. Typical American diets are quite high in fat (40%-45% of total calories). Recommendations from the U.S. Senate Select Committee on Nutrition and Human Needs are 12% protein, 30% fat and 58% carbohydrates.

Directions: Use the following formula and example to assist you in computing your own percentages:

$$\text{PERCENT OF TOTAL CALORIES} = \left(\frac{\text{calories from energy nutrient}}{\text{TOTAL CALORIES}}\right)100$$

Example: A diet of 100 grams protein (4 cal/gm), 145 grams fat (9 cal/gm) and 300 grams carbohydrates (4 cal/gm) is evaluated as follows:

calories from protein	= 100 × 4 = 400 calories
calories from fat	= 145 × 9 = 1305 calories
calories from carbohydrates	= 300 × 4 = 1200 calories
TOTAL CALORIES = 2905	

$$\text{percent from protein} = \left(\frac{400}{2905}\right)100 = 13.77\%$$

$$\text{percent from fat} = \left(\frac{1305}{2905}\right)100 = 44.92\%$$

$$\text{percent from carbohydrates} = \left(\frac{1200}{2905}\right)100 = 41.31\%$$

Make computations using your data from the previous page.

Grams of protein _____, Grams of fat _____, Grams of carbohydrates _____

calories from protein	=	_____
calories from fat	=	_____
calories from carbohydrates	=	_____
percent from protein	=	_____
percent from fat	=	_____
percent from carbohydrates	=	_____

How do your percentages compare to recommendations of the U.S. Senate Select Committee? Rate your diet as "equal," "over," or "below" for each nutrient.

	PROTEIN	FAT	CARBOHYDRATE
U.S. Dietary Goals	12%	30%	58%
Your Diet	%	%	%
Your Rating			

FORM 6.   CHOLESTEROL — SATURATED FAT INDEX (CSI)

Daily total of: A.   Saturated Fat _____ grams (g.)

B.   Cholesterol _____ milligrams (mg.)

Formula: CSI = Saturated Fat (1.01) + Cholesterol (.05)

= _____ g. (1.01) + _____ mg. (.05)

CSI for Daily Intake: = _____

RISK OF CARDIOVASCULAR DISEASE

	Low Risk "Healthy" Diet	High Risk Average American Diet
Women & Children	CSI = 16–19	CSI = 51–60
Men & Teenagers	CSI = 23–26	CSI = 69–82

From Connors, S. & Connors, W. *The New American Diet: The Lifetime Family Eating Plan for Good Health.* Simon & Schuster, 1986.

FORM 7.   COMPARISON OF NUTRIENT INTAKE TO RDA'S

Directions: Compare your daily intake of nutrients to the recommended dietary allowances listed for your sex and age in Appendix 7. Note foods which were consumed and could be consumed that provide high levels of each nutrient.

	Calories	Protein (gm)	Calcium (mg)	Iron (mg)	Vitamin A (I.U.)	Thiamin (Vit. B_1) (mg)	Riboflavin (Vit. B_2) (mg)	Niacin (mg)	Ascorbic Acid (Vit. C) (mg)
Daily Total of nutrients in your 24 hour period									
Recommended Daily Allowance (RDA)									
Evaluation of your totals ("Below" "Equal" or "Above" the RDA)									
Food in your diet that is highest in each nutrient									
List another food in each column which would add significantly to that nutrient.									

References

Andresky, J. 1985. *Vitamins in nutrition and health*. Englewood, CO: Morton Publishing.

Brody, J. 1981. *Jane Brody's nutrition book*. New York: Bantam.

Calories and weight: U.S.D.A. pocket guide. 1970. U.S. Department of Agriculture. *Department of Health & Human Services Home and Garden Bulletin #153*. Washington, D.C.: Government Printing Office.

Diet, nutrition and cancer prevention: A guide to food choices. 1984. Public Health Service. Department of Health & Human Services. NIH publication #85-2711. Washington, D.C.: Government Printing Office.

Dietary goals for the United States, 2nd ed. 1977. Select Committee on Nutrition & Human Needs, U.S. Senate. Washington, D.C.: Government Printing Office.

Dietary guidelines for Americans. 1980. U.S. Department of Agriculture, Department of Health & Human Services. Home & Garden Bulletin #232. Washington, D.C.: Government Printing Office.

Dubick, M. and Rucker, R. 1983. Dietary supplements and health aids: A critical evaluation. *Journal of Nutrition Education* 15 (2 and 3).

Dusek, D. 1982. *Thin and fit: Your personal lifestyle*. Belmont, CA: Wadsworth.

Guthrie, H. 1986. *Introductory nutrition*. St. Louis, MO: C. V. Mosby Publishing.

Hui, Y. 1985. *Principles and issues in nutrition*. Monterey, CA: Wadsworth.

Hunter, B. 1985. Risky cooking practices: Don't get burned. *Consumer's Research* 68(May):29.

King, J. et al. 1978. Evaluation and modification of the basic four food guide. *Journal of Nutrition Education* 10:27.

Marshall, G. 1985. *Vitamins and minerals: Help or harm?* Philadelphia, PA: George F. Stickley.

New American eating guide. Washington, D.C.: Center for Science in the Public Interest.

Nutritive Value of Foods. 1981. U.S. *Department of Agriculture. Department of Health & Human Services Home and Garden Bulletin #72*. Washington, D.C.: Government Printing Office.

Recommended dietary allowances. 9th ed. 1980. Committee on Dietary Allowances, Food & Nutrition Board. Washington, D.C.: National Academy of Science.

Retkin, A. 1986. Eat like a peasant, feel like a king. American Health 5(March):37.

Rinzler, C. 1985. The chemistry of cooking. *American Health* 4(December):42.

Simko, M., Cowell, C. and Gilbride, J. 1984. *Nutrition assessment*. Rockville, MD: Aspen Systems.

Simonopoulos, A. 1982. Assessment of nutritional status. *American Journal of Clinical Nutrition* 35 (supplement), 1095.

Solomons, N. and Allen, L. 1983. Functional assessment of nutritional status: Principles, practice and potential. *Nutrition Reviews* 41:33.

The ABC's of taking supplements. 1985. *Tufts University Diet and Nutrition Letter* 3(May):7.

The ABC's of vitamins. 1981. *Consumer's Digest* 20(July)–August).

Vegetarianism: Can you get by without meat? 1980. *Consumer Reports* 45(June):357.

Whitney, E. and Hamilton, E. 1984. *Understanding nutrition*. 3d ed. New York: West Publishing.

Why sugar continues to concern nutritionists. 1985. *Tufts University Diet and Nutrition Letter* 3(May):3.

Wrap-up: Minerals. 1986. *University of California, Berkeley Wellness Letter* 2(January):4.

10

Stress and Stressors

What is stress?

What causes stress in your life?

What is the relationship between stress and illness?

Is stress always harmful?

Is the environment or your personality the more important cause of stress?

Introduction

This chapter presents an overview of stress, discussing how it is manifested in the body, the effect of stress on health, and the common causes of stress. The next chapter will present a well-rounded holistic stress management program. The basic components of the stress management program presented in these two chapters are outlined in Figure 10.1.

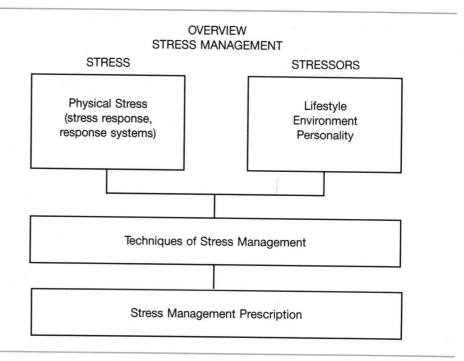

FIGURE 10.1
An overview of stress management.

Basic Definitions

Stress: The body reacting; the buildup of pressure, the strain of muscles tensing; psychophysiological arousal that can fatigue the body systems to the point of malfunction and disease.

Stressor: Any condition or event that causes a stress response. These may be physical, social, or psychological—including imagination.

Stress management: Understanding of the stress response; recognition of stressors; development of stress reduction skills; and the regular incorporation of these into one's lifestyle.

The difficulty in studying and managing stress is that it permeates every aspect of life. Physically, the body responds to stress in a variety of ways. However, the physical effects of stress are influenced by behavior, which in turn is determined by factors such as psychology, emotions, personality, social learning, and habituation. Philosophical and spiritual influences also play a role in the development of and response to stress.

Defining stress as one-dimensional (physical, social, etc.) is limiting. The definition of stress should be holistic and include the physical domain as well as the social, psychological, and philosophical domains. If one starts with a holistic definition of stress, the management of stress will more likely be holistic and include the same four domains.

Physical Stress

In physical terms, *stress* means strain, pressure, or force on a system. In the context of the human organism it describes the effects of the body reacting to the environment through the buildup of internal pressure and the strain of muscles tensing for action. When we discuss stress we rely on the basic premise that in the final analysis stress is *physical*. It is the physical pressure and strain which, if prolonged, can fatigue or damage the body to the point at which health is adversely affected. However, the concept of stress as a physical phenomena needs further elaboration.

Stress is physical in nature. It is a natural defense mechanism that has allowed our species to survive. Without it we would not survive even the relatively tame world in which most of us live today. Stress is a physical response to protect our physical lives. We need stress and do not want to, nor can we, eradicate our stress response. The goal is to *manage* our stress by diminishing the *excess* stress in our lives—the stress that is inappropriate for accomplishing our objectives. To illustrate this point, allow yourself to imagine a cave man with a club in his hand, dripping with blood, and a slain sabertooth tiger in the background. Your imaginary X-ray vision allows you to view inside the man's stomach, which reveals a peaceful scene representative of a calm state. Now picture modern man or woman in a business suit, clenched jaw, squinting eyes, forehead furrowed, and shaking a fist at his/her boss in the background. Your ability to see inside the stomach shows a raging inferno, indicative of pressure. The principle of an appropriate stress response becomes clear. Cave man was able to handle, or dissipate, his stress more appropriately because when he was aroused by fear for his life he battled with the tiger to kill or be killed. Or, he could choose to run and escape with his life. Either option resulted in the use and dissolution of his internal stress buildup.

Walter B. Cannon defined stress as the "fight or flight syndrome." He noted that when one becomes stressed, the proper use of that stress is to either fight off the threat or run from it. In order to do either, the body prepares itself through a myriad of physiological mechanisms, and the mechanisms endowed to modern humans are the same as those used by our cave-dwelling ancestors. The difference is that in our modern society our options for dissipating stress usually do not include a physical response. In our imagined scene, the "threat" was the boss. We cannot hit the boss with a club, or shout angrily at him/her. We cannot "run" from the threat, and in many cases we can not even talk about our grievances. Nonetheless, the stress response has been activated. Pressure builds up, half the muscles strain to strike out, the other half strain to hold back our natural response. Externally, nothing happens. Internally, the body is a raging inferno of stress and tension.

The stress response of modern man and woman is often inappropriate to the situation and inappropriate in its level of intensity. While physical stressors still exist, most often the stresses of modern society are primarily ego or social related. When stress is ego related or is in response to a social situation, it cannot be solved by a physical response. Additionally, these stressors may not be alleviated for long periods

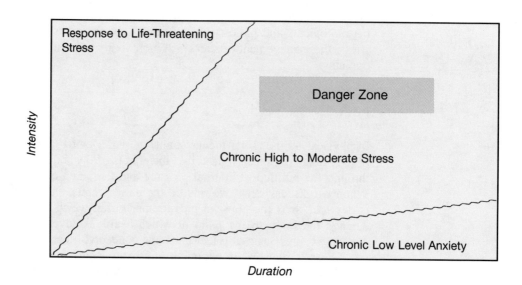

FIGURE 10.2
The relationship
between intensity and
duration in the stress
response.

of time. The stress response described above is thus inappropriate for the degree of threat involved; in addition, it is also innapropriate in intensity, which refers to the magnitude and duration of the stress. Figure 10.2 depicts the intensity–duration relationship.

In Figure 10.2 the zone labeled "Response to Life-Threatening Stress" illustrates the appropriate use of the stress response. This means that such intense stress is at times necessary, and is usually not detrimental to one's health unless repeated too often. After an intense response, the elevated physiological parameters usually drop to normal within twenty-four to forty-eight hours. The stressors that might stimulate such an intense response include a very strenuous bout of exercise, a physical attack, an automobile accident or near miss, or a medical procedure that involved harsh drugs or surgery. The stress goes up during the event, it comes down afterwards, and then it is gone.

The other extreme, labeled "Chronic Low Level Anxiety" in Figure 10.2, is characterized by a low level anxiety that persists, but to such a low degree it is tolerated by the body. The "Danger Zone" is the moderate to moderately high intensity of stress response that persists over a long period of time. It is this ongoing intensity of stress that results in system fatigue, system breakdown, and eventual health problems.

The explanation of physical stress would not be complete without the presentation of another basic concept first presented by the father of the modern study of stress, Hans Selye. The concept is that of *Eustress,* which is positive, action-enhancing stress, and *Distress,* which is negative, debilitating, or harmful stress. *Optimal stress* is a point between eustress and distress. At this point the stress is intense enough to motivate and physically prepare one to perform optimally yet not intense enough to cause the body to overreact, to become confused, or to sustain harmful effects. Figure 10.3, an often-seen diagram of optimal stress, illustrates this concept.

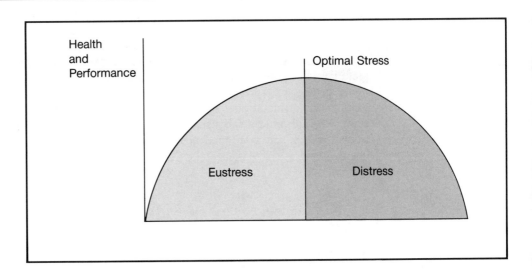

FIGURE 10.3
The point of optimal stress.

Eustress helps us overcome lethargy. It is what gives the athlete the competitive edge and the public speaker the enthusiasm to project optimally. Distress produces overreaction, confusion, poor concentration, performance and test anxiety, and usually results in a generally below par performance. Prolonged distress moves the organism into the health danger zone discussed previously.

An optimal level of stress may be defined as the point at which stress increases health and performance. Distress or overload begins when stress continues to increase and performance begins to suffer. At this point, though this effect may be difficult to recognize, health also begins to suffer. This brings us to the next major concept in the study of stress, which concerns recognizing the signs and symptoms of stress arousal.

One of the primary goals of this chapter is to increase your awareness of what stress is and how it affects you. The best way to find and use your optimal stress level and, conversely, to recognize and prevent debilitating distress is to develop the ability to recognize the signs and symptoms of distress and then reduce them. While that sounds simple enough, in actuality it isn't. The human organism characteristically becomes accustomed to its level of arousal, which after a period of time becomes the body's normal state. In other words, people become immune to their stress arousal if it lasts for a period of time (a few weeks). This is because the body's sensitivity to the awareness of stress arousal may become dulled. However, lack of awareness does not mean the effects of the stress arousal are any less problematic.

The solution to this problem is to increase your sensitivity to the signs of distress. It can be said that stress is a phenomenon that is unique to each individual. The final product, "your stress arousal," is unique to you. That uniqueness lies in the particular stress symptoms you happen to manifest. Researchers in the field of psychophysiology have identified hundreds of physiological and behavioral effects of excessive stress arousal, and the ones you experience represent your unique pattern of response. Some people always respond with the same system, such as the muscle system. Every time they become stressed they get the same type of tension headache or a spasm in the same muscle. For reasons not well understood at this time, their muscle system has become sensitized, and has become their depot for storage of excess nervous impulses.

Those individuals who respond to stress with the same predictable kind of stress response in one or two systems of their body are referred to as *rigid responders*. Others who do not respond in such a predictable pattern are referred to as *random responders*.

It is hoped that this discussion will motivate you to increase your awareness of your own signs and symptoms of distress. To begin developing that awareness, complete Exercise I below, which illustrates some of the potential signs of arousal in three major categories. Check the symptoms you usually experience and then list (on the lines provided) additional symptoms you may also experience. When these signs or symptoms are present this usually means you have gone beyond the optimal point of stress arousal and continued arousal will be detrimental to your performance and health.

The Stress Response

The signs and symptoms of stress arousal occur when a physiological system of the body becomes excessively stimulated. The normal functioning of a particular system has been altered and if the condition persists for an extended period of time damage may result. Prolonged over-activation of an organ system can eventually fatigue that system and result in temporary or permanent pathological change or disease. Additionally, prolonged stimulation may alter resistance to disease.

The noted stress researcher Hans Selye observed the detrimental effects of stress arousal after he exposed laboratory animals to various stressors. Selye was among the first to recognize the relationship between stress and disease and he formulated a model that helped to illustrate the body's response to stress. This model has become known as the General Adaptation Syndrome (GAS). The three stages of the GAS are: (1) the alarm reaction, (2) the state of resistance, and (3) the stage of exhaustion (Selye 1956).

In the *alarm stage* the body shows generalized stress arousal. No specific organ system is affected, although most, and in some cases all, of the body systems show measurable changes.

The second stage, called the *resistance phase*, is marked by channeling the arousal into one or several organ systems. Some researchers describe this process as *adaptation to stress*. This is because the organism adapts to the stress arousal by "absorbing" the arousal in a less responsive or sensitive system. For example, stress arousal in some parts of the nervous or cardiovascular systems can produce life-threatening debilitation in a short period of time. The human body, which is programmed to survive, seems to channel the arousal into less sensitive systems, such as the muscular system, thereby reducing the immediate danger to the body. This is the concept of stress adaptation. However, Selye realized that this adaptation process can contribute to the development of stress-related illness. "Disease by adaptation" forms the basis of the modern concept of the psychosomatic disease process. The specific organ or system to which stress arousal has been channeled may eventually fatigue and malfunction. Chronic resistance may eventually diminish the ability of that system to function and disease will result. Your responses to Exercise 1 may indicate the systems in your body that are likely to be subjected to stress arousal and may become weakened.

EXERCISE I
Check if usually experienced.

Musculoskeletal Signs

_____ stiffness in neck
_____ fingers and hands tremble or shake
_____ twitch in muscles (specific muscle _____)
_____ difficulty standing still or sitting quietly
_____ stuttering or stammering speech
_____ frequent headaches (location on head _____)
_____ muscles feel tense (specific muscles _____)
_____ voice quivers
_____ nervous mannerisms; e.g., biting nails, pulling hair, tapping feet, etc.
_____ other _____

Visceral Signs

_____ heart pounding
_____ light headed or faint
_____ cold chills
_____ cold hands
_____ cold feet
_____ dry mouth
_____ profuse sweating (location _____)
_____ upset stomach
_____ sinking feeling in stomach
_____ frequent digestive disturbance
_____ moist or sweaty palms
_____ flushed or hot face
_____ other _____

Mood and Disposition

_____ preoccupied
_____ frequent insomnia
_____ feeling uneasy or uncomfortable
_____ nervous or shaky
_____ feel confused
_____ forgetful
_____ feel insecure
_____ overexcited
_____ feel angry
_____ irritated
_____ worried
_____ anxious
_____ exhausted
_____ other _____

The resistance or adaptive process is limited, and exhaustion may eventually occur. This forms the basis of the third phase of the GAS called the *exhaustion phase*. The exhaustion of a weakened system may force another system to become involved in the resistance phase or the entire body may exhaust its ability to control the arousal and collapse. Usually the body can resist stress arousal for long periods of time. However, in the process of resisting, systems deteriorate. Systems such as the cardiovascular system become particularly vulnerable. Chronic heart disease, hypertension, and so on, can indicate exhaustion and result in death.

The Response Systems

Each one of the system responses discussed here is a natural response that is necessary for the fight or flight response. When taken to excess, especially when prolonged over a long period of time, the responses become debilitating. The specific ways in which long-term stress affects different systems are discussed below.

The Nervous System

The nervous system is the initiator of the complex and complete stress response, but it is also a response organ since stress increases neural excitability. A small amount of stress produces just enough arousal to get people "up," to get them excited, to really get them motivated to do what they have to do. Too much stress makes them jittery or nervous and often results in difficulty in concentrating and making decisions. Performance anxiety, the inability to make decisions, and/or emotions like fear and anger can cause further physiological stress. A vicious cycle develops when the physiological arousal of the nervous system causes increased anxiety and increased hostility, which in turn cause greater nervous system arousal.

The Muscular System

The system that most people associate with the effects of stress is the muscular system. There are two muscular systems in the body, the voluntary and the involuntary. The voluntary system is the one that allows us to move our muscles. Again, a slight increase in tension helps to improve performance because it gets our muscles ready to act. However, excessive muscle tension causes a variety of muscular problems, such as tension headaches, which are a widespread complaint in our society today. Tension headaches seem to be caused by increased muscle tension in the neck muscles, the muscles around the head, and especially the muscles of the upper back (the trapezius muscles). These are muscles that are involved in what is normally called the "defense posture." When people are threatened, they prepare themselves for battle, which causes them to tense up in readiness. Chronic "readiness" is usually not noticed until that tension causes a great deal of pain. Chronic tension headache and chronic muscle spasm are very common responses of the voluntary muscle system to stress.

The involuntary muscle system deals primarily with the gastrointestinal system. Changes in the tonus and mobility of the gastrointestinal system cause many difficulties. Problems include difficulty swallowing, and changes in the tonus of the colon that often result in diarrhea, constipation, and spastic colon. Stress problems in other involuntary muscle areas might include bronchial spasms, breathing difficulty, and perhaps stress-precipitated asthma attacks.

The Gastrointestinal System

In the stomach stress reactions cause an increase in hydrochloric acid and a decrease in the protective mucus which lines the stomach (and the small intestine). The mucus layer normally protects these areas from peptic enzymes and hydrochloric acid. Harold Wolf (1947) was one of the first individuals to study gastric response to stress, using a famous research subject named Tom. Through a natural hole in Tom's stomach, researchers were able to see that when Tom became aroused (especially when he was angered), blood filled the tissues in the lining of his stomach, the lining became frail, and at times hemorrhaging would even occur. It was easy to deduce that ulceration could and would occur as a result of these effects. Researchers also measured increases in the production of hydrochloric acid during times of stress.

Stress also causes changes in metabolic activity. For example, an overall mobilization of protein and fat occurs. The protein mobilization causes various difficulties; for example, if the stress reaction lasts over a prolonged period of time, there is a decrease in antibody production. If the situation is prolonged, the individual may have immune reaction difficulties and an increased susceptibility to normal viral and bacterial illnesses. Another aspect of protein mobilization is that of *muscle wasting*. Remember that the flight or fight response is an *immediate* reaction designed to save the individual's life *right now*. The body is not worried about what is going to happen later—it has to live through the stress event now. Therefore, available proteins are used to produce enzymes for metabolic activity, and very few go into the production of structure. Over time, such protein allocation causes overall muscle wasting.

Fat metabolism during the stress response is simply a mechanism for getting usable energy into the cells of the body. During a stress situation, glucose (which is normally available at some level to all body cells) is shunted into the central nervous system. This is because the central nervous system can burn only glucose, and fat must be mobilized so that cells of the body have something to burn. Since modern man rarely uses physical movement as a response to stress, this output of fat is not needed, and the fat circulates in the system until it is finally reabsorbed into storage tissue. Evidence shows that this circulating fat may be deposited along arterial walls in the development of atherosclerosis.

The Cardiovascular System

In the cardiovascular system, stress brings about an overall increase in activity. If you are going to run away or fight, you are going to need more blood, especially in the muscles. To accommodate this need, the heart rate increases. Individuals who are anxious and/or who have a higher level of chronic stress tend to have an increased heart rate, even at rest. In addition to increased heart rate, increases in stroke volume and cardiac output also occur, which means that there is more blood being pumped out of the heart with each beat. At the same time there is generalized vasoconstriction in the already busy cardiovascular system in order to get more blood to the muscles. This vasoconstriction increases blood pressure and may eventually be responsible for vascular headaches, exacerbation of atherosclerotic condition, and for aggravating diseases such as Raynaud's disease and Berger's disease.

Other Responses

Several other minor physiological responses occur during stress arousal. One is increased sodium retention, which can feed back and aggravate the increase in blood pressure. Another is increased neurological sweating in the areas of the underarms, the palms of the hands, and the soles of the feet. If these areas are constantly wet, it is a sign that you are responding to a situation with anxiety or stress.

The Causes of Stress: Stressors

Why does a person become stressed? What are the causes? How does one's personality influence his or her stress arousal? For each person the answers to these questions are different. The causes of stress are unique—that is even though there are a dozen common causes of stress, your response is unique depending upon your stressors and how they interact with your personality and are affected by your lifestyle.

STRESS = ENVIRONMENT/LIFESTYLE + PERSONALITY

In this stress equation lifestyle, personality, and environment are all variables. The table below outlines the factors that make up these general categories of stressors for each of us. The rest of this chapter is devoted to discussions of each of these factors.

Table 10.A The major classification of stressors.

LIFESTYLE/ PSYCHOSOCIAL	PERSONALITY	ENVIRONMENT
Adaptation	Self-concept	Biological rhythms
Overload	Anxious–reactivity	Nutrition
Frustration	Time-urgency	Noise
Deprivation	Anger–hostility	Drugs

Lifestyle/Psychosocial

Lifestyle refers to how one lives in the socio-cultural environment, and is often mentioned as the most important determinant of stress. Lifestyle encompasses the events of our lives, as well as our daily work and play activities. Lifestyle includes what we eat or otherwise ingest, and other factors of our physical environment including the noise, the rush, and the pressure we encounter every day. Lifestyle also includes those people with whom we interact, and human interaction is possibly the most potent stressor of all. Even people we don't know can act as significant stressors in our lives. For example, we have all had our stress aroused by politicians or editorialists with views that oppose our own. All of these factors will be discussed in more detail below.

Adaptation

The stress response exists to help us adapt to change. Consequently, the more change we experience in our lives the more stress we experience. Major events and abrupt changes in our lives can throw us off balance. Biologists refer to this as being out of our natural equilibrium or homeostasis. In order to survive, we must adapt to these events and changes, and adaptation consumes energy as the body fights to restore balance. Some events require major adaptation while others require only minor adjustments. Two decades ago researchers Thomas Holmes and Richard Rahe (1967) compiled a list of life events, both positive and negative, that required their subjects to change their lives or adapt to some degree. The result of their efforts was the *Social Readjustment Rating Scale*, a simple paper and pencil test that assigns a numerical value to life events. A higher score (life events are assigned a point value based on the severity or degree of the change involved) on this test was found to be positively correlated with subsequent illness rates in those individuals, making this test an important tool for the study of adaptive stress. Based on this work, other similar scales have been developed that validate this precept for specific populations. However, while the majority of studies do show that individuals with a greater number of severe life change events do experience more stress and more illness, many people who experience the same life events do not experience ill effects. Reasons for this lie in the difference in coping abilities, the influence of individual perception of the life event, past experience, susceptibility and other factors that are currently being investigated.

This chapter contains a self-scoring test called the *Stressor Self Test*, designed to give you an indication of the aspects of your lifestyle that may be causing you stress. Complete each part of the test as you encounter it in this chapter, and read the accompanying explanation. As you do, remember that this test is an educational tool and is designed to promote awareness. It in no way substitutes for the diagnostic procedures used by physicians or psychologists. Any concerns about your physical or mental health should be directed to your physician. Stressor Self-Test Part 1, presented below, is a variation of the Social Readjustment Rating Scale and will give you an indication of the events in your life that require your adaptive energy.

The higher scores indicate an increased vulnerability to stress due to a drain of adaptive energy. However, you must take into consideration that the importance of life events lies not so much in whether the change is positive or negative, a major life event or a minor one, but more on your perception of the significance of the event to your life.

STRESSOR SELF-TEST, PART 1

Below are a list of some common life events usually perceived as stressful. Check the ones you have experienced in the last twelve months.

Major change in work or school:

_____ increase in hours per week
_____ increase in responsibility
_____ increase in authority
_____ decrease in pay 25% or more
_____ increase or decrease in autonomy
_____ shift change (long term)
_____ loss of job or suspension from school
_____ problems with superiors
_____ change of job or school
_____ change of school major
_____ *Total number of checks x 2 = _____*

Major change in interpersonal relationships:

_____ marriage
_____ divorce or break up of long-term relationship
_____ serious problems with partner; e.g., infidelity, arguments
_____ serious restriction of social life
_____ major disagreements with family
_____ *Total number of checks x 4 = _____*

Major change in life style:

_____ change of residence of more than 100 miles away
_____ incurrence of a large debt
_____ problems with the law
_____ death of a close friend or family member
_____ serious illness of a close friend or family member
_____ *Total number of checks x 4 = _____*

Major change in health status:

_____ injury or illness resulting in loss of time at work or school
_____ problems with drugs or alcohol
_____ unwanted pregnancy (male or female partner)
_____ premature end of a pregnancy
_____ birth of a child
_____ *Total number of checks x 4 = _____*

Add the sum of the four sections to arrive at a score for this test.

Total score _____   A score between 0–20 is low risk
                                              20–40 low to moderate risk
                                              40–60 moderate to high risk
                                              60+   high risk

Overload

Our body has the ability to respond to stress, and as it does it becomes conditioned to be increasingly sensitive to stress. When our lives become overloaded our stress response system eventually becomes over responsive and overstressed. Overload is defined as a state in which the demands of life exceed your capacity to meet them. The term *overstimulation* is often used to describe overload. Most of us occasionally feel that the pressures of life are building up faster than our ability to deal with them, or that there are simply not enough hours in the day or days in the week to accomplish what needs to be done. This is overload. As a result of overload, you might become tired and irritable, experience more colds or other illness symptoms, begin to feel fatigued and less sociable, and become increasingly less enthusiastic about life.

STRESSOR SELF-TEST, PART 2

Choose the most appropriate answer for each of the following statements and place the letter of your response in the space to the left of the statement.

_____ 1. I find myself with not enough time to do the activities I really enjoy.
      (a) almost always   (b) often   (c) seldom   (d) almost never

_____ 2. I feel people expect too much from me.
      (a) almost always   (b) often   (c) seldom   (d) almost never

_____ 3. I feel less competent than I think I should.
      (a) almost always   (b) often   (c) seldom   (d) almost never

_____ 4. I find myself getting anxious about my work or school.
      (a) almost always   (b) often   (c) seldom   (d) almost never

_____ 5. I feel that I have too much responsibility.
      (a) almost always   (b) often   (c) seldom   (d) almost never

_____ 6. I have difficulty falling asleep because I have too much on my mind.
      (a) almost always   (b) often   (c) seldom   (d) almost never

_____ 7. I feel when I make a mistake it is usually due to being rushed.
      (a) almost always   (b) often   (c) seldom   (d) almost never

Scoring - a = 4, b = 3, c = 2, d = 1

Total score is _____
      7–13 low vulnerability to stress from overload.
      14–20 moderate vulnerability
      21–28 high vulnerability

Overload can come from many aspects of your life. The most prevalent source of stress due to overload in most people's lives is their work, which can include school. There are several common causes of work stress. One of these is referred to as *quantitative overload*, which means that an individual tries to do too many things at one time, tries to meet too many deadlines, and tries to be in too many places at the same time. Another cause of work stress is referred to as *qualitative overload*, which occurs when individuals find themselves in situations where the work is beyond their ability, such as after a promotion or during training for a new task. Qualitative overload has become more prevalent in this age of computers and high technology: individuals who have been doing the same job for many years may suddenly find that their job has changed and evolved beyond their present ability level. Time pressures, deadlines, decision-making, and performance anxiety are also stress producers. Performance anxiety can be especially stressful to those who, in their jobs, are responsible for other people's lives and well-being, or for large sums of money.

If your work is being a student, you may experience similar forms of overload. Our society's demand for higher education has created a highly competitive academic environment reaching back into primary grades. Students are pressured to do well academically to ensure admission to college. College students must then compete for honor status to be considered for graduate or professional schools. It is little wonder that test anxiety is a major problem in college and that academic overload leads to poor self-concept, emotional disturbances, and to students dropping out of school.

In addition to work overload, other areas in our lives contribute to overload stress. For instance, we may experience *urban overload*, which arises from having too many people in too small a space. Cities generate overload stimulation in the forms of stress-producing noise, pollution, crowding, and competition for everything from parking places to restaurant tables. One must move faster just to keep pace in an environment of unfamiliar, seemingly uncaring faces. Even your home may be a source of overload: for some people, crowding, noise, lack of privacy, cooking, cleaning, and repair work make leaving the house to go to work the most pleasant part of the day.

Frustration

Closely related to overload is the stress engendered by the frustration that occurs when we are blocked from doing what we want to do. We may often have the feeling that with all those people getting in the way we are being kept from accomplishing those goals we set for ourselves. Our work and/or our personal lives have the potential to cause us great frustration, whether due to time restraints, competition, disappointed expectations, or other factors. Some common aspects of work that may result in job-related frustration are:

1. *Job ambiguity:* Not knowing exactly what the job entails, or not knowing what is expected of you or how you will be evaluated.

2. *Role conflicts:* Needing to play a role that does not fit your beliefs or values.

3. *Bureaucracy:* Dealing with complex rules, excessive paperwork, stifled creativity, and/or poor communication.

4. *Discrimination and prejudice:* Having to submit to these factors, which have the potential to stifle anything from day-to-day activities to long-range opportunities and dreams.

5. *Socio-economic opportunities:* Experiencing the powerlessness and hopelessness of the disadvantaged, and perhaps being held back from playing a meaningful role in life.

STRESSOR SELF-TEST, PART 3

Choose the most appropriate answer for each of the following statements and place the letter of your response in the space to the left of the statement.

_____ 1. I feel stifled or held back in my personal life or at work.
   (a) almost always   (b) often   (c) seldom   (d) almost never

_____ 2. I find myself upset because things have not gone according to my plan.
   (a) almost always   (b) often   (c) seldom   (d) almost never

_____ 3. I find myself frustrated.
   (a) almost always   (b) often   (c) seldom   (d) almost never

_____ 4. I feel that I am in a rut.
   (a) almost always   (b) often   (c) seldom   (d) almost never

_____ 5. I perceive myself as lost, or in the wrong job or school.
   (a) almost always   (b) often   (c) seldom   (d) almost never

_____ 6. I feel as though I am a victim of discrimination.
   (a) almost always   (b) often   (c) seldom   (d) almost never

_____ 7. I feel like pushing people or things out of my way.
   (a) almost always   (b) often   (c) seldom   (d) almost never

Scoring - a = 4, b = 3, c = 2, d = 1

Total score is _____   7–13 low vulnerability to stress from frustration
                            14–20 moderate vulnerability
                            21–28 high vulnerability

Deprivation

Deprivational stressors are just the opposite of overload, and may be just as stressful. Deprivation is the boredom engendered from living a lifestyle or working at a job that is not demanding or challenging. Deprivation is not always related to the performance of highly repetitive tasks; deprivation may also exist when an individual is simply not active enough over a long period of time. Too much passive entertainment (such as television viewing), over-indulgence in antisocial or antimotivational alcohol or drugs, too much time alone, or being out of work are all examples of deprivation. Research on loneliness, lack of activity, and lack of purpose indicates that these factors are associated with diminished self-esteem, decreased social stimulation, and spiritual disintegration. All of these social indicators of excessive stress arousal have been associated with increased susceptibility to illness and accidents (Lynch, 1977).

STRESSOR SELF-TEST, PART 4

Choose the most appropriate answer for each of the following statements and place the letter of your response in the space to the left of the statement.

_____ 1. I find myself bored.
   (a) almost always   (b) often   (c) seldom   (d) almost never

_____ 2. I feel that my life and/or work are not stimulating enough.
    (a) almost always   (b) often   (c) seldom   (d) almost never
_____ 3. I find myself becoming restless.
    (a) almost always   (b) often   (c) seldom   (d) almost never
_____ 4. I wish my life was more exciting.
    (a) almost always   (b) often   (c) seldom   (d) almost never
_____ 5. I find myself daydreaming.
    (a) almost always   (b) often   (c) seldom   (d) almost never
_____ 6. I find myself with nothing to do.
    (a) almost always   (b) often   (c) seldom   (d) almost never
_____ 7. I feel over qualified to be doing what I am doing.
    (a) almost always   (b) often   (c) seldom   (d) almost never

Scoring - a = 4, b = 3, c = 2, d = 1

Total score is _____   7–13 low vulnerability to stress from deprivation
    14–20 moderate vulnerability
    21–28 high vulnerability

Personality

It is not impossible to change our environment and reduce the stimulation we receive from change, overload, and frustration. However, if the required changes involve other people, they may be very difficult. In some cases it is more efficient to change *ourselves*, reducing stress by modifying our stressful personality traits. Thus, personality is perhaps the most important variable in the stress equation presented earlier. Personality may be interpreted as the influence of personal characteristics, attitudes, and values on the behavior patterns we formulate while interacting with our environment. Certain personality characteristics may cause us to be more susceptible to stress—in other words, our personalities may make us more or less prone to stress caused by environment and lifestyle. Low stress arousal can be achieved by manipulating the environment to try to eliminate or avoid most major stressors. However, in our modern, fast-paced society it is difficult to completely eliminate stressors. Therefore, the most efficient path is usually to develop low stress personality characteristics.

Self-Concept

One important stress-related personality variable is *self-concept*, often called self-perception or self-regard. Everyone has an opinion of themselves and that opinion is based on a great many different factors, experiences, and self evaluations. The causes and effects of low self-concept or self-esteem are too complex to discuss in detail here. In fact, we are faced with a "chicken and egg" problem since low self-esteem is both the cause and reinforced result of social interaction problems. In other words, there is a cyclical nature to this problem. People tend to like other people who are out-going, assertive, creative, interesting, and who can make decisions about what they want and how to achieve it. We like these qualities in ourselves, also. Low self-esteem usually prevents a person from asserting him- or herself, from getting ideas heard, and so on. Low self-esteem leads to poor performance and subsequently to a reinforcement of the problem. Frustration, anxiety, and hostility—psychological manifestations of stress—often result. A person who recognizes him- or herself in this description may feel helpless to escape the cycle, but it is important to realize that help is available and that the cycle can be broken. Counseling is an important first step. It is most important to recognize the stress-inducing aspects of this problem and to seek to reduce the stress.

STRESSOR SELF-TEST, PART 5

Choose the most appropriate answer for each of the following statements and place the letter of your response in the space to the left of the statement.

_____ 1. I feel I do not have much going for me.
   (a) almost always   (b) often   (c) seldom   (d) almost never
_____ 2. I am uncomfortable around members of the opposite sex.
   (a) almost always   (b) often   (c) seldom   (d) almost never
_____ 3. I am uncomfortable around my superiors.
   (a) almost always   (b) often   (c) seldom   (d) almost never
_____ 4. Whenever something goes wrong I tend to blame myself.
   (a) almost always   (b) often   (c) seldom   (d) almost never
_____ 5. I shun new endeavors because of fear of failure.
   (a) almost always   (b) often   (c) seldom   (d) almost never
_____ 6. I have a strong need for recognition and approval.
   (a) almost always   (b) often   (c) seldom   (d) almost never
_____ 7. I frequently boast about myself.
   (a) almost always   (b) often   (c) seldom   (d) almost never

Scoring - a=4, b=3, c=2, d=1

Total score is _____   7–13 low vulnerability to stress from low self-concept
                            14–20 moderate vulnerability
                            21–28 high vulnerability

Time Urgency

Our society's race against the clock is a major source of stress. Virtually every organization imposes some form of time pressure over those within that organization, whether it is a business, a family, or a classroom. Stressful as such organizational time restraints can be, it is our *internal clocks* that cause the most significant stress arousal, especially for those exhibiting a time-urgency personality trait. These individuals tend to have an excessive sense of time, and are almost always worried about how long something is going to take. The time urgency personality trait has been extensively studied as part of the famous cardiovascular "Type A" prone personality construct that was originally formulated by Friedman and Rosenman (1974). Time urgency as a behavior and other closely-related personality factors such as anger and hostility are definite stress producers. Such personality characteristics are also the most significant characteristics of the Type A pattern in relation to developing cardiovascular disease. Thus far, research has not sufficiently explained how and why any one person develops Type A characteristics, although it is obvious our society is time-conscious and does reward hard work and achievement. However, one can work hard and be very successful without being excessively hard driving and competitive.

Choose the most appropriate answer for each of the following statements and place the letter of your response in the space to the left of the statement.

_____ 1. I catch myself rushing when there is no need to do so.
      (a) almost always   (b) often   (c) seldom   (d) almost never

_____ 2. I hate to wait.
      (a) almost always   (b) often   (c) seldom   (d) almost never

_____ 3. I try to make my activities competitive.
      (a) almost always   (b) often   (c) seldom   (d) almost never

_____ 4. I feel guilty when I am not being productive.
      (a) almost always   (b) often   (c) seldom   (d) almost never

_____ 5. I tend to lose my temper or get irritable.
      (a) almost always   (b) often   (c) seldom   (d) almost never

_____ 6. When frustrated I feel like hitting something.
      (a) almost always   (b) often   (c) seldom   (d) almost never

_____ 7. I seem to eat and/or walk faster than most people.
      (a) almost always   (b) often   (c) seldom   (d) almost never

Scoring - a = 4, b = 3, c = 2, d = 1

Total score is _____   7–13 low vulnerability to stress from time urgency
                              14–20 moderate vulnerability
                              21–28 high vulnerability

Research has shown that the Type A person is likely to have a lower than average self-esteem, which may account for the "I need to do more, faster, to be as good" attitude. Type As also seem to have a higher degree of general hostility, which may stem from resentment at having to pedal faster to keep up. Interestingly, the Type A person usually feels comfortable with these characteristics, values them, and feels no strong need to change until they cause health problems. Usually their family and co-workers are most anxious to see a change, as a hostile person is often difficult to live and work with.

If you think back to the section of this chapter on the physiology of stress, the anger reaction was characterized by the build up of pressure. Sometimes that pressure results in an explosion, sometimes it is suppressed to such a degree that it damages internal structures. In any case, an excessive sense of time urgency and the resultant anxiety and hostility are major stress-producers in our modern society. Those wishing to reduce stress in their lives will need to assess and modify their excessive tendencies in this area.

Anxiety and Anxious-Reactivity

Anxiety is a well-documented *reaction* to stress, and being anxiety-prone is also a *cause* of excessive stress. Some individuals exhibit an extreme anxiety reaction to stress that persists long after the stressor has been eliminated. In these individuals, the body's reaction to stress *becomes* the stress—they do not seem to possess the feedback-dampening mechanisms normally used to cope with stress anxiety. It is almost as if the body becomes so conditioned to react with anxiety that with the slightest amount of stress the body immediately assumes the maximum anxiety response, which is then prolonged.

A complete explanation of anxiety can be read in Speilberger (1972). He defines the anxiety reaction, also called state anxiety, as a stimulus that is perceived as threatening. It is important to remember our earlier discussion of the appropriateness of stress, and that the way we perceive a threat is unique to each of us. Our perception of a "threat" is given meaning in several parts of the brain, including the subconscious. Fears are not always grounded in logic, nor can logic alone explain them away or diminish the stress response. The feeling of fear or insecurity activates the parts of the body that control arousal of endocrine and sympathetic nervous systems, which are needed to carry out protective action.

Anxiety and fear produce similar responses in the body and are in many ways the opposite of anger. Anger fills the body with blood and excessive pressure, as if to prepare us for the fight. The anxiety reaction is one of fear, of diminshed blood to organs, lowered internal pressure, and a sense of hiding or being frozen in position hoping not to be seen by the threat. The anger response is to strike back while the fear response is to hide. The body prepares for both. Anxiety has been described as chronic fear, and anxious reactivity is the body becoming increasingly stressed when the fear arousal is sensed. For example, the anxious response may produce an awareness of hands trembling, heart pounding, or stomach gurgling. This "awareness," whether it is conscious or subconscious, further exacerbates the anxious stress response and subsequently the stress response increases in severity. One of the most important stress reduction techniques is to reduce the body's reaction to the situations that cause anxiety and to reduce the tendency of the body to be over sensitive to stress arousal. The relaxation techniques presented in the next chapter are designed for this purpose.

STRESSOR SELF-TEST, PART 7

Choose the most appropriate answer for each of the following statements and place the letter of your response in the space to the left of the statement.

_____ 1. I tend to imagine the worst things happening in any situation.
     (a) almost always   (b) often   (c) seldom   (d) almost never

_____ 2. I re-live instances or situations over and over in my mind.
     (a) almost always   (b) often   (c) seldom   (d) almost never

_____ 3. I feel my stomach sinking, or my heart pounding.
     (a) almost always   (b) often   (c) seldom   (d) almost never

_____ 4. I have a difficult time falling asleep at night.
     (a) almost always   (b) often   (c) seldom   (d) almost never

_____ 5. I have difficulty speaking or notice my hands and fingers trembling.
     (a) almost always   (b) often   (c) seldom   (d) almost never

_____ 6. I am tense.
     (a) almost always   (b) often   (c) seldom   (d) almost never

_____ 7. I feel difficulties are piling up.
     (a) almost always   (b) often   (c) seldom   (d) almost never

Scoring - a = 4, b = 3, c = 2, d = 1

Total score is _____

    7–13 low vulnerability to stress from anxiety and anxious reactivity
    14–20 moderate vulnerability
    21–28 high vulnerability

Environmental Stress

The concept of environmental stress stems from the relationship that the human organism has with its environment. This type of stress is only somewhat influenced by an individual's personality or thought process. As we discuss below, however, there is a definite relationship between one's behavior and the stress "imposed" by the environment. The four general classes of environmental stimuli that can contribute to distress are:

1. Biological rhythms
2. Nutritional habits
3. Environmental pollution, especially noise
4. Drugs

Biological Rhythms

Time has always been recognized as one of our greatest stressors. Most people associate time-induced stress with *society's* deadlines and time restrictions. However, other aspects of "time" also influence our lives. The natural world runs on time: solar or light time, lunar time, and seasonal time are but a few examples. The human body also runs on time: temperature time, metabolic time, energy time, and hormonal time just to mention a few. Social, cultural, technological man and woman have arrogantly ignored their biological time or rhythm for the sake of convenience and conformity. We try to synchronize work and recreation schedules with what is socially and economically efficient. We utilize artificial light and we speed through time zones. All of these things and more act to change the body's natural tempo and rhythm. The result of being out of synchrony with our bodies may be undue irritability, emotional instability, and increased susceptibility to illness.

Someday synchronization of internal rhythm or body time may dictate work and social schedules, but for the present, learning about your own body rhythm will at least allow you to minimize the potential stressors involved. Stress arousal can be diminished by your understanding of fluctuation in body weight, muscle tone, energy, strength, hunger, sleep, excretion demands, motivation, attention, and productivity.

Biological rhythms are naturally-recurring cycles of biological activities governed by the nervous and hormonal systems. Some of these activities are completely internal, stubbornly resisting change; others are greatly influenced by external stimulation, such as exposure to light. Still others, such as eating, adapt themselves to clock time and social activities. Biological rhythms recur in periods of time that may be minutes, hours, days, or years.

The most researched cycle is the 24-hour cycle, called the *circadian* (Latin for "about a day") rhythm. Some of the body processes that fluctuate in a circadian rhythm are body temperature, blood pressure, respiration rate, blood sugar, hemoglobin levels, adrenal hormone levels, amino acid levels, and urine production. As these fluctuate, so do strength and energy levels, attention span, and motivation. As strength changes, so do vulnerabilities. Drugs taken at one time of the day may produce a mild effect whereas the same dose taken later in the day may produce a more profound effect. The same holds true for reactions to various emotional and physical stressors.

Another rhythm or cyclic variation that has received much attention in recent years is the *infradian*, or longer than circadian, rhythm. These cycles may last for days, weeks, or even months. The female menstrual cycle is an infradian cycle during which hormonal, structural, and functional changes occur in a stubbornly systematic manner, month after month. This cycle has been so thoroughly researched and written about that its patterns have become familiar to most adults in the world. Other infradian rhythms are now thought to control the ebb and flow of emotional responses and moods. These rhythms have also been related to fluctuations in motivation, hunger, and performance. While these rhythms are basically set, they can be changed. However, the body cannot make the necessary adjustment in the short time usually allowed. For example, we would expect a night worker's body temperature cycle to be opposite that of a day worker's, but this usually is not the case unless the night shift schedule has been maintained for several weeks—long enough for the body to adapt to a new schedule. In many companies workers may continually rotate shifts working nights one week and days the next, giving them an inadequate time to adapt to the change.

The recent interest in jet lag or jet fatigue has spurred several studies, and researchers have found that jet lag is characterized by the following symptoms: headache; gastrointestinal problems, including loss of appetite; increased sweating; blurred vision; and alteration of sleep patterns (nightmares, insomnia); in addition, female flight attendants may experience menstrual difficulties. Concerned companies have increased layover time for airline crews and business travelers, correctly reasoning that the extra cost of room and board is a good investment when weighed against the potential costliness of accidents, poor business decisions, or illness.

In summary, we now have enough information regarding the health aspects of biological rhythms to realize that they may help to explain mood and behavior fluctuations, changes in immunity, incidences of illness, variability in toxicity of drugs, changes in body weight, appetite, motivation, activity levels, changes in sexual interest and performance, sensitivity to stress, and, in general, the development of stress-related disease. Knowledge of bio-rhythms should help us to eliminate stress by reducing the frustration and self-doubt that often accompany normal fluctuations in mood and performance.

Nutrition and Stress

The consumption of certain foods or other substances (such as nicotine or drugs) can add to the stress of everyday life, either by stimulating the sympathetic stress response directly, or by contributing to its stimulation by creating a state of fatigue and increased nervous irritability. Either condition greatly lowers our tolerance to the common stress of day-to-day living. In this section we examine some of the more common nutritional habits that are thought to be related to stress.

Sympathomimetic agents are chemical substances that mimic the sympathetic stress response. Many foods contain these sympathomimetic substances naturally. Consumption of these foods triggers a response in your body proportional to the amount consumed and your individual susceptibility to the chemical.

The most common of these sympathomimetic stressors in the American diet is caffeine, a chemical that belongs to the xanthine group of drugs. Xanthines are powerful amphetamine-like stimulants that increase the metabolism rate and create a highly awake and active state. They also trigger the release of stress hormones, which are capable of increasing heart rate, blood pressure, and oxygen demands upon the heart. Extreme or prolonged stress hormone secretion can even initiate myocardial necrosis, that is, destruction of heart tissue.

Generally speaking, six to eight ounces of coffee can overstimulate the metabolic system of children, and more than three cups of coffee within one hour for adults will adversely affect their behavior and increase the possibility of stomach upset or irritation. For the child, more than two cola beverages a day may be considered excessive, while for the adult more than four such beverages a day would be excessive.

Another nutritional factor related to stress is that of vitamin depletion. Especially during stressful times, high levels of certain vitamins are needed to maintain the proper functioning of the nervous and endocrine systems; these are Vitamin C and the vitamins of the B complex, particularly Vitamins B-1 (thiamine), B-2 (riboflavin), niacin, B-5 (pantothenic acid), B-6 (pyridoxine hydrochloride), and choline. The B-complex vitamins are especially important components of the stress response since deficiencies of Vitamins B-1, B-5, and B-6 can lead to anxiety reactions, depression, insomnia, and cardiovascular weaknesses. Deficiencies of Vitamins B-2 and niacin have been known to cause stomach irritability and muscle weakness. The depletion of these essential vitamins lowers tolerance to, and ability to cope with, stressors.

Vitamins also play important roles in the actual mechanics of the stress response. Vitamins B-1, B-2, and niacin are used up at far greater rates during the stress response because of their roles in carbohydrate metabolism. In addition, Vitamins B-5, C, and choline are necessary elements in the production of adrenal hormones secreted during the stress response. Therefore, excessive stress over prolonged periods of time will deplete these vitamins, making you more prone to stress and other problems caused by B-complex deficiencies.

Another way in which diet may predispose an individual to distress is through a hypoglycemia phenomenon. Hypoglycemia is a state of low blood sugar. Symptoms may include anxiety, headache, dizziness, trembling, and increased cardiac activity. These symptoms may cause normal stimuli to become severe stressors by making the individual highly irritable and impatient. In effect, they lower the individual's stress tolerance.

The conscious manipulation of nutritional behavior to control stress may be referred to as *nutritional engineering*. When used as one of the social engineering strategies, it can prove to be a powerful addition to the holistic program for stress management.

Nicotine is the final substance we will consider in this section. A discussion of smoking may seem out of place in a section on nutritional habits, but for smokers eating and smoking share many psychosocial characteristics. Tobacco contains nicotine. Like caffeine, nicotine is a sympathomimetic chemical, and as such it is capable of all the adverse reactions of the sympathetic nervous system noted earlier. Thus nicotine can trigger a stress response.

You may take nicotine into your body by smoking tobacco, by inhaling the tobacco smoke of others, or by chewing tobacco. Nicotine stimulates the adrenals, releasing hormones that elicit the stress response of accelerated heart rate, blood pressure, respiration rate, and release of fatty acids and glucose into the blood, among other body reactions. Ironically, the chronic smoker's body is continuously elevated to the point where this arousal state becomes the "normal" state. Thus, being deprived of the stimulating effect of nicotine (often referred to as an adrenalin high) will create a mild depression and an uneasy feeling, which in turn will lead to the desire for additional nicotine for the pickup.

Stress and Drugs

Although people take drugs (and we refer also to alcohol) for various reasons, a common motivation is to get "high" or experience an altered state of consciousness, often in an attempt to reduce stress. An "altered" state can be defined as a deviation from the "normal" state of consciousness, in which most of us communicate, are goal-directed, and have rational, cause-and-effect thinking.

To alter the normal ego-consciousness, one must move from the "planning-doing" state to a "feeling-experiencing" state, sometimes termed the *egoless state*. In the egoless state of consciousness the environment is perceived as nonthreatening; clothes, cars, colleges, and vacation spots are not important. Impressions do not have to be made, images protected, nor feelings guarded. One does not think in terms of cause and effect; thus the significance of subjective experiences or ideas is also changed. In many altered states one loses the feeling of needing to control the environment. In fact, there may be a diminished sense of where the self ends and the environment begins. Self-centered daydreams diminish, a sense of depersonalization occurs, and inhibitions are diminished. The sense of time changes with the reduction of attention to time-dictated events. The perception of body, self, and reality often changes, and many times visual imagery is experienced.

Altered states of consciousness provide glimpses of ego- or self-transcendence and enlightenment. *Self-transcendence* is said to be egolessness and freedom from anxiety and defenses; it allows for expansion of experiences and feelings and for increased knowledge of self. Ego, time, and space are transcended, giving rise to peace and tranquility.

Being in an altered state of consciousness means that one has shifted from the normal, taking-care-of-business state to some other level of consciousness. This other level may be as basic as daydreaming or as spiritual as cosmic consciousness, but be assured that we all wander in and out of normal consciousness many times throughout the day and night. The frequency of these occurrences depends a great deal on our external and internal environment—especially the level of stimulation around us—but the frequency can also be planned or allowed by one's own mind.

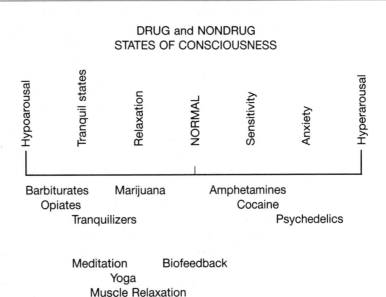

FIGURE 10.4
Drug and nondrug
states of consciousness.

A *drug-induced* altered state of consciousness is often a pleasant experience. The intensity or quality of the experience depends on such factors as when and even where one takes the drug. The quantity and quality of the drug are important, as are one's mood when taking the drug, one's motivation for taking the drug, one's general state of health (especially emotional well-being), one's knowledge about drugs, and one's personality and expectations. Frustration and disappointment may develop when expectations are not met; and fear, apprehension, and injury can result if the drug is too strong or dangerously adulterated. Either way, one is not really in control of the experience and is in a sense imprisoned in an altered state of consciousness until the drug has been metabolized. More importantly, drugs change but do not stop the flood of sporadic thoughts that bombard the consciousness; thus, the goal of quieting the mind is not usually realized.

The sense of unreality and lack of ego that result from some forms of drug use may be calming in the sense that the drug creates a temporary block that prevents one from actively thinking about a problem. Unfortunately, the problem still exists. It is stored in parts of the brain, and is producing feelings and other body alterations that continue to exist even though one is not actively aware of them. The psychoactive drugs, both legal and illegal, that we typically consume to promote relaxation do not change body physiology. Our problems are still present and continue to stress the system. The only difference is that we have temporarily blocked the situation from active, here-and-now thoughts.

Drugs do create temporary blocks, and altered states of consciousness are glimpses of ego- or self-transcendence. When the drugs wear off, however, the feelings are gone and can only be regained by repeated use of the drug. There is little positive carry-over, little is learned in the drug state, and few people are changed. Their world, their problems, and their coping mechanisms are the same as before. Drugs have fulfilled a limited goal, an altered state of consciousness, but they have not fulfilled the dream—that the experience would somehow grant the user greater insights and the ability to naturally transcend the ego and live a calmer, more relaxed and enlightened life.

Herein lies the crux of the problem: a lack of understanding of what constitutes self-transcendence. In order to gain inner awareness—an *active* process from *within*—one must have control of one's thoughts, feelings, and thinking processes. Drugs, which are uncontrollable to a lesser or greater degree, promote the feeling that this experience is a *passive* process, externally induced.

The passivity of the drug experience is in itself a drawback. Passive experiences in which the individual just rides along, seeing, feeling, and experiencing are somehow not as satisfying as those in which the individual is the active, creative center of the experience. Creative activities increase one's feelings of self-esteem, and in a circular pattern increase motivation and readiness for future unknown ventures.

Altered states can be induced through such activities as meditation, daydreaming, or drug taking. They can be brought on by hypoarousal or hyperarousal of the central nervous system. It is healthier to induce these states by mind direction rather than by using drugs. There are many currently popular techniques that aim at inducing a self-transcendent, altered state of consciousness through mind direction or control. Yoga, meditation, muscular relaxation, autogenic training, and biofeedback are but a few examples. These are a more positive approach than drugs, not only because they are less dangerous, more socially acceptable, and more controllable, but also because they are active and creative, requiring and promoting self-control and self-discipline. These are learning exercises that result in temporary feelings of self-transcendence, thus providing the foundation and motivation needed to re-educate one's thoughts and coping processes. If mastered, they lead to an even higher state—that of conscious self-transcendence, an egoless, or ego-expanded state in which ego boundaries are infinitely extended. This is a higher state because it is integrated with ongoing life, and provides benefits to the individual, society, and humankind in general.

Noise

The study of noise as a stressor is somewhat complex. Noise impacts us both psychosocially and biologically, and can produce a stress response in one or more of the following ways:

1. By causing physiological reaction, that is, by stimulating the sympathetic nervous system;
2. By being annoying and subjectively displeasing;
3. By disrupting ongoing activities.

As item (2) indicates, noise can act as a stressor in a strictly psychological way (apart from any physical impact). This occurs when noise is perceived as unwanted or somehow inappropriate. This reaction—and the accompanying stress response— can occur at any frequency level, because it depends upon the particular situation. For example, a conversation at a distance of three feet generates only about 60dB, far below the pain threshold; but if you are trying to figure out your income tax or study for a final exam, this conversation could become stressful because it disrupts your activity. Similarly, what may be "music" to you may be "noise" to someone else. Thus, the music that one person plays every day and finds relaxing might be very annoying, and thus stressful, to another. Noise consists of biological and psychosocial components—both capable of causing distress. Regardless of certain adaptive characteristics, noise in excessive quantity or quality is distressful (Girdano and Everly 1986).

Summary

The stress response is a natural physical response that accelerates the body's defenses when the body is threatened. In prehistoric times before egos, bosses, traffic, and time deadlines, threats were physical and sporadic. Now the threats that may trigger a stress response are social-psychological and constant. The primary stressors for modern humans are lifestyle factors such as adaptation to change, overload, frustration, and deprivation; personality factors such as self-concept, time urgency and anxiety; and environmental factors such as noise, nutrition, and drugs. Each of us responds to the presence of these stressors in a slightly different way determined by our lifestyle, experience, and coping ability. If coping abilities are not adequate and the stress response lasts too long, the body's defenses can fatigue, organ systems can deteriorate, and physical illness can result. Now that you have an awareness of what causes stress, use the techniques presented in Chapter 11 to construct a program for stress management.

References

Friedman, M. and R. Rosenman. 1974. *Type A behavior and your heart*. New York: A. A. Knopf.

Girdano, D. A. and G. S. Everly. 1986. *Controlling stress and tension: A holistic approach*. 2d ed. Englewood Cliffs: Prentice Hall.

Holms, T. H. and R. H. Rahe. 1967. The social readjustment rating scale. *Journal of Psychosomatic Research:* 231–218.

Lynch, J. J. 1977. *The broken heart: The medical consequences of loneliness*. New York: Basic Books.

Selye, H. 1956. *The stress of life*. New York: McGraw-Hill.

Speilberger, C. D. 1972. *Anxiety: Current trends in theory and research*. Vol. 1. New York: Academic Press.

Wolf, S., and H. G. Wolff. 1947. *Human gastric function*. 2d. New York: Oxford University Press.

11

Techniques of Stress Management

Can your stress response be changed?

How do drugs affect stress and stress reduction?

Can you modify a stressful environment?

Can you change personality traits that may contribute to stress?

Can you change beliefs or life philosophies that may contribute to stress?

Introduction

As can be seen from Figure 11.1, the basic model of developing a healthy life-style, which consists of positive health behaviors and self-care techniques, starts with awareness and proceeds through behavior change.

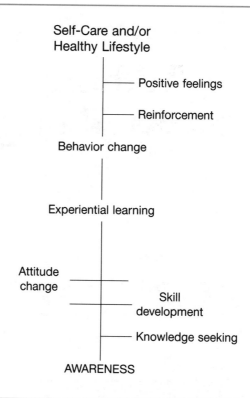

FIGURE 11.1
Developing a healthy lifestyle.

Stress management is one of the best examples of this model in action. Management begins with awareness that stress exists and that it can be detrimental to your health. You can then increase your knowledge about the stressors that exist in your life. This will help you develop an attitude that will motivate you to learn the skills necessary to manage stress. Once developed, these skills can influence changes in behavior which, if properly reinforced, may be adapted into a lifestyle that is stress reducing.

The awareness aspect of this program can be presented in a relatively few words and represents the rationale for this chapter. The skills of relaxation are not difficult to learn but do take time and are significantly enhanced by personal interaction with an instructor. One chapter in a book cannot provide a *comprehensive* discussion of all aspects of stress management. However, the final section of this chapter will outline the components of a stress management program and describe some stress reduction techinques.

The components of a stress management program can be divided into three categories: (1) Activities designed to quiet the external environment in order to reduce the stressors in your life; (2) activites designed to quiet your internal environment to reduce the stimulation of the nervous system; and (3) activities designed to condition the mind to reduce stress-inducing thoughts.

Quieting the External Environment

These activities are designed to quiet the external environment in order to reduce the stressors in your life. They should produce a cognitive awareness of life events and then be utilized in restructuring your environment, thought patterns, and behavior (Girdano and Everly, 1986). Some representative techniques are outlined below.

Social Engineering

For Adaptive Stress
> a. Establish routines.
> b. Use time management techniques.
> c. Establish a consistent "mental health" day.
> d. Minimize other changes during periods of large change.

For Frustration
> a. Find new alternatives to the frustrated goal.

For Overload
> a. Practice time management and set priorities.
> b. Avoid over commitments—learn to say no.
> c. Determine optimal stress level.
> d. Reduce tasks to manageable parts.
> e. Delegate responsibility.

For Deprivation
> a. Plan activities.
> b. Challenge yourself.

For Environmental Stress
> a. Avoid noise.
> b. Regulate diet.
> c. Try to live with your natural rhythms.

Personality Engineering

For Poor Self-Esteem and Depression
> a. Learn and practice assertiveness.
> b. Verbalize your positive qualities.
> c. Accept compliments.

For Time Urgency
> a. Use time management.
> b. Use goal alternatives.
> c. Practice concentration.
> d. Practice thought stopping.

Quieting Your Internal Environment

These activities are designed to quiet your internal environment to reduce the stimulation of the nervous system. They decrease sensory stimulation, produce a relaxation response, and condition that response. Some representative techniques are:

Breathing exercises	Visual imagery
Hatha Yoga	Biofeedback
Muscle relaxation	Physical exercise

A brief description of each technique will be presented to help you choose the one that has best potential for meeting your needs and interests (Girdano, 1980, 1981).

Breathing Exercises

There seems to be a physiological relationship between the centers that control respiration and the centers that control our general nervousness or reactivity. From the ancient yogis to recent researchers one basic recommendation for calming the body has been the use of some kind of breathing technique, specifically diaphragmatic breathing. We know that a stressed person breathes differently than a relaxed person. A person who is stressed will breathe shallowly and rapidly, while a person who is relaxed will breathe deeply, as though from the abdomen. In diaphragmatic breathing, you can actually feel the abdomen move in and out when you breathe. Simply sitting down for a few minutes several times a day and controlling your breathing teaches your body to respond in a relaxing manner. If you breathe like a relaxed person, you will *be* more relaxed, for at least a short period of time.

A more complete description of breathing exercises can be found below, in the section "Relaxation Exercises."

Hatha Yoga

The word yoga is derived from the Sanskrit root meaning "union" or "reunion" and is a method of physical, mental, and spiritual development based on the philosophies of Lord Krishna. Knowledge was passed from enlightened master to student, generation after generation for thousands of years before the first written record of this technique appeared around 200 B.C. in Patangali's *Sutras*. Since then, thousands of books have been written describing the many types of yoga, called "paths," that have developed into spiritual schools and in many instances have become distinctly separate schools in themselves. Raja-yoga, or royal yoga, the path to self-realization and enlightenment, is very similar to meditation. The most popular path in the Western world is hatha yoga, which uses positions and exercises to promote physical and mental harmony. Most yoga practice starts with hatha yoga, since it is said to provide the body with the health and endurance needed to learn more advanced forms of yoga. Hatha yoga is practiced for its own rewards, which include strength, flexibility, and reduction of muscle tension; it is also used as a technique to quiet the body in preparation for quiet mental states.

It is important to remember that yoga masters come from a different culture, in which both physical structure and physical activity patterns are significantly different from those in Western cultures. Sometimes it is difficult for Westerners to master all of the positions completely. Nevertheless, positive results can be derived from yoga, especially if the exercises are chosen for specific groups of people with specific outcomes in mind.

Muscle Relaxation

Neuromuscular relaxation training is a program of systematic exercises that train not only the muscles but also the nervous system components that control muscle activity. The objective is to reduce the tension in the muscles. The muscles make up such a large portion of the body's mass that muscle relaxation leads to a signficant reduction in total body tension as well. There are literally hundreds of techniques, and almost every relaxation program utilizes some form of neuromuscular relaxation. The basic objective is to teach the individual to relax the muscles at will by first developing a thinking-feeling awareness of what it feels like to be relaxed. If you are able to distinguish between tension and relaxation, control over tension will easily follow. To accomplish this you must learn to center on the task or problem and control the mind's tendency to wander aimlessly in daydreams.

Neuromuscular relaxation requires concentration. However, the concentration must be passive and must not add to the tension level. Thoughts should be centered on techniques and awareness of tension levels and must not become ego or goal-centered. As you perfect your ability, these exercises can be practiced anywhere, even in short periods of usually "wasted" time, such as when you have stopped for a red light, or while waiting for an appointment.

Visual Imagery

Visual imagery is the use of self-directed mental images of relaxed states. This simple technique centers around conditioned patterns of responses that become associated with particular thoughts. Recall a moment when you allowed your mind to run away and catastrophize a potentially threatening event. You may have been worried about losing your job, a change in company policy, or perhaps problems with a partner or spouse. You get chills and the hair rises on the back of your neck. This represents a conditioned physiological response to that particular association. The opposite effect can also be generated, producing an equally dramatic but very different physiological response. If you imagine yourself in your favorite relaxation spot, perhaps sitting on a quiet beach with the sun warming your body or fishing your favorite stream, physiologically a relaxation response is triggered. The technique of visual imagery simply helps condition relaxation through self-generated recall of relaxed body states and memories of relaxed times in your life. It is a method in which you talk to your body and tell it to relax. It helps if you are able to imagine a scene or a "feeling state" vividly and have already achieved a quiet physical state.

One of the common techniques used in this form of relaxation capitalizes on the body's ability to follow the commands of the conscious centers of the brain. If you can imagine warmth, the body has the tendency to reproduce that sensation. Blood flow, responding to the conscious demand, will increase to the desired areas, thereby creating the desired warmth. Such a physiological change would be impossible without a change in the "tone" of your nervous system, and through such a change relaxation is facilitated and gradually conditioned.

Biofeedback

The appearance of most biofeedback instruments, which look like sophisticated stereo systems with additional wires and cables, and the science-fiction-like accounts of results obtained using biofeedback probably make this technique seem somewhat mysterious and magical. However, there is no magic involved in biofeedback—it follows accepted scientific principles. The only real mystery of biofeedback is our seemingly unlimited abilities to regulate and influence our own psychophysiology.

The simple principle of biofeedback is *awareness of body function*. This is the first and most important ingredient in changing the behavior that causes the stress reaction. Biofeedback is best understood as an educational tool that provides information about behavior or performance in much the same manner that a congratulatory letter from superiors gives feedback on job performance or the bathroom scale gives information about the success of weight reduction efforts. If we learn to listen, our bodies will tell us a lot about their functioning. Biofeedback magnifies the subtle signals so they become more noticeable. It can be used simply as a device that trains or attunes our awareness of body language. For example, thermal measurements of skin temperature can be used to indicate blood flow changes to a particular region of the body. Then after only a few training sessions one can usually learn to feel the changes without the instrument. The contraction of skeletal muscle can also be measured in order to detect muscle action before it reaches the state of producing pain and discomfort. Through training one can then learn to sense even the most minute change in muscle tension. Likewise, monitoring brain waves can tell us much about states of consciousness and information processing, which can then aid in the voluntary control of consciousness. The possibilities are as numerous as the systems that can be measured.

In another sense biofeedback is much more than just a self-monitoring system. It can be used to promote self-exploration, self-awareness, and self-control. Relaxation and tranquility condition the tone of the nervous system to be less reactive, and gradually you begin to change behavior by "becoming" a more tranquil person. This process disciplines the mind to reduce the constant chatter of imagination and anticipation, allowing for greater problem-centered concentration and often leading to revealing insights and creativity. What started out as an exercise in relaxation quickly turns into a development of self-awareness and self-control.

Physical Exercise

The primary stress response is the "fight or flight" response. This reaction has always helped ensure human survival and continues to do so today; in fact, no amount of relaxation training can diminish the intensity of this innate reflex. Stress is physical, intended to make possible a physical response to a physical threat. However, any threat, either physical or symbolic, can bring about this response. Once the stimulation of the event penetrates the psychological defenses, the body prepares for action. Increased hormonal secretion, energy supply, and cardiovascular activity, signify a state of stress, a state of extreme readiness to act as soon as the voluntary control centers decide what action to take. Usually the threat is not physical, but holds only symbolic significance; our lives are not in danger, only our egos. Physical action is not warranted and must be subdued, but for the body organs it is too late—what took only minutes to start will take hours to undo. The stress products are flowing through the system and will activate various organs until these by-products are reabsorbed back into storage or gradually used by the body. While this gradual process is taking place, the body organs suffer.

The simple solution is to use the physical stress arousal for its intended purpose— physical movement. The increased energy intended for fight or flight can be used to run or swim or ride a bike. In this way one can accelerate the dissipation of the stress products, and if the activity is vigorous enough, it can cause a rebound or overshoot after exercise into a state of deep relaxation.

It is important to note that exercise is a stressor and competition adds substantially to that arousal level. While the stress of the exercise is usually absorbed by the exercise, the stress of competition often sets in motion thoughts and feelings that linger. These thoughts may even become the stimulus for prolonged emotional arousal with the rehash of missed points, social embarrassment, and self-doubt. We often confuse recreation with relaxation—they are not necessarily the same. In fact, for most people they are usually not the same. Recreation can be stressful, especially if it is competitive. Ideally, exercise to reduce stress should be devoid of ego involvement. Though strenuous, it should be a time of peace and of the harmonious interaction of mind and body. In that sense, it may be the most natural of stress reduction techniques.

Conditioning the Mind

These activities are designed to condition the mind to reduce stress-inducing thoughts. They reduce stress-arousing memories and anticipations, and instead direct thoughts to produce a peaceful and tranquil state. Representative techniques include many varieties of meditation.

Meditation

Modern meditative practices represent a mixture of philosophies and techniques descended from ancient Yoga and Zen Buddhism. Regardless of their ancestry, all meditative techniques have two common phases, which include a quiet body and a quiet mind. One cannot relax or quiet the mind if the brain is being bombarded with stimulation of tense muscles and hyperactive glands. Elaborate exercises, postures, and other rituals were developed in an attempt to slow the body activities to a point at which the mind would also be allowed to become quiet. The primary goal is to reduce what is referred to as the *surface chatter* of the mind, that is, the constant thinking in the form of planning, remembering, and fantasizing. Surface chatter seems to occupy our every waking moment and keeps us implanted in our ego consciousness. If you can reduce the surface chatter—or in other words reduce the thoughts of self—anxiety will be reduced, general arousal will be reduced, and the mind can periodically achieve peace and quiet.

Research has shown that during meditation the activity of most physical systems is reduced. At the same time, the meditator is in complete control of the experience and has control over emotions, feelings, and memories. Although meditation is a passive state of mind, it is an active process that takes thought, preparation, and practice.

Meditation is a simple, natural process that can produce results if it is used. For some reason it is difficult for Westerners to maintain the discipline of continued practice. Even though it is easy to learn, meditation has not been as effective as it could be for Westerners since it requires a different mental set than we have been conditioned to use. The Western mind is used to being occupied and stimulated. We are not taught to sit quietly without reading or watching television. When meditation techniques are used, however, they provide an effective means of stress reduction.

Relaxation Exercises

After you have learned some of the powerful relaxation techniques, you then have to refine your use of them so as to be able to relax at will. The following exercises do not represent a complete stress management program; however, they can be easily learned and when perfected represent an excellent first step.

Breathing exercises

During the course of an average day, many of us find ourselves in anxiety-producing situations. Our heart rates increase, our stomachs may become upset, and our thoughts may race uncontrollably through our minds. It is during such episodes as these that we require fast-acting relief from our stressful reactions. The brief exercise described below has been effective in reducing most of the stress reaction we suffer during acute exposures to stressors—in effect, it is a quick way to "calm down" in the face of a stressful situation.

The basic mechanism for stress reduction in this exercise involves deep breathing. The procedure is as follows:

Step 1. Assume a comfortable position. Rest your left hand (palm down) over your navel. Now place your right hand so that it comfortably rests on your left. Your eyes should remain open.

Step 2. Imagine a hollow bottle, or pouch, inside your body beneath your hands. Begin to inhale. As you do, imagine that the air is entering through your nose and descending to fill that internal pouch. Your hands will rise as you fill the pouch of air. As you continue to inhale, imagine the pouch being filled to the top with air. Your rib cage and upper chest will continue the rise that began at your navel. The total length of your inhalation should be three seconds for the first week or so, and then lengthen to four or five seconds as you progress in skill.

Step 3. Hold your breath. Keep the air inside the pouch. Repeat to yourself, "My body is calm."

Step 4. Slowly begin to exhale, to empty the pouch. As you do, repeat to yourself, "My body is quiet." As you exhale, you will feel your chest and then abdomen fall.

Repeat this four-step exercise four to five times in succession. Should you begin to feel light-headed, stop at that point. If light-headedness remains a problem, consider shortening the length of the inhalation and/or decreasing the total number of repetitions of this exercise.

Practice this exercise five to ten times a day. Make it a habit in the morning, afternoon, and evening, as well as during stressful situations. After a week or two of practice, you may want to omit Step 1, which was for teaching the technique only. Because this form of relaxation is a skill, it is important to practice at least five to ten times a day.

At first you may not notice any on-the-spot relaxation. However, after a week or two of regular practice you will increase your capabilities to relax "on-the-spot." Remember—you must practice regularly if you are to master this skill. Regular, consistent practice of these daily exercises will lead to the development of a more calm and relaxed attitude—a sort of anti-stress attitude—and when you do have stressful moments, they will be far less severe.

Another exercise to promote relaxation and increase your power of concentration is breath counting. You may do this sitting or lying down. As before, you will use quiet, normal diaphragmatic breathing. Concentrate on your breathing. As you breathe in, think "in." Let the air out and think "out." Think "In . . . Out . . . In . . . Out." Now each time you breathe out, count the breaths. Count the consecutive breaths without missing a count. If you happen to miss one, start over. When you get to ten, start at one again. Do this ten times as you sit quietly, concentrate, anticipate the breath, and block all other thoughts from your mind.

Relaxation–Recall Exercises

One of the physical responses that accompanies relaxation is *vasodilation,* an expansion of the arteries in the skin of the extremities. This produces a warm, heavy sensation as blood flow increases in that area.

Generally speaking, relaxed individuals tend to have warmer hands, and anxious or stressed individuals tend to have cooler hands. If one can imagine warmth, or, on a feeling level, can reproduce the heavy sensation in the limbs, the body has the tendency to "relive" or "reproduce" that state. A shift in blood flow is impossible without a change in nervous system tone, thus facilitating relaxation. After a degree of proficiency has been obtained, you can add a more complex imagination process by utilizing personal visual imagery of a time and place that was particularly relaxing to you. If your "feeling memory" is pretty good and if you have developed some body control and concentration abilities, the memory of the beautiful times in your life can be one of your keys to controlling stress and tension.

The exercises in this section are quiet concentration activities that can be done either sitting or lying down. The object is to tell yourself to reproduce feelings of heaviness and warmth in the legs. If you are successful, a heavy, warm, sensation will occur as blood flow increases in that area. The body will "relive" or "reproduce" that state, thus facilitating relaxation.

You must be quiet and undistracted. You must concentrate.

Part 1.   Start by taking three deep breaths. Repeat the following phrases quietly to yourself: "I am relaxed." "I am calm." "I am quiet."

Go slowly; allow the time between each phrase to feel the sensations. Say quietly to yourself,

> *"My right leg is heavy . . . My right leg is heavy and warm . . . My right leg is warm and relaxed . . . I am calm and quite relaxed . . . My left leg is heavy . . . My left leg is heavy and warm . . . My left leg is warm and relaxed . . . I am calm and quite relaxed . . . I am quiet and at peace . . . I am relaxed."*

This activity should take about five minutes.

Part 2. For this exercise, concentrate on the trunk area of the body. You are to try to imagine warmth being emitted from the nerve plexis that lies behind the stomach right above the navel. Focus your attention on what you feel is the exact center of your body. The nerves there form the Solar Plexis. Softly, slowly, and quietly say to yourself,

> *"I am relaxed . . . I am calm . . . I am quiet . . . My solar plexis is warm . . . I can feel the heat radiating throughout my entire body . . . My body is warm and relaxed . . . I am quiet and at peace . . . I am relaxed."*

This activity should take about five minutes.

Part 3. By now you should be familiar with the procedure for this exercise. It will be quiet concentration of heaviness and warmth in the arms and hands. If you had any success with the first two parts, you will do very well on the next. If you have had difficulty with those previous exercises, this one should provide you with a breakthrough. The reason for this is that you have finer control over your hands and arms than over your legs and trunk. More nerves innervate fewer muscles and you have more practice in using the upper extremities. You may sit or lie down. Start with a few deep breaths. Center yourself. Close your eyes and concentrate on your hands and arms. Repeat to yourself, slowly and quietly,

> *"I am relaxed . . . I am calm . . . I am quiet . . . My right arm is heavy . . . My right arm is heavy and warm . . . My right arm is warm . . . My right arm is warm and relaxed . . . I am calm and quite relaxed . . . My left arm is heavy . . . My left arm is heavy and warm . . . My left arm is warm . . . My left arm is warm and relaxed . . . I am calm and quite relaxed . . . My body is warm and relaxed . . . I am quiet and at peace . . . I am relaxed."*

Breathing and Relaxation—Recall Together

Step 1. In a quiet room and in a comfortable chair, assume a restful position and a quiet, passive attitude. Take four deep breaths. Make each one deeper than the one before. Hold the first inhalation for four seconds, the second one for five seconds, the third one for six seconds, and the fourth one for seven seconds. Pull the tension from all parts of your body into your lungs and exhale it with each expiration. Feel more relaxed with each breath.

Step 2. Count backward from ten to zero. Breathe naturally, and with each exhalation count one number and feel more relaxed as you approach zero. With each count you descend a relaxation stairway and become more deeply relaxed until you are totally relaxed at zero.

Step 3. Now go to a favorite relaxation place (in your memory). Stay there for five minutes. Try to recall, vividly but passively, the feelings of that place and time that were very relaxing.

Step 4. Bring your attention back to yourself. Count from zero to ten. Energize your body. Feel the energy, vitality, and health flow through your system. Feel alert and eager to resume your activities. Open your eyes.

Relieving Muscle Tension

The last group of exercises we will present in this area is perhaps the most important. It is essential that you become aware of muscle tension and learn ways to counteract that tension.

Most experts in the relaxation field feel that reducing excess muscle tension not only directly reduces total body tension and anxiety but also indirectly helps eliminate the psychological forerunner of the muscle tension. It is no wonder that muscles are the one organ system that is included in almost every relaxation program. We know that one cannot relax the mind or concentrate fully if the brain is being bombarded by muscle tension impulses. Whether muscle tension reduction is considered an end in itself, or a means to an end, it is an essential step in this procedure.

Much of the harmful, stress-producing muscle tension is extremely subtle and very difficult to detect. If you are thinking defensive thoughts, you start to assume a defensive posture. It is practically impossible to think of an action and not have your muscles prepare for the potential action. The tense individual who is defensive and who is constantly imagining action creates a situation in which the body becomes very efficient at being tense, and adapts by maintaining a chronic state of muscle tension.

If such a condition is permitted to exist for an extended period of time, a wide variety of physical disorders may be produced or exaggerated. A few of the more common disorders are tension headaches, muscle cramps and spasms (such as writer's cramp), limitation of range of movement and flexibility, susceptibility to muscle injuries such as tears and sprains, insomnia, and a wide variety of gastrointestinal maladies (constipation, diarrhea, colitis), renal system problems, dysmenorrhea. This list seems endless, but remember that the muscular system is involved in every body process and in every expression of emotion.

Exercises that relieve muscle tension are the ones that fully contract the muscles and then allow full relaxation, and the ones that stretch the muscles.

For Your Lower Extremities

Toe Raise, Sitting. As you sit in your seat, lean forward and place your hands or elbows on your knees. Then raise up on your toes, using your upper body for as much resistance as you want. Do at least ten of these.

Toe Touch. You need not make a big production out of this exercise. Simply bend down and tie your shoe or get something out of your purse or briefcase while it rests on the floor. Do only a few repetitions, but stay in the down position for five seconds.

The Knee and Thigh Stretch. Sit with your legs positioned under you so that your buttocks are resting on your ankles. Your toes should be pointed backward. Place your hands on the floor outside and behind your feet. Supporting your weight on your arms and legs, straighten your body with your head raised high. Hold this position for a count of ten; relax and repeat five times.

For Your Trunk

The Back Stretch. As its name implies, you will feel this stretch in different parts of your back as the exercise progresses. Lie on the floor. Slowly tensing your stomach muscles, raise your trunk through the sitting position to a point where your head is as close to your knees as possible. Once there, place your hands on your *knees,* thumb on the inside of your leg, elbow held as high as possible. Hold for ten counts and return to the lying position. Move very slowly. Feel the stomach muscles contract as they raise and lower your upper body. Feel the stretch in the lower back.

On the second repetition, place your hands *halfway between your knees and ankles.* Try to get your head to your knees; however, go only as far as your flexibility allows. Don't force it, you will get there. Hold for a count of ten and relax back to the lying position. Feel the stretch and subsequent relaxation in the back slightly higher than in repetition one.

On the third repetition, try for your *ankles.* Go slowly, feel the stretch a little higher on the back. Try to get your head to your knees. Hold for a count of ten and relax. For the fourth repetition, try to place your hands on the *bottoms of your feet.* Draw the trunk toward your legs. Allow your elbows to rest on the floor. Hold for a count of ten and slowly return to the lying position. Relax, feel the tension release.

Standing Trunk Bend. Stand with your feet together, legs straight. The first motion will be a side bend. Stretch your arms over your head and then bend your trunk as far as possible to the right. Try to achieve a right angle to your lower body. Go only as far as you can, hold for a count of ten, and return to an erect position. Then repeat to the left. Hold for ten seconds and return. Then bend backward as far as you can, hold for ten and return. The final move is forward. Bend to a right angle and hold for ten and return. Move very slowly, feel the stretch. After all four moves, bring your arms to your sides and relax.

For Your Upper Extremities

Reach for the Wall. Stand in front of a wall so that your outstretched arms just reach the wall. Place the palms of your hands against the wall. Now remove your hands from the wall and *step back* about six inches. Extend your arms primarily from the shoulders and reach for the wall. At the same time, spread your fingers and extend them backward. When you make contact with the wall, your shoulders, elbows, wrists, and finger joints should be at full extension and stretch. Hold the stretch for a count of six and return. Repeat five times.

The Shoulder Roll. While you are standing, do the second exercise in this group, the shoulder roll. Clasp your hands behind your back. The object is to roll your shoulders by first dropping them to the lowest possible point, rolling them back, then up, as in a shoulder shrug, and then forward before you lower them once again. Complete five circles and return to an erect standing position. Do this five times.

Shoulder Elevation. The next exercise is done either sitting on the floor or standing. Clasp your hands behind your back, allowing them to rest comfortably against your buttocks. Keeping your back straight, raise your arms as high as possible. Hold in the farthest position for a count of five and return to the resting position. Repeat five times.

Back Reach. Raise your arms above your head and clasp your hands together. Bend your arms back so that your hands touch the back of your neck. Once there, pause and then stretch so that your hands touch a point further down your back. Hold the extreme position for a count of five. Repeat at least three times.

For Your Head and Neck

Backward, Forward, and Side Neck Stretch. Move your head slowly back toward your spine until your nose is pointed straight up in the air. Feel the stretch in the front of the neck. Feel the muscles and skin pull tight from the chin. By the way, this will help that saggy double chin problem. Hold for a count of five and slowly move your chin toward your chest. Try to get your chin to your chest, but be sure to keep your back straight, don't cheat. When you get as far forward as you can, try to completely relax and let the weight of the head stretch the neck muscles. Allow the head to dangle loose. Hold for a count of five and return to an upright position by slowly contracting your neck and back muscles. (No fast, jerky movement should be made during any of these exercises.) Return to center, rest for a breath, and then rotate the head so as to look over the right shoulder. Return to center, rest for a breath, and then look over the other shoulder. Hold each of these for a count of five.

For Your Face

Facial Exercises. To take the tight feeling from your face muscles, take a moment in front of the mirror and open your mouth wide, stick your tongue out, raise your eyebrows, and stretch all the muscles of your face. Hold for six counts and then relax. Repeat the exercise five times and notice where you've been holding some of your stress throughout the day.

The Role of Play in Stress Reduction

Hans Selye was only one of the wise men who has said that you cannot be stressed and laugh at the same time. If we turn that around and assume that if you are laughing and having fun, you cannot be stressed, then we can also assume that having fun and playing are good stress-reduction techniques. That sounds simple enough, but it isn't, not by a long shot. Most adults have lost their ability to play. Oh, we go on vacations, we belong to clubs, we play tennis, handball, and golf, we spend a lot of time pursuing recreation, but there is a big difference between recreation and relaxing play.

Play is the spontaneous expression of our naturalness and is the guru of our "right brain." Playfulness is spontaneity, self-confidence, attunement to life, joy, the ability to be focused and immersed or to be in flow, forgetting time and responsibilities; it's the ability to obtain pleasure, to be silly, and to see and experience the less serious side of life.

Imposed structure and organized games also frequently block play behavior. Whenever we are told how to play, whom to play with, and how long to play, our naturally playful responses are blocked. Structure implies right and wrong ways of doing things, which heightens the possibility of making mistakes and makes work out of play.

Stress Management Prescription

1. Reread the previous chapter and gain awareness of what stress is and how it can be harmful to your health, decrease your performance, and reduce your happiness.
2. Make a list of your stress-related symptoms, both physical and emotional.
3. Go back to your stress profiles and identify the stressors to which you seem most vulnerable.
4. Plan a program to reduce stressors and eradicate your negative stress-related symptoms. This will involve:

   a. Establishing desired outcomes. Be specific (for example, deciding to stop biting your fingernails).
   b. Learning about specific stress reduction techniques. This must include both social engineering and personality engineering techniques and relaxation procedures.
   c. Matching techniques to your specific needs.
   d. Developing a plan of action complete with practice schedules.
   e. Writing a contract with yourself complete with the evidence of, and rewards for, success.
   f. Carrying out the program, including monitoring for progress, changing any program that is not working, evaluating success, and giving rewards.

Summary

Relaxation training reinforced by such techniques as meditation, neuromuscular and autogenic relaxation, and biofeedback-aided relaxation helps reduce emotional reactivity. Not only does relaxation training promote voluntary control over some central nervous system activities associated with arousal, it promotes a quiet sense of control that eventually influences attitudes, perception, and behavior. Relaxation training will foster interaction with your inner self and you will learn by actually feeling (visceral learning) that what you are thinking influences your body processes, which in turn influences your thought processes. You will come to know your feelings and emotions as a part of your thinking experience. More and more your behavior will come from what is within you rather than merely being made up of responses triggered by the people and the environment around you.

One essential to mental health, productivity, and happiness is the ability to experience each current situation in *real terms*, without imagining consequences that could or should occur. The effects of such expectations are usually negative, and perhaps the primary therapeutic benefit of a relaxation program is the development of the ability to concentrate attention on the present, to quiet the imagination, and to distinguish reality from fantasy. You can develop the ability to direct your thoughts away from the ego self, the primary source of stress, and direct it to the problem at hand. You can become more problem-centered and less ego-centered. As you become less stressed, you automatically become more efficient; they go hand in hand.

Stress is a blocker. It blocks and consumes your energy. When you free yourself from stress, you create a void that can be filled with a sense of energy and power needed to take a risk, pursue a different path, throw off your fixed stress-causing belief system, to find peace, tranquility, happiness—enlightenment. Stress is the bottled-up energy that becomes blocked when you stuff yourself into a restricted life, tricking yourself into giving up what you truly need for nourishment and growth. When you start using any or all of these techniques, you begin to know yourself and to be directed by your inner feelings. The energy that has been freed by such techniques can then be used to empower you into the natural flow of life.

References

Carrington, Patricia. 1984. "Modern forms of meditation." In *Principles and Practice of Stress Management,* Woolfolk, R., and Lehrer, P. M. (eds.). New York: The Guilford Press.

Everly, G. S. and D. A. Girdano. 1980. *The stress mess solution.* Englewood Cliffs, NJ: Prentice-Hall.

Girdano, D. A. 1980. *Better late than never: How to avoid a midlife fitness crisis.* Englewood Cliffs, NJ: Prentice-Hall.

Girdano, D. A. and G. S. Everly. 1986. *Controlling stress and tension: A holistic approach.* Second edition, Englewood Cliffs, NJ: Prentice-Hall.

12

Your Self: Your Choice

Are you experiencing "quality living"?

How healthy are you in each aspect of your life?

How much effort are you making to become all you can be?

What are your goals for each dimension of your life and what must you do to reach them?

What can you do *now* to get started?

Introduction

This chapter is for you to write. It is about you: How you are right now, how you would like to be, and what you can do to start becoming the person you want to be. In Chapters 1 and 3 you learned what comprises and what jeopardizes quality living. In Chapter 2, you learned about a process that can help you decide how you want to be and determine how to pursue your goal. In Chapters 4–11, you actually began that process by learning about behaviors that contribute to high level functioning in all dimensions of life, and you learned how to engage in these behaviors safely and effectively.

To *really* evaluate your status regarding quality living, however, you need to bring all of your knowledge and assessment data together in one "big picture." The forms and exercises in this chapter will help you accomplish this.

Assessing Your Current Functional Status

To begin, estimate your current functional level in each dimension of life using Form 12.1, the *Functional Status Worksheet*, as a guide. This worksheet provides a checklist of criteria that reflect healthy functioning in each dimension of life, as defined in Chapter 1. It might be helpful to review these definitions at this point. For your convenience, they are restated here:

Physical Health — The ability to carry out daily tasks with energy remaining for unforeseen circumstances; biological integrity.

Emotional Health — The ability to control emotions and express them appropriately and comfortably.

Social Health — The ability to interact well with people and the environment; having satisfying interpersonal relationships.

Mental Health — The ability to learn, including intellectual capabilities.

Spiritual Health — The belief in some unifying force such as nature, scientific laws, or a godlike entity.

FORM 12.1 FUNCTIONAL STATUS WORKSHEET

Directions: This table is designed to assist you in assessing your functional status in each of the five dimensions of life. Criteria to consider in determining your status are offered for each dimension, and spaces are provided for you to add your own criteria if desired. Circle the number that best describes your current level of functioning for each criterion listed, using the following scale:

0 = Unknown   1 = Low level of functioning   2 = Average functioning

3 = Above average functioning   4 = High level of functioning

For example, if your muscular strength/endurance is above average, circle the 3 for that category. If your cholesterol level is well within safe limits, circle the 4 for that category (this means if you have a dangerously high cholesterol level, you should circle 1, which would indicate a low level of functional status for that category). Since many of the self assessments that you have done while reading this book are relevant, you may want to review your results on those that you completed before doing this profile.

Dimension	Criteria to Consider	Current Functional Status				
PHYSICAL	Overall fitness level	0	1	2	3	4
	Cardiorespiratory fitness	0	1	2	3	4
	Muscular strength/endurance	0	1	2	3	4
	Body Composition (% fat)	0	1	2	3	4
	Body chemistry profile:					
	Total cholesterol	0	1	2	3	4
	HDL	0	1	2	3	4
	LDL	0	1	2	3	4
	Glucose level	0	1	2	3	4
	Iron intake	0	1	2	3	4
	Heart function:					
	Heart rate	0	1	2	3	4
	Blood pressure	0	1	2	3	4
	Daily rest/relaxation	0	1	2	3	4
	Energy level	0	1	2	3	4
	Recommended nutritional intake:					
	Cholesterol	0	1	2	3	4
	Complex carbohydrates	0	1	2	3	4
	Protein	0	1	2	3	4
	Sodium	0	1	2	3	4
	Calcium	0	1	2	3	4
	Total fat	0	1	2	3	4
	Saturated fat	0	1	2	3	4
	Unsaturated	0	1	2	3	4
	Fiber	0	1	2	3	4
	Other criteria (specify)					
	_____	0	1	2	3	4
	_____	0	1	2	3	4

(Continued)

EMOTIONAL	Self-esteem:	0	1	2	3	4
	Positive self talk	0	1	2	3	4
	Self-confidence	0	1	2	3	4
	Self image	0	1	2	3	4
	Body image	0	1	2	3	4
	Honest expression of emotions	0	1	2	3	4
	Appropriate expression of feelings/desires	0	1	2	3	4
	Other criteria (specify)					
	_____	0	1	2	3	4
	_____	0	1	2	3	4
SOCIAL	Stress level	0	1	2	3	4
	Interpersonal relationships:					
	Comfort level with others	0	1	2	3	4
	Number of close friends	0	1	2	3	4
	Satisfying intimate relationships	0	1	2	3	4
	Enjoy interactions with other people	0	1	2	3	4
	Engage in a variety of activities	0	1	2	3	4
	Other criteria (specify)					
	_____	0	1	2	3	4
	_____	0	1	2	3	4
MENTAL	Informed/aware regarding:					
	World events	0	1	2	3	4
	National events	0	1	2	3	4
	Local events	0	1	2	3	4
	Technical information for job	0	1	2	3	4
	Personal growth issues	0	1	2	3	4
	Intellectual abilities:					
	Quick to learn	0	1	2	3	4
	Perceptive	0	1	2	3	4
	Analytical	0	1	2	3	4
	Performance:					
	Quality	0	1	2	3	4
	Productivity	0	1	2	3	4
	Creativity	0	1	2	3	4
	GPA or job evaluations	0	1	2	3	4
	Other criteria (specify)					
	_____	0	1	2	3	4
	_____	0	1	2	3	4
SPIRITUAL	Personal life philosophy:					
	Well-defined ideas about meaning/purpose					
	of life/death	0	1	2	3	4
	Feel at peace with self/life	0	1	2	3	4
	Positive outlook on life	0	1	2	3	4
	Strong identity with self/values	0	1	2	3	4
	Other criteria (specify)					
	_____	0	1	2	3	4
	_____	0	1	2	3	4

Assessing Your Current Efforts

Since *how* you are living your life, and your goals, plans, and progress—that is, what you are "becoming"—are also part of experiencing quality living, your "big picture" is not complete until you have indicated your *efforts* to develop your capacities in each dimension of life. You can do this by using the lifestyle circle described in Chapter 1.

Your lifestyle circle will help you determine how balanced your efforts currently are to develop each dimension of your life — that is, to live a *wellness lifestyle*. It will help you identify those dimensions of your life in which a greater effort might result in higher levels of functioning and more satisfaction in living. Or, your lifestyle circle might show that you *are* doing the best you can, even though your functional status might not reflect it due to illness or some other type of limitation, *or* simply because of the delay that sometimes exists between efforts and results, such as when you try to lose weight, lower blood cholesterol levels, or increase fitness.

Use Form 12.2, the Lifestyle Worksheet, to determine your current effort level or lifestyle. First make a list of the efforts you have made during the last week to develop your capacity in each dimension of life. Use Table 12.A as a guide; it provides examples of efforts that comprise a wellness lifestyle.

After completing your "effort list" for each dimension, use a scale of "0" to "10" to rate the intensity of your efforts, with "0" representing no effort and "10" representing your best effort. Then use these numbers to shade in the lifestyle circle in Form 12.2. (You may find it helpful to refer back to Figure 1.3 in Chapter 1, which shows examples of lifestyle circles.)

Evaluating Your Current Functional Status and Efforts

After completing the Functional Status Worksheet and your Lifestyle Circle, evaluate what your assessments indicate. Does your personal worksheet describe you as functioning in each dimension at a level with which you are satisfied? Is your health status where you would like it to be? Does your lifestyle circle indicate you are operating at as high a level of effort as you're able? Are your efforts balanced among the dimensions?

If your answer is "yes" to all of these questions, then you are to be congratulated; you undoubtedly are experiencing a high level of quality living. However, many, if not most, of us are not satisfied with our status in one or more areas. We know we could expend more effort at developing ourselves. Nonetheless, we would like to be somehow magically transformed and not have to struggle through the changes that would enable us to alter our functional status. Unfortunately there is no magic. There are only small steps, which, if arranged appropriately so they fit into a meaningful sequence, can lead to larger steps and eventually to large and permanent changes. Remember, nothing is static. Everything is in process. You are who you are now *only* at this moment, and you can choose in the next moment to launch yourself in a new direction.

FORM 12.2 LIFESTYLE WORKSHEET

1. List your efforts (deliberate choices) during the last week to develop your capabilities in each dimension of your life:

   Physical   *Emotional*   *Social*   *Mental*   *Spiritual*

2. Level of Effort

   Estimate your overall level of effort in each dimension using a scale of "0" (NO EFFORT) to "10" (BEST EFFORT).

   _____   _____   _____   _____   _____

   Physical   *Emotional*   *Social*   *Mental*   *Spiritual*

3. Shade in your effort levels on the Lifestyle Circle. This will allow you to actually *see* how you are living now. (Figure 1.5 in Chapter 1 shows examples of shaded lifestyle circles.)

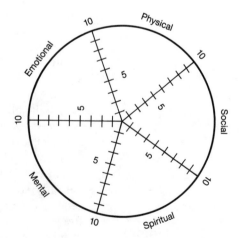

Table 12.A   Examples of efforts comprising a wellness lifestyle.

PHYSICAL DIMENSION	SOCIAL DIMENSION

PHYSICAL DIMENSION

Efforts to be physically fit:
- Regular aerobic exercise
- Regular strength and flexibility exercise
- Adequate rest
- Maintaining appropriate weight and lean body mass

Efforts to eat well:
- Low fat/high carbohydrate/diet/high fiber
- Variety of nutritious foods
- Meeting RDA standards
- Following U.S. Dietary Goals

Efforts to protect self from physical hazards:
- Avoiding ingestion, abuse of, and/or exposure to harmful substances such as cigarette smoke, pollution, drugs, radiation, and so on.
- Observing safety precautions, such as wearing seat belts, not drinking and driving, wearing appropriate clothing for the weather, keeping any equipment in good repair.

SOCIAL DIMENSION

Efforts to manage stress:
- Saying "no" if already overburdened
- Planning time for self
- Delegating responsibilities
- Making a daily plan
- Developing interests and engaging in a variety of activities

Efforts to establish satisfying interpersonal relationships
- Acknowledging and respecting the concerns and feelings of others
- Caring about and helping others
- Identifying others you enjoy doing things with
- Taking time to learn/care about another on an intimate basis

MENTAL DIMENSION

Efforts to expand knowledge/awareness:
- Reading/listening to news and talking with others about local, national and world concerns
- Reading and taking classes/seminars to gain technical information for job and/or personal growth and life management skills

Efforts to be self-reliant and productive:
- Using skills and knowledge to be creative and perform capably on job and in personal life

EMOTIONAL DIMENSION

Efforts to promote/maintain self-esteem:
- Acknowledging personal qualities and accomplishments
- Establishing reasonable expectations of self (stress management)
- Seeking companionship with people who care for and about you
- Expressing feelings honestly

Efforts to control and express emotions appropriately:
- Being assertive, but not aggressive
- Listening as well as telling
- Expressing desire without demanding
- Loving without possessing

SPIRITUAL DIMENSION

Efforts to develop personal philosophy:
- Read, talk with others, take classes regarding established approaches to life philosophy as from science, religion, and philosophy
- Trying out various philosophical/religious options
- Identifying personal beliefs and feelings about life

Deciding How You Want To Be

The next step is to *decide* whether your current functional status and effort levels are where you want them to be. Using Form 12.3, the Long-Term Goal Worksheet, record the goals you wish to fulfill in each area of your life. Be as specific as you can.

FORM 12.3 LONG-TERM GOAL WORKSHEET: "How I Would Like To Be"

Directions: First review your completed Functional Status Worksheet. Then, for each dimension indicate how you would like to be as compared to what your Functional Status Worksheet indicates. Use the worksheet to help you be specific. If you are satisfied with your current functional status in any dimension, simply place a checkmark in the designated column. Finally, rank the goals in each dimension in terms of their importance to your overall health and well-being.

GOALS

Dimension of Life	I would like to be:	Importance	I am how I want to be
Physical			
Emotional			
Social			
Mental			
Spiritual			

Reviewing the Functional Status Worksheet you used earlier in this chapter will help you recall specific weaknesses and strengths. If you are satisfied with your current functioning in a given dimension, simply indicate that in the appropriate column.

Once you have completed this worksheet you have, in effect, listed your *long-term goals* for becoming the "you" you want to be. Chances are your list of goals to be accomplished may seem rather overwhelming. To make "overwhelming" into "achievable," prioritize the goals in each dimension in terms of their importance to your overall health and well being. Your #1 long-term goal in each dimension will then be your focus in planning how to *start* becoming the person you want to be.

Formulating Short-Term Goals

Having identified your most important goal in each dimension, the next step is to break that goal down into smaller, short-term goals or actions that you believe you can actually achieve. The Short-Term Goal Worksheet (Form 12.4) is designed to help you do this.

Focusing only on your #1 goal in each dimension, make a list of possible actions you could take to start becoming more like your goal describes you. It is especially important that each action on your list be stated as specifically as possible in measurable or observable behaviors. For example, "I will walk 30 minutes, three times per week" can be observed and recorded precisely. "I'll start doing some exercise" is too vague. You haven't said how much "some exercise" is or even what "exercise" means. Similarly, "I can eat a piece of fruit instead of my usual afternoon candy bar" is sufficiently specific to be measurable, but "I want to eat better" is not.

Use what you've learned in this book to help you formulate your list of short-term goals. The preceding chapters offered many recommendations regarding what you could do to improve your health and well-being and how you could do it safely and effectively. These suggestions ranged from simply gathering more information (through behavior diaries or talking with others who have made changes in their lives, for example) to actually attempting a behavior change (such as substituting 10 minutes of deep breathing at times when you snack, hungry or not). More than likely your short-term goals will include a similar range of possible actions since considering and attempting are the first two steps in the behavior change process (see Figure 1.6, Chapter 1). If you have already achieved your ideal functional status in any one dimension, then your list of short-term goals will consist of the actions you need to take to *maintain* your capacities.

When you have finished your "action list" for each of your priority long-term goals, you will have created an array of possible steps you might undertake in the process of becoming how you want to be. The next step is to prioritize these short-term goals according to their importance to your health and well-being *and* your readiness to do them. The instructions for doing this are given on the Short-Term Goal Worksheet.

If many of the goals you are most ready to attempt are also ranked as most important to you, you are at a somewhat advanced stage of the "consideration process" of behavior change. Probably you have been thinking about trying a different behavior for some time; perhaps you have even attempted it once or twice. If, on the other hand, the actions you are most ready to attempt are not the goals you rated as most important, you may simply be at an earlier point in the "consideration process," or perhaps some of your short-term goals need to be stated in smaller steps to become "accomplishable." You may also find the action for which you *do* feel ready is actually

FORM 12.4 SHORT-TERM GOAL WORKSHEET: "The Small Steps to Success"

Directions: For each dimension, first list your #1 long-term goal (from Long-Term Goal Worksheet) and then list *specific actions* you think you could do now to start achieving your #1 goal. State your short-term goals in a way that allows you to measure or record your progress. Finally, rank your goals according to their importance to your health and well-being and according to your readiness to start doing the specified action *now.*

PHYSICAL DIMENSION

#1 Long-Term Goal _____

_____

Short-Term Goals	*Importance*	*Readiness*
1. _____	_____	_____
_____		
2. _____	_____	_____
_____		
3. _____	_____	_____
_____		
4. _____	_____	_____
_____		

EMOTIONAL DIMENSION

#1 Long-Term Goal _____

_____

Short-Term Goals	*Importance*	*Readiness*
1. _____	_____	_____
_____		
2. _____	_____	_____
_____		
3. _____	_____	_____
_____		
4. _____	_____	_____
_____		

SOCIAL DIMENSION

#1 Long-Term Goal _____

_____

Short-Term Goals	*Importance*	*Readiness*
1. _____	_____	_____
_____		
2. _____	_____	_____
_____		
3. _____	_____	_____
_____		
4. _____	_____	_____
_____		

MENTAL DIMENSION

#1 Long-Term Goal _____

_____

Short-Term Goals	Importance	Readiness
1. _____	_____	_____
_____		
2. _____	_____	_____
_____		
3. _____	_____	_____
_____		
4. _____	_____	_____
_____		

SPIRITUAL DIMENSION

#1 Long-Term Goal _____

_____

Short-Term Goals	Importance	Readiness
1. _____	_____	_____
_____		
2. _____	_____	_____
_____		
3. _____	_____	_____
_____		
4. _____	_____	_____
_____		

a step *toward* your important goals even if it is not the most direct step. Whatever the case, make your top priority that action you are most ready to take at this point in time. It is the step with which you are most likely to succeed, and accomplishing one change may give you the confidence and incentive to try another, perhaps your most important one.

Taking Action: Making a Contract with Yourself

At this point you have identified at least one long-term goal and one short-term goal you feel ready to pursue in each dimension of your life. While it is possible that you could succeed at making all of these changes at the same time, successful change is more likely if you use the *one step at a time* approach. Thus, to give yourself the best chance to succeed, select just one dimension of your life to work on for the moment. Use the same criteria to prioritize the dimensions as you used for prioritizing and selecting goals within each dimension—that is, prioritize according to the importance of that aspect to your health and well-being and according to your readiness to try the action specified.

Once you have identified that dimension of your life most important to you right now, it is time to take action. As suggested in Chapter 2, making a contract with yourself is one of the best ways to do this because it helps you to plan for all the things that seem to increase your chances for success. A good contract form asks you to specify exactly what you will do and when, how you will avoid potential pitfalls, who will be your support person or group, how you will reward yourself, and when you will evaluate and revise your action plan. An example of a completed contract form like the one just described was shown and discussed in detail in Chapter 2, should you wish to review it more thoroughly.

Your contract form is provided below. Filling it out can be your key to action—action that leads to becoming and being all you can be. Before you close this book and lay it aside, choose to do that for yourself.

Choosing to grow is valuing and honoring your life. It is quality living. It is your choice — your life. Give it your best.

> *Each of us experiences life in our own context,*
> *but for all of us there is a struggle to balance the*
> *reality of life with our needs and our dreams.*
> *Perhaps the most difficult thing of all is to value*
> *our life and who we are, and to direct our life in*
> *a manner that honors it . . .*
> *Laurie Harper,* A Taste for Life

A CONTRACT WITH MYSELF

I, _____, hereby declare that I am ready and willing to commit myself to the following goals and activities. I realize that to achieve my long term goals I must be willing to work for small gains, I must seek support and I must be adequately prepared. Therefore, for the next week I resolve to myself to do the following:

1. Long term goal(s):_____

_____

2. Specific goal: During the next week, I plan to: _____

_____

_____

3. I will ask my helper to assist me by: _____

_____

_____

4. I realize I can easily avoid fulfilling my action plan by: _____

_____

_____

5. So I plan to avoid doing this by: _____

_____

_____

6. My reward to myself when I fulfill the terms of my action plan each day will be: _____

_____

_____

TODAY'S DATE: _____   SIGNATURE: _____

REVIEW DATE: _____   HELPER: _____

7. Action Plan Evaluation/Revision

   a. After working on my action plan for one week, I found that: _____

      _____

      _____

      _____

      _____

      _____

      _____

      _____

      _____

   b. To continue working toward my goal in small steps during the next week, I plan to:

     _____   Follow the same action plan because: _____

           _____

           _____

           _____

     _____   Expand my action plan to include: _____

           _____

           _____

           _____

     _____   Cut back on my original plan for now because: _____

           _____

           _____

           _____

1

Tests of Cardiorespiratory Fitness

A. Queen's College Step Test

Instructions

This test involves (1) Stepping up and down at a fixed rhythm from a gymnasium bleacher for three minutes, and (2) Taking a 15-second pulse count afterwards to see how hard your heart beats after doing this amount of exercise. Although the test can be done by anyone of any age, the available norms are based on the results of college-age males and females. Persons of other ages may use this test without referring to the norms by testing periodically and comparing personal results over time. Specific instructions are as follows:

1. Step height: 16¼ inches (This is the height of a standard gymnasium bleacher or stadium bleacher).
2. Rhythm: Females: 22 steps/minute
   Males: 24 steps/minute
   Note: The stepping procedure requires both feet to step up and both feet to step down using an UP UP DOWN DOWN procedure. A metronome for establishing the rhythm is set at a rate of four times as fast so that each step may be counted against a beat. Thus, the metronome rhythm is:
   Females: 88 beats/minute
   Males: 96 beats/minute
3. At a signal to go, begin stepping up and down from the bleacher in time to the metronome using the UP UP DOWN DOWN procedure. After three minutes, stop the test and find your pulse at the radial or temporal artery (as described in Chapter 5). Starting five seconds after stopping the test, take a 15-second pulse count. Multiply this by 4 to convert the count into a minute rate (that is, the number of beats/minute).

4. Find your predicted aerobic capacity ($\dot{V}O_2$ max) in Table A below. Also determine your percentile when compared to a sample of people of the same sex and a similar age. Table 5.C in Chapter 5 provides a method of classifying individuals based on aerobic capacity.

Table A   Percentile rankings for recovery heart rate and predicted maximal oxygen consumption for male and female college students.

PERCENTILE RANKING	RECOVERY HR, FEMALE	PREDICTED MAX VO$_2$ (ML/KG · MIN)	RECOVERY HR, MALE	PREDICTED MAX VO$_2$ (ML/KG · MIN)
100	128	42.2	120	60.9
95	140	40.0	124	59.3
90	148	38.5	128	57.6
85	152	37.7	136	54.2
80	156	37.0	140	52.5
75	158	36.6	144	50.9
70	160	36.3	148	49.2
65	162	35.9	149	48.8
60	163	35.7	152	47.5
55	164	35.5	154	46.7
50	166	35.1	156	45.8
45	168	34.8	160	44.1
40	170	34.4	162	43.3
35	171	34.2	164	42.5
30	172	34.0	166	41.6
25	176	33.3	168	40.8
20	180	32.6	172	39.1
15	182	32.2	176	37.4
10	184	31.8	178	36.6
5	196	29.6	184	34.1

From Katch, F. I. and McArdle, W. D. (1983). *Nutrition, Weight Control and Exercise*, Philadelphia: Lea & Febiger. Used with permission.

B.   Canadian Step Test[1]

General Instructions

This test may be used by adults of any age because the stepping tempo and termination point are adjusted according to age and fitness status. The test consists of three different 3-minute stages at successively faster and faster rates. Each stage is separated by a brief 30-second rest during which a 10-second pulse count is taken. The step bench must be constructed in accordance to the specifications outlined in the technical manual for this test, namely a 2-step bench with 20 cm steps (see Figure 1 below). Specific instructions taken from the operation manual provided by the Canadian government

[1]From: *Standardized test of fitness: Operations manual*. (1985). Hull, Quebec, K1A0S9, Fitness and Amateur Sport, Canada.

Step testing sequence and cadence:
Demonstrate and have the subject
practice the stepping sequence
described below.

START:

Stand in front of the first step,
feet together.

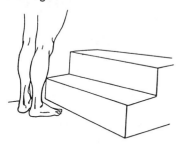

1. STEP:

Place your right foot up on the
first step.

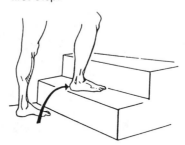

2. STEP:

Bring your left foot up to the
second step.

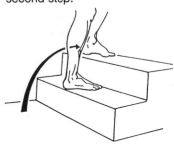

3. UP:

Bring your right foot up on the
second step, feet together.

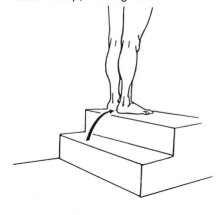

4. STEP:

Start down with your left foot to
the first step.

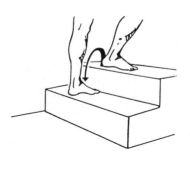

5. STEP:

Bring your right foot down to
the ground level.

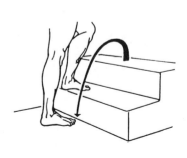

6. DOWN:

Bring your left foot to the
ground level, feet together.

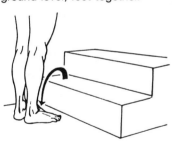

STEP-STEP-UP!
STEP-STEP-DOWN!

UP-2-3! DOWN-2-3!

UP-2-3! DOWN-2-3!

FIGURE 1   Stepping sequence for Canadian Step test.

are provided in Box 1 below. They assume that a tape recording of the tempo is being used. If it is not available, the test can be administered using a standard metronome. The instructions also assume that an assistant will administer this test to aid you in attaining accurate results.

On completion of the test, aerobic capacity (in ml/kg/min) can be predicted using the aerobic calculator which is supplied free by the Canadian Government, or by using the following equation:

$$\dot{V}O_2 \text{ max} = 42.5 + (16.6)\,(\dot{V}O_2) - (.12)\,(W) - (.12)\,(H) - (.24)\,(A)$$

where $\dot{V}O_2$ = the average energy cost of the last stage of exercise you completed (see Table B to determine this value).

W   = body weight in kg

H   = post-exercise pulse rate (in beats/min) following the last stage completed. (This should be measured from 5–15 seconds after stopping, with the number of beats then multiplied times 6.)

A   = age in years

Table B   Average energy cost in L/min of completing different stages on the Canadian step test.

STAGE	MALES	FEMALES
1	1.1391	.9390
2	1.3466	1.0484
3	1.6250	1.3213
4	1.8255	1.4925
5	2.0066	1.6267
6	2.3453	1.7867
7	2.7657	

Inexperienced persons have a tendency to measure post-exercise pulse rate inaccurately, underestimating by 1 beat or more on the average. Therefore, care should be taken to obtain accurate results or have an experienced assistant measure you with a stethoscope.

Norms and percentiles of aerobic capacity for both sexes and all ages based on the results of this test are provided in Table C. The standard error of estimate for predicted aerobic capacity on this test is 4.08 ml/kg/min.

Table C Norms and percentiles by age groups and sex for predicted maximal oxygen consumption (ml/kg/min).

AGE (YRS.)	15–19		20–29		30–39		40–49		50–59		60–69	
SEX	M	F	M	F	M	F	M	F	M	F	M	F
Excellent	≥60	≥43	≥57	≥40	≥48	≥37	≥42	≥35	≥38	≥30	≥30	≥25
Good	58–59	40–42	52–56	37–39	46–47	34–37	40–42	32–34	36–38	27–29	29–30	24–25
Average	54–57	37–39	43–51	35–37	42–45	31–33	37–39	26–31	34–35	25–27	27–28	22–23
Below Average	44–53	35–37	40–42	32–34	38–41	29–31	34–37	24–25	31–33	22–25	26–27	20–22
Poor	≤43	≤34	≤40	≤31	≤37	≤29	≤33	≤23	≤30	≤21	≤26	≤19

AGE (YRS.)	15–19		20–29		30–39		40–49		50–59		60–69	
SEX	M	F	M	F	M	F	M	F	M	F	M	F
Percentiles												
95	62	45	59	43	51	39	44	36	40	31	32	26
90	61	43	58	41	50	38	43	35	39	30	31	26
85	60	43	57	40	48	37	42	35	38	30	30	25
80	59	42	56	39	47	37	42	34	38	29	30	25
75	59	41	55	39	47	36	41	33	37	28	29	24
70	58	40	54	38	46	35	40	33	36	28	29	24
65	58	40	52	37	46	34	40	32	36	27	29	24
60	57	39	48	37	45	33	39	31	35	27	28	23
55	57	38	44	36	44	32	38	30	35	26	28	23
50	56	38	43	35	43	32	38	28	34	26	28	22
45	54	37	43	35	42	31	37	26	34	25	27	22
40	52	37	42	34	41	31	37	25	33	25	27	22
35	47	36	42	34	40	30	36	25	33	24	27	21
30	46	35	41	33	39	30	35	24	32	23	27	21
25	44	35	40	32	38	29	34	24	31	22	26	20
20	43	34	40	31	37	29	32	23	28	21	26	19
15	42	34	39	31	36	28	31	22	26	20	25	19
10	41	33	38	30	34	28	30	22	25	19	24	18
5	40	32	37	29	33	27	29	21	24	18	23	17

From *Standardized Test of Fitness,* 2nd Edition, Fitness and Amateur Sport, Canada, 1981.

BOX 1	SPECIFIC INSTRUCTIONS FOR CANADIAN STEP TEST

Equipment: Stethoscope, sphygmomanometer, tape recorder and CST tapes (or record player and CST record), timer, steps.

Procedure: Preliminaries: Have the subject remove his/her shoes, sit and rest for five minutes. Use a comfortable chair with arm rests. During this time, briefly explain how the test is to be conducted and for what purposes.

Starting exercise. Determine the starting exercise of the subject, based on age, using the following table:

Age	Starting Exercise	
	Males	**Females**
60 and over	1 (66)*	1 (66)
50–59	2 (84)	1 (66)
40–49	3 (102)	2 (84)
30–39	4 (114)	3 (102)
20–29	5 (132)	3 (102)
15–19	5 (132)	4 (114)

*(Stepping Tempo in steps per minute.)

The subject should then be informed that the first stepping exercise is three minutes in duration. The subject will cease to step when the music stops and remain motionless. Indicate that upon completion of this first stage you will inform the subject if he/she is to stop or continue for a second stage.

Post-exercise heart rate — first stage only. Start the tape recorder (or record player) and have the subject perform the first stage of the test. Observe the subject for signs of intolerance.* After three minutes have the subject remain motionless. Determine the post-exercise heart rate with the stethoscope. Start counting on the command word COUNT and continue counting until the command word STOP. (A 10-second timing sequence).

DO NOT stop the tape (or record player) during the test. Pulse counting pauses have been recorded on the tape. It is imperative that the tape (or record player) continue operating for the duration of the test. Pulse counting and determination of the subject's ability to complete the next stage must be accomplished during the time interval *between* the musical stepping tempos.

The determination of an accurate post-exercise heart rate is the critical measurement for deciding if the subect should continue to another stage and to predict maximum oxygen consumption ($\dot{V}O_2$ max.). Quickly determine if the subject is to continue or stop the test. The subject is not to continue if the heart rate is equal to or exceeds these Ceiling Post-Exercise Heart Rates (10 second count):

	Ceiling Post-Exercise Heart Rates (10 sec.)	
Age	**After 1st stage**	**After 2nd stage**
60 and over	24	23
50–59	25	23
40–49	26	24
30–39	28	25
20–29	29	26
15–19	30	27

Completing a second or third stage. If there are no contraindications, have the subject complete a second stage. Repeat the measurements as for the first stage. Determine if the subject is to continue for a third and final stage. The tempos for these stages are listed below:

Subjects Being Tested (by age)		Tempos (beats/min.)
Males:	60s	66; 84; 102
Females:	60s, 50s	
Males:	50s	84; 102; 114
Females:	40s	
Males:	40s	102; 114; 132
Males:	30s	114; 132; 144
Males:	20s; 15–19	132; 144; 156
Females:	30s; 20s	102; 114; 120
Females:	15–19	114; 120; 132

Final post-exercise heart rates. After the subject has completed a third and final stage of stepping, or when the test has been terminated on the basis of post-exercise heart rate measurement (while standing), have the subject sit down.

Discontinuation of the test. The examiner will discontinue the step test if the subject begins to stagger, complains of dizziness, extreme leg pain, nausea, chest pain, or shows facial pallor. Have the subject lie down and check his/her heart rate and blood pressure. Request assistance from a nurse or physician if the subject does not seem to recuperate after a few minutes. If necessary, have someone call an ambulance.

If it becomes obvious that the subject is unable to maintain the proper cadence after the first minute of stepping, step with the subject. If the difficulty in stepping appears to be related to some physiological disfunction discontinue the test. Suggest that the CST could be retaken later at a mutually convenient time.

*dizziness, unusual fatigue, angina, staggering, distressful breathing, nausea, and facial expressions that indicate difficulty in maintaining the cadence.

C. Submaximal Bicycle Ergometer Test[2]

Instructions

This test involves four successive 2-minute stages on a bicycle ergometer (not to be confused with a stationary bicycle designed for exercise). Workload is adjusted based upon body weight and previous activity status. Pulse rate is measured during the last 15 seconds of each stage and then used to predict maximum aerobic capacity (max $\dot{V}O_2$). Specific instructions are as follows:

1. Determine which test protocol to use according to your body weight and activity status in Tables D and E below. You are defined as being "very active" if you have been participating regularly in vigorous activity for at least 15 minutes, 3 days per week, for the last 3 months.

Table D   Selecting a protocol to use.

VERY ACTIVE YES	NO	BODY WEIGHT IN KG (LBS)
Protocol A	Protocol A	< 73 (160)
Protocol B	Protocol A	74–90 (161–199)
Protocol C	Protocol B	< 91 (200)

ACTIVITY STATUS

Table E   Test protocols.

MINUTES OF THE TEST

PROTOCOL	1–2 STAGE I	3–4 STAGE II	5–6 STAGE III	7–8 STAGE IV
A	*25 (150)	50 (300)	75 (450)	100 (600)
B	*25 (150)	50 (300)	100 (600)	150 (900)
C	*50 (300)	100 (600)	150 (900)	200 (1200)

*Workload is in watts (kilogram-meters/min)

[2]Adapted from American College of Sports Medicine. (1986). *Guidelines for exercise testing and prescription,* 3rd. Ed. Philadelphia: Lea and Febiger.

2. Complete the protocol, having an assistant measure your pulse rate during the last 15 seconds of each stage with a stethoscope or by palpation. Stop the test when you heart rate reaches 65–70% of your age-adjusted maximal heart rate (see Table F). Heart rate should be measured for at least two and preferably three stages.

3. A rough estimate of your maximal aerobic capacity can be attained by plotting your heart rates as a function of workload and then extrapolating the line of best fit to your maximum heart rate. Figure 2 illustrates such a technique with sample data.

4. Table 5.2 provides a method of classifying individuals based on aerobic capacity.

Table F Heart rates for terminating ergometer test.

AGE (YEARS)	HEART RATE (BEATS/MIN)
< 20	140
20–29	135
30–39	130
40–49	120
50–59	115
60–65	110

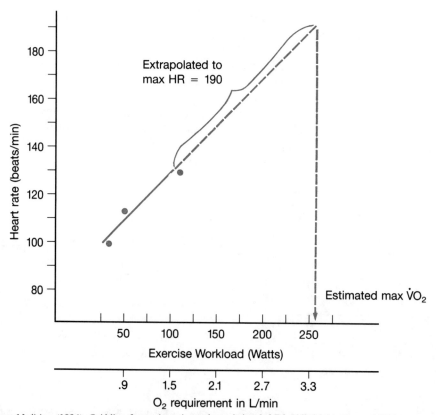

FIGURE 2
Method of determining aerobic capacity based on heart rates on bicycle ergometer test.

Adapted from American College of Sports Medicine, (1986). *Guidelines for exercise testing and prescription,* 3rd Ed. Philadelphia: Lea and Febiger.

D. Cooper 12 Minute Run and 1.5 Mile Run Tests[3]

Instructions for the 12 Minute Run Test

This test involves determining how far you can run/walk in 12 minutes. Since it is a test of maximal performance and thereby one in which you push yourself to your limits, it is not advisable for anyone who has one or more of the major risk factors for cardiovascular disease (see Chapter 5) to take this test until proper medical clearance has been given by a physician. In addition, if you have been previously sedentary, a preconditioning program focusing on developing cardiorespiratory endurance lasting for three weeks or more is strongly advised before endeavoring to take this test. Practice at pacing yourself while running for 12 minutes will also help assure that your score correctly reflects your fitness status. Specific instructions are as follows:

1. After a proper warm-up of 5–10 minutes, run/walk on a measured track for 12 minutes. Record the number of laps covered, including the last one to the nearest ⅛th mile.
2. Using Tables G and H below, determine the percentile into which you fall for your age and sex.

Instructions for the 1.5 Mile Run Test

This test is virtually the same as the 12 Minute Run Test except that you measure how long it takes you to run/walk 1.5 miles. The precautions mentioned above should be followed when preparing for this test also. Specific instructions are as follows:

1. After a proper warm-up of 5–10 minutes, run/walk on a measured track for 1.5 miles (i. e., 6 laps on a standard ¼mile track). Record your time to the nearest second.
2. Using Tables G and H below, determine the percentile into which you fall for your age and sex.

---

[3]Used with permission from Institute for Aerobics Research, 12330 Preston Rd., Dallas, TX 75230.

Table G Percentiles for Cooper 12-minute run and 1.5 mile tests: FEMALE.

%	AGE 20–24		AGE 30–39		AGE 40–49		AGE 50–59		AGE 60+		
	12 MIN. RUN DISTANCE (MILES)	1.5 MILE RUN (TIME)	12 MIN. RUN DISTANCE (MILES)	1.5 MILE RUN (TIME)	12 MIN. RUN DISTANCE (MILES)	1.5 MILE RUN (TIME)	12 MIN. RUN DISTANCE (MILES)	1.5 MILE RUN (TIME)	12 MIN. RUN DISTANCE (MILES)	1.5 MILE RUN (TIME)	
99	>1.78	<8:33	>1.66	<10:05	>1.61	<10:47	>1.48	<12:28			S
95	1.61	10:47	1.53	11:49	1.45	12:51	1.33	14:20	1.35	14:06	
90	1.54	11:43	1.45	12:51	1.41	13:22	1.29	14:55	1.29	14:55	
85	1.49	12:20	1.43	13:06	1.35	14:06	1.24	15:29	1.21	15:57	E
80	1.45	12:51	1.38	13:43	1.32	14:31	1.21	15:57	1.18	16:20	
75	1.41	13:22	1.35	14:08	1.29	14:57	1.20	16:05	1.17	16:27	
70	1.37	13:53	1.33	14:24	1.25	15:76	1.17	16:27	1.13	16:58	G
65	1.35	14:08	1.29	14:50	1.23	15:41	1.14	15:51	1.09	17:29	
60	1.33	14:24	1.27	15:08	1.21	15:57	1.13	16:58	1.07	17:46	
55	1.31	14:35	1.26	15:20	1.19	16:12	1.11	17:14	1.05	18:00	
50	1.29	14:55	1.25	15:26	1.17	16:27	1.10	17:24	1.03	18:16	F
45	1.27	15:10	1.22	15:47	1.16	16:34	1.09	17:29	1.01	18:31	
40	1.25	15:26	1.21	15:57	1.13	16:58	1.06	17:54	.99	18:44	
35	1.22	15:48	1.17	16:23	1.12	16:59	1.04	18:09	.98	18:54	
30	1.21	15:57	1.16	16:35	1.10	17:24	1.02	18:23	.97	18:59	P
25	1.17	16:26	1.13	16:58	1.09	17:29	1.01	18:31	.97	19:02	
20	1.16	16:33	1.11	17:14	1.05	18:00	.98	18:49	.94	19:21	
15	1.13	16:58	1.09	17:29	1.02	18:21	.97	19:02	.93	19:33	
10	1.10	17:21	1.05	18:00	1.01	18:31	.93	19:30	.89	20:04	VP
5	1.03	18:14	1.01	18:31	.96	19:05	.90	19:57	.86	20:23	
1	<.94	>19:25	<.93	>19:27	<.89	>20:04	<.83	>20:47	<.81	>21:06	
N	764	764	2049	2049	1630	1630	878	878	202	202	

Table H Percentiles for Cooper 12-minute run and 1.5 mile tests: MALE.

%	AGE 20–24 12 MIN. RUN DISTANCE (MILES)	AGE 20–24 1.5 MILE RUN (TIME)	AGE 30–39 12 MIN. RUN DISTANCE (MILES)	AGE 30–39 1.5 MILE RUN (TIME)	AGE 40–49 12 MIN. RUN DISTANCE (MILES)	AGE 40–49 1.5 MILE RUN (TIME)	AGE 50–59 12 MIN. RUN DISTANCE (MILES)	AGE 50–59 1.5 MILE RUN (TIME)	AGE 60+ 12 MIN. RUN DISTANCE (MILES)	AGE 60+ 1.5 MILE RUN (TIME)	
99	>1.94	<6:29	>1.89	<7:11	>1.85	<7:42	>1.77	<8:44	>1.71	<9:30	S
95	1.81	8.13	1.77	8:44	1.71	9:30	1.62	10:40	1.57	11:20	
90	1.74	9:09	1.71	9:30	1.65	10:16	1.57	11:18	1.49	12:20	
85	1.69	9:45	1.65	10:16	1.57	11:18	1.49	12:20	1.41	13:22	E
80	1.65	10:16	1.61	10:47	1.54	11:44	1.45	12:51	1.37	13:53	
75	1.62	10:42	1.57	11:18	1.53	11:49	1.41	13:22	1.33	14:24	
70	1.61	10:47	1.55	11:34	1.47	12:34	1.38	13:45	1.29	14:53	G
65	1.57	11:18	1.53	11:49	1.45	12:51	1.35	14:03	1.26	15:19	
60	1.54	11:41	1.49	12:20	1.42	13:14	1.33	14:24	1.24	15:29	
55	1.53	11:49	1.47	12:38	1.41	13:22	1.31	14:40	1.21	15:55	
50	1.50	12:18	1.45	12:51	1.37	13:53	1.29	14:55	1.19	16:07	F
45	1.49	12:20	1.41	13:22	1.35	14:08	1.26	15:78	1.17	16:27	
40	1.45	12:51	1.39	13:36	1.33	14:29	1.25	15:26	1.15	16:43	
35	1.43	13:06	1.37	13:53	1.30	14:47	1.22	15:53	1.13	16:58	
30	1.41	13:22	1.35	14:08	1.29	14:56	1.21	15:57	1.11	17:14	P
25	1.37	13:53	1.33	14:24	1.25	15:26	1.17	16:23	1.08	17:32	
20	1.34	14:13	1.29	14:52	1.23	15:41	1.15	16:43	1.05	18:00	
15	1.33	14:24	1.25	15:20	1.21	15:57	1.13	16:58	1.01	18:31	
10	1.27	15:10	1.21	15:52	1.17	16:28	1.09	17:29	.95	19:15	VP
5	1.19	16:12	1.17	16:27	1.10	17:23	1.01	18:31	.89	20:04	
1	<1.06	>17:48	<1.13	>18:00	<.98	>18:51	<.92	>19:36	<.82	>20:57	
N	1675	1675	7094	7094	6837	6837	3808	3808	1005	1005	

2

Strength Percentiles for Females and Males

Adult Females and Males of All Ages:[1]

The norms seen below are broken into age categories for adults of both sexes. They are applicable only to 1 repetition maximum (1 RM) tests for the *bench press exercise* and the *leg press exercise* on a Universal Gym machine. To standardize the norms for body weight, your strength score in pounds should be divided by your body weight and then compared to the appropriate table and age category.

[1]Norms are used with permission from the Institute for Aerobics Research, 12330 Preston Rd., Dallas, TX 75230.

Absolute strength: 1 Repetition Maximum Bench Press: FEMALE.*

BENCH PRESS-WEIGHT RATIO <u>WEIGHT PUSHED IN LBS.</u>
                         BODY WEIGHT IN LBS.

%	<20	20-29	30-39	40-49	50-59	60 +		
				AGE				
99	>.88	>1.01	>.82	>.77	>.68	>.72		S
95	.88	1.01	.82	.77	.68	.72		
90	.83	.90	.76	.71	.61	.64		
85	.81	.83	.72	.66	.57	.59		E
80	.77	.80	.70	.62	.55	.54		
75	.76	.77	.65	.60	.53	.53		
70	.74	.74	.63	.57	.52	.51		G
65	.70	.72	.62	.55	.50	.48		
60	.65	.70	.60	.54	.48	.46		
55	.64	.68	.58	.53	.47	.46		
50	.63	.65	.57	.52	.46	.45		F
45	.60	.63	.55	.51	.45	.44		
40	.57	.59	.53	.50	.44	.43		
35	.56	.58	.52	.48	.43	.41		
30	.56	.56	.51	.47	.42	.40		P
25	.55	.53	.49	.45	.41	.39		
20	.53	.51	.47	.43	.39	.39		
15	.52	.50	.45	.42	.38	.36		
10	.50	.480	.42	.38	.37	.33		VP
5	.41	.436	.39	.35	.305	.26		
1	<.41	<.436	<.39	<.35	<.305	<.26		
N	20	191	379	333	189	42	TOTAL 1154	

Absolute strength: 1 Repetition Maximum Bench Press: MALE.*

BENCH PRESS-WEIGHT RATIO <u>WEIGHT PUSHED IN LBS.</u>
                         BODY WEIGHT IN LBS.

%	<20	20-29	30-39	40-49	50-59	60 +		
				AGE				
99	>1.76	>1.63	>1.35	>1.20	>1.05	>.94		S
95	1.76	1.63	1.35	1.20	1.05	.94		
90	1.46	1.48	1.24	1.10	.97	.89		
85	1.38	1.37	1.17	1.04	.93	.84		E
80	1.34	1.32	1.12	1.00	.90	.82		
75	1.29	1.26	1.08	.96	.87	.79		
70	1.24	1.22	1.04	.93	.84	.77		G
65	1.23	1.18	1.01	.90	.81	.74		
60	1.19	1.14	.98	.88	.79	.72		
55	1.16	1.10	.96	.86	.77	.70		
50	1.13	1.06	.93	.84	.75	.68		F
45	1.10	1.03	.90	.82	.73	.67		
40	1.06	.99	.88	.80	.71	.65		
35	1.01	.96	.86	.78	.70	.65		
30	.96	.93	.83	.76	.68	.63		P
25	.93	.90	.81	.74	.66	.60		
20	.89	.88	.78	.72	.63	.57		
15	.86	.84	.75	.69	.60	.56		
10	.81	.80	.71	.650	.57	.53		VP
5	.76	.72	.65	.590	.53	.49		
1	< .76	<.72	<.65	<.590	<.53	<.49		
N	60	425	1909	2090	1279	343	TOTAL 6106	

*When using the Universal DVR machine, use the number on the *right* side of the weight plate to determine maximum lift.

Absolute strength:　1 Repetition Maximum Leg Press: FEMALE.*

LEG PRESS-WEIGHT RATIO <u>WEIGHT PUSHED IN LBS.</u>
　　　　　　　　　　　　　BODY WEIGHT IN LBS.

%	<20	20-29	30-39	40-49	50-59	60+		
				AGE				
99	>1.88	>1.98	>1.68	>1.57	>1.43	>1.43		S
95	1.88	1.98	1.68	1.57	1.43	1.43		
90	1.85	1.82	1.61	1.48	1.37	1.32		
85	1.81	1.76	1.52	1.40	1.31	1.25		E
80	1.71	1.68	1.47	1.37	1.25	1.18		
75	1.69	1.65	1.42	1.33	1.20	1.16		
70	1.65	1.58	1.39	1.29	1.17	1.13		G
65	1.62	1.53	1.36	1.27	1.12	1.08		
60	1.59	1.50	1.33	1.23	1.10	1.04		
55	1.51	1.47	1.31	1.20	1.08	.99		
50	1.45	1.44	1.27	1.18	1.05	.99		F
45	1.42	1.40	1.24	1.15	1.02	.97		
40	1.38	1.37	1.21	1.13	.99	.93		
35	1.33	1.32	1.18	1.11	.97	.90		
30	1.29	1.27	1.15	1.08	.95	.90		P
25	1.25	1.26	1.12	1.06	.92	.86		
20	1.22	1.22	1.09	1.02	.88	.85		
15	1.19	1.18	1.05	.97	.84	.80		
10	1.09	1.14	1.0	.94	.78	.72		VP
5	1.06	.99	.96	.85	.72	.63		
1	<1.06	<.99	<.96	< .85	<.72	< .63		
							TOTAL	
N	20	192	381	337	192	44	1166	

Absolute strength:　1 Repetition Maximum Leg Press: MALE.*

LEG PRESS-WEIGHT RATIO <u>WEIGHT PUSHED IN LBS.</u>
　　　　　　　　　　　　　BODY WEIGHT IN LBS.

%	<20	20-29	30-39	40-49	50-59	60+		
				AGE				
99	>2.82	>2.40	>2.20	>2.02	>1.90	>1.80		S
95	2.82	2.40	2.20	2.02	1.90	1.80		
90	2.53	2.27	2.07	1.92	1.80	1.73		
85	2.40	2.18	1.99	1.86	1.75	1.68		E
80	2.28	2.13	1.93	1.82	1.71	1.62		
75	2.18	2.09	1.89	1.78	1.68	1.58		
70	2.15	2.05	1.85	1.74	1.64	1.56		G
65	2.10	2.01	1.81	1.71	1.61	1.52		
60	2.04	1.97	1.77	1.68	1.58	1.49		
55	2.01	1.94	1.74	1.65	1.55	1.46		
50	1.95	1.91	1.71	1.62	1.52	1.43		F
45	1.93	1.87	1.68	1.59	1.50	1.40		
40	1.90	1.83	1.65	1.57	1.46	1.38		
35	1.89	1.78	1.62	1.54	1.42	1.34		
30	1.82	1.74	1.59	1.51	1.39	1.30		P
25	1.80	1.68	1.56	1.48	1.36	1.27		
20	1.70	1.63	1.52	1.44	1.32	1.25		
15	1.61	1.58	1.48	1.40	1.28	1.21		
10	1.57	1.51	1.43	1.35	1.22	1.16		VP
5	1.46	1.42	1.34	1.27	1.15	1.08		
1	<1.46	<1.42	<1.34	<1.27	<1.15	<1.08		
							TOTAL	
N	60	424	1909	2089	1286	347	6115	

*When using the Universal DVR machine, use the number on the *left* side of the weight plate to determine maximum lift.

Grip Strength for Males and Females of All Ages

Using a grip dynamometer (see Figure 6.5) adjusted for your hand size, squeeze as hard as you can for 1–2 seconds with each hand. Record your sum of scores.

Norms and Percentiles by Age Groups and Sex for Combined Right and Left Hand Grip Strength (kg)

AGE	15–19		20–29		30–39		40–49		50–59		60–69	
SEX	M	F	M	F	M	F	M	F	M	F	M	F
Excellent	≥ 113	≥ 71	≥ 124	≥ 71	≥ 123	≥ 73	≥ 119	≥ 73	≥ 110	≥ 65	≥ 102	≥ 60
Above Average	130–112	64–70	113–123	65–70	113–122	66–72	110–118	65–72	102–109	59–64	93–101	54–59
Average	95–102	59–63	106–112	61–64	105–112	61–65	102–109	59–64	96–101	55–58	86–92	51–53
Below Average	84–94	54–58	97–105	55–60	97–104	56–60	94–101	55–58	87–95	51–54	79–85	48–50
Weak	≤ 83	≤ 53	≤ 96	≤ 54	≤ 96	≤ 55	≤ 93	≤ 54	≤ 86	≤ 50	≤ 78	≤ 47

AGE (YRS.)	15–19		20–29		30–39		40–49		50–59		60–69	
SEX	M	F	M	F	M	F	M	F	M	F	M	F
Percentiles												
95	125	78	136	78	135	80	128	80	119	72	111	67
90	119	74	127	74	127	76	123	76	114	69	106	62
85	113	71	124	71	123	73	119	73	110	65	102	60
80	110	69	120	70	120	71	117	71	108	63	99	58
75	108	67	118	68	117	69	115	69	105	62	96	56
70	105	65	115	67	115	68	112	67	103	60	94	55
65	103	64	113	65	113	66	110	65	102	59	93	54
60	101	63	111	64	111	65	108	64	100	58	91	53
55	99	61	109	63	109	63	106	62	99	57	89	52
50	97	60	107	62	107	62	104	61	97	56	88	52
45	95	59	106	61	105	61	102	59	96	55	86	51
40	93	58	104	59	104	60	100	58	94	54	84	50
35	90	57	102	58	101	59	98	57	92	53	82	49
30	87	56	100	56	99	58	96	56	90	53	81	49
25	84	54	97	55	97	56	94	55	87	51	79	48
20	81	53	95	53	94	55	91	53	85	50	76	47
15	77	51	91	52	91	53	89	51	83	48	73	45
10	73	49	87	50	87	51	84	49	80	46	69	43
5	67	45	81	47	81	48	76	46	74	42	62	39

Canada Fitness Survey 1981. From *Standardized Tests of Fitness,* 2nd Ed., Fitness and Amateur Sport, Canada, 1981.

College-Age Females:[2]

The norms seen below were developed from data on 221 female college-age students collected at the end of a ten-week beginning weight training class. These norms represent 1 repetition maximum (1 RM) scores using free weights and are organized by weight categories. Comparisions to these norms must only be done using free weights. Descriptions of the exercises are as follows:

1. *Bench Press:* In a supine position, the subject receives the weight from a spotter with arms extended vertically, lowers the weight until it touches the chest, and then lifts the weight upward until the arms are extended again.

2. *Half Squat:* The subject straddles a narrow bench which is positioned between her legs, lifts the weight from a supporting rack to behind her shoulders, steps one step backward and squats until the buttocks touch the bench, and then returns to a stand.

3. *Bent Arm Pullover:* From a supine position on a bench (with the top of the shoulders at the end of the bench), the subject lifts a weight from the floor behind the head to the chest and returns it to the floor.

4. *Dead Lift:* With the weight placed in front of the feet, the subject bends at the waist and hips, keeping the back as close to vertical as possible, picks up the weight and then stands up.

5. *Military Press:* With the weight on the floor in front of the feet, the subject lifts the weight to the shoulder ("high clean") and then presses the weight to full arm extension above the head without allowing the knees to extend.

[2]From Kindig, L. E., Soares, P. L., Wisenbaker, J. M., NS Mrvos, S. R. (1984) Standard scores for women's weight training. *Physician Sptsmed.* 12, 67–74. (Reprinted by permission of *The Physician and Sportsmedicine*, a McGraw-Hill publication.)

Bench-Press Norms and Reliability Estimates by Weight Classification (lb.)*

PERCENTILE	Z		95-104	105-114	115-124	125-134	135-144	145-154	155 +
		N	11	28	58	55	31	19	15
		MEAN	69.09	76.536	77.07	80.36	79.19	88.42	109.00
		SD	12.613	15.60	16.78	18.10	16.33	23.34	24.44
99	2.33		98 (7.9)	112 (7.3)	116 (5.6)	123 (8.1)	117 (6.7)	143 (14.1)	166 (11.0)
90	1.28		85 (5.3)	96 (5.1)	99 (3.8)	104 (5.3)	100 (4.8)	118 (9.9)	140 (8.45)
80	.85		80 (4.4)	89 (4.3)	91 (3.1)	96 (4.3)	93 (4.0)	108 (8.2)	130 (7.6)
70	.52		76 (3.9)	84 (3.7)	86 (2.6)	90 (3.6)	88 (3.5)	101 (7.0)	122 (7.0)
60	.25		72 (3.6)	79 (3.3)	81 (2.3)	85 (3.0)	83 (3.1)	94 (6.0)	115 (6.6)
50	0		69 (3.5)	76 (3.0)	77 (2.0)	80 (2.5)	79 (2.8)	88 (5.2)	109 (6.3)
40	−.25		66 (3.5)	72 (2.7)	73 (1.9)	76 (2.2)	75 (2.5)	83 (4.5)	103 (6.0)
30	−.52		63 (3.7)	67 (2.5)	68 (1.8)	71 (2.1)	71 (2.3)	76 (4.0)	96 (6.0)
20	−.85		58 (4.1)	62 (2.5)	63 (1.9)	65 (2.3)	65 (2.3)	69 (3.6)	88 (5.9)
10	−1.28		53 (5.0)	56 (2.8)	56 (2.2)	57 (3.0)	58 (2.6)	59 (4.0)	78 (6.2)

Half-Squat Norms and Reliability Estimates by Weight Classification (lb.)*

PERCENTILE	Z		95-104	105-114	115-124	125-134	135-144	145-154	155 +
		N	10	29	59	54	30	19	15
		MEAN	132.5	155.69	157.97	163.70	170.83	175.00	201.33
		SD	29.838	29.27	34.57	34.834	32.986	33.953	42.947
99	2.33		202 (15.6)	224 (11.3)	239 (10.3)	245 (9.9)	248 (9.1)	254 (13.1)	301 (28.0)
90	1.28		171 (11.5)	193 (8.0)	202 (7.2)	208 (7.1)	213 (7.0)	231 (9.3)	256 (18.6)
80	.85		158 (10.2)	180 (6.9)	187 (6.1)	193 (6.2)	199 (6.4)	204 (8.3)	238 (15.1)
70	.52		148 (9.6)	171 (6.1)	176 (5.3)	182 (5.6)	188 (6.1)	193 (8.0)	224 (12.7)
60	.25		140 (9.3)	163 (5.6)	167 (4.8)	172 (5.2)	179 (6.0)	183 (7.9)	212 (11.1)
50	0		132 (9.2)	156 (5.3)	157 (4.5)	164 (5.0)	170 (6.0)	175 (8.1)	201 (10.0)
40	−.25		125 (9.4)	148 (5.1)	149 (4.3)	155 (4.9)	163 (6.1)	167 (8.5)	191 (9.3)
30	−.52		117 (9.7)	140 (5.1)	140 (4.2)	146 (4.9)	154 (6.2)	157 (9.1)	179 (9.4)
20	−.85		107 (10.4)	131 (5.3)	129 (4.5)	134 (5.2)	143 (6.6)	146 (10.1)	165 (10.4)
10	−1.28		94 (11.7)	118 (6.0)	114 (5.2)	119 (5.8)	129 (7.3)	132 (11.6)	146 (12.9)

Dead-Lift Norms and Reliability Estimates by Weight Classification (lb.)*

PERCENTILE	Z		95-104	105-114	115-124	125-134	135-144	145-154	155 +
		N	11	29	58	54	29	20	15
		MEAN	138.64	135.86	147.41	155.56	165.34	171.500	214.33
		SD	23.032	30.621	32.663	32.718	23.066	43.622	32.451
99	2.33		192 (9.2)	207 (8.8)	224 (7.7)	232 (6.6)	219 (6.5)	273 (12.5)	290 (12.7)
90	1.28		168 (6.8)	175 (6.7)	189 (5.4)	197 (5.0)	195 (5.0)	227 (9.4)	256 (10.1)
80	.85		158 (6.3)	162 (6.1)	175 (4.8)	183 (4.6)	185 (4.6)	209 (9.1)	242 (9.3)
70	.52		151 (6.1)	152 (5.8)	164 (4.5)	173 (4.4)	177 (4.4)	194 (9.2)	231 (8.8)
60	.25		144 (6.0)	144 (5.7)	156 (4.3)	165 (4.3)	165 (4.3)	182 (9.5)	222 (8.4)
50	0		139 (6.2)	139 (5.6)	147 (4.5)	156 (4.3)	160 (4.4)	171 (10.1)	214 (8.2)
40	−.25		133 (6.5)	128 (5.8)	139 (4.6)	147 (4.3)	153 (4.6)	161 (10.7)	206 (8.0)
30	−.52		127 (6.8)	120 (6.0)	130 (4.9)	139 (4.5)	149 (11.6)	197 (8.0)
20	−.85		119 (7.5)	110 (6.4)	120 (5.5)	128 (4.8)	146 (4.9)	134 (12.8)	187 (8.2)
10	−1.28		109 (8.5)	106 (7.0)	106 (6.3)	114 (5.3)	136 (5.5)	116 (14.6)	173 (8.5)

*Standard errors reported in parentheses.

Bent-Arm Pullover Norms and Reliability Estimates by Weight Classification (lb.)*

PERCENTILE	Z		95-104	105-114	115-124	125-134	135-144	145-154	155+
		N	11	28	56	54	30	20	15
		MEAN	53.64	58.75	61.70	65.37	68.50	74.25	79.33
		SD	7.103	11.108	13.324	15.717	20.050	18.937	21.784
99	2.33		70 (4.3)	85 (5.0)	93 (3.8)	102 (6.5)	115 (12.1)	118 (14.7)	130 (14.8)
90	1.28		63 (3.2)	73 (3.5)	79 (2.7)	85 (4.3)	94 (8.1)	98 (9.7)	107 (10.1)
80	.85		60 (2.8)	68 (3.0)	73 (2.3)	79 (3.5)	86 (6.5)	90 (7.6)	98 (8.4)
70	.52		57 (2.5)	65 (2.5)	69 (2.1)	74 (2.9)	79 (5.3)	84 (6.2)	91 (7.2)
60	.25		55 (2.3)	62 (2.3)	65 (1.9)	69 (2.5)	74 (4.4)	79 (5.0)	85 (6.4)
50	0		54 (2.1)	59 (2.0)	62 (1.8)	65 (2.2)	69 (3.6)	74 (4.0)	79 (5.8)
40	−.25		52 (2.0)	56 (1.8)	58 (1.8)	61 (1.9)	63 (3.0)	70 (3.6)	74 (5.4)
30	−.52		50 (1.9)	53 (1.7)	55 (1.9)	57 (1.9)	58 (2.7)	64 (2.6)	68 (5.4)
20	−.85		48 (1.9)	49 (1.7)	50 (2.0)	52 (2.0)	51 (2.9)	58 (2.8)	61 (5.7)
10	−1.28		45 (1.9)	45 (1.9)	45 (2.3)	45 (2.6)	43 (3.8)	50 (4.1)	51 (6.8)

Military-Press Norms and Reliability Estimates by Weight Classification (lb.)*

PERCENTILE	Z		95-104	105-114	115-124	125-134	135-144	145-154	155+
		N	11	28	57	55	31	19	15
		MEAN	54.55	63.93	62.81	65.91	65.81	76.05	92.000
		SD	11.057	15.656	13.693	13.645	15.005	16.715	19.346
99	2.33		80 (5.5)	100 (5.3)	95 (2.6)	98 (3.4)	101 (7.2)	115 (6.8)	137 (7.0)
90	1.28		69 (3.7)	84 (3.6)	80 (1.9)	83 (2.5)	85 (4.9)	97 (4.4)	117 (5.4)
80	.85		64 (3.3)	77 (3.1)	74 (1.8)	78 (2.3)	79 (4.0)	90 (3.8)	108 (5.0)
70	.52		60 (3.0)	72 (2.8)	70 (1.7)	73 (2.1)	74 (3.5)	84 (3.5)	102 (4.8)
60	.25		57 (3.0)	68 (2.7)	66 (1.7)	69 (2.0)	70 (3.0)	80 (3.5)	97 (4.9)
50	0		55 (3.0)	64 (2.7)	63 (1.8)	66 (1.9)	66 (2.8)	76 (3.6)	92 (4.9)
40	−.25		52 (3.1)	60 (2.8)	59 (2.0)	62 (1.9)	62 (2.6)	72 (3.9)	87 (5.1)
30	−.52		49 (3.4)	56 (2.9)	56 (2.1)	59 (1.9)	58 (2.6)	67 (4.3)	82 (5.4)
20	−.85		45 (3.7)	51 (3.3)	51 (2.3)	54 (2.0)	53 (2.8)	62 (4.9)	76 (5.7)
10	−1.28		40 (4.4)	44 (3.8)	45 (2.6)	48 (2.1)	47 (3.3)	55 (5.9)	67 (6.5)

*Standard errors reported in parentheses.

College-Age Males:[3]

The norms seen below were developed from data on college age males enrolled in a beginning weight training course. They represent 1 RM scores taken after two weeks of preconditioning and instruction on a Universal Gym Gladiator/SR series weight machine and are only applicable if measurements are made on a similar apparatus. The norms are organized by weight categories. Descriptions of the exercises are as follows:

1. *Bench Press:* In the supine position, the subject lifts the handles of the machine upward vertically until the arms are extended and then returns to the starting position.

2. *Sitting Press:* Sitting on a seat, the subject lifts the handles of the machine upward vertically until the arms are extended and then returns to the starting position.

3. *Leg Press:* Sitting on the leg press seat with hips and knees in a flexed position, the subject extends the legs and then returns to the starting position.

4. *Biceps Curl:* Standing or sitting in front of the machine with the back kept straight, the subject grasps the pulley attachment to the machine with the arms extended, flexes the elbow, and returns to the starting position.

Bench press

			BODY WEIGHT						
T-SCORE	Z-SCORE	%	125-139	140-149	150-159	160-169	170-179	180-189	190-209
87	3.70	100	216	271	254	262	289	311	289
63	1.28	90	165	194	190	197	215	222	212
59	.85	80	156	180	179	186	201	207	199
55	.52	70	150	170	170	177	191	195	188
53	.25	60	144	161	163	169	183	185	180
50	.00	50	139	153	156	163	175	175	172
47	−.25	40	133	145	149	156	168	166	164
45	−.52	30	128	136	142	148	159	156	155
41	−.85	20	121	126	134	139	149	144	145
37	−1.28	10	112	112	122	128	136	129	131

[3]Used with permission from Gregory, L. W. (1981). Some observations on strength training and assessment. *J. Sports Med. and Physical Fitness* 21, 130–137.

Sitting press

T-SCORE	Z-SCORE	%	BODY WEIGHT						
			125-139	140-149	150-159	160-169	170-179	180-189	190-209
87	3.70	100	174	196	210	218	219	233	212
63	1.28	90	139	153	159	169	172	177	168
59	.85	80	133	145	150	160	164	168	160
55	.52	70	128	139	143	153	157	160	154
53	.25	60	124	134	138	148	152	154	149
50	.00	50	121	130	132	143	147	148	145
47	−.25	40	117	126	127	138	142	142	140
45	−.52	30	113	121	121	132	137	136	135
41	−.85	20	108	115	115	125	131	129	129
37	−1.28	10	102	107	106	117	122	119	121

Leg press

T-SCORE	Z-SCORE	%	BODY WEIGHT						
			125-139	140-149	150-159	160-169	170-179	180-189	190-209
87	3.70	100	424	399	454	466	478	510	498
63	1.28	90	331	328	363	371	388	401	411
59	.85	80	314	316	347	355	372	382	395
55	.52	70	301	306	334	342	360	367	383
53	.25	60	291	298	324	331	349	354	373
50	.00	50	281	291	315	321	340	343	364
47	−.25	40	271	284	305	311	331	332	355
45	−.52	30	261	276	295	301	320	319	345
41	−.85	20	248	266	283	288	308	305	333
37	−1.28	10	231	254	266	271	292	285	318

Biceps curl

T-SCORE	Z-SCORE	%	BODY WEIGHT						
			125-139	140-149	150-159	160-169	170-179	180-189	190-209
87	3.70	100	106	117	114	119	121	135	133
63	1.28	90	86	91	92	96	97	106	104
59	.85	80	82	86	88	91	93	101	99
55	.52	70	79	82	85	88	90	98	95
53	.25	60	77	79	82	86	88	94	92
50	.00	50	75	76	80	83	85	91	89
47	−.25	40	72	74	77	81	83	88	86
45	−.52	30	70	71	75	78	80	85	83
41	−.85	20	67	67	72	75	77	81	79
37	−1.28	10	63	62	68	71	73	76	74

3

Exercises for Special Purposes

Static Strength Exercises:[1]

These exercises require no specialized equipment other than objects typically found within a household. Taken together these exercises focus on most of the important muscles of the body. Creative adaptations can be used to develop modifications for particular needs. See Chapter 6 for a discussion of general guidelines for using static exercises and their limitations.

1. *Shoulder pull:* Grasp hands together with elbows facing outward; pull outward with the shoulder and arm muscles.
2. *Shoulder push:* Standing in a doorway, place hands on doorjam and push outward.
3. *Chest push:* Lock hands together with elbows facing outward; push inward with chest and arm muscles.
4. *Elbow flexion:* While seated at a heavy desk, place hands underneath middle drawer and lift upward with arms.
5. *Elbow extension:* While seated at a desk, place hands on top of desk and press downward with arms.
6. *Grip:* Grip a tennis ball or folded towel and squeeze.
7. *Knee extension:* While seated on a chair, place feet under the edge of a heavy bed and extend knee.
8. *Knee squeeze:* With a big pillow placed between legs, squeeze legs together. (Alternative: Cross arms and place hands on inside of knees to push against while squeezing legs.)
9. *Leg spread:* Cross arms and place hands on outside of knees; resist as legs are spread apart.
10. *Leg curl:* While seated in chair, wrap legs to the outside of front legs of chair and pull legs backward.

[1]Adapted from Heyward, V. H. (1984). *Designs for Fitness*, Minneapolis, Minn.: Burgess.

11. *Leg press:* While seated sideways in a doorway, place legs against doorjam and extend legs.
12. *Pelvic tilt:* While in a supine position with arms raised overhead, tighten abdominal muscles while pressing lower back into the floor.
13. *Gluteal squeeze:* While lying prone, tighten and squeeze gluteal muscles together.

The Y's Way to a Healthy Back (Abbreviated)[2]

The following exercises are taken from the successful YMCA program which focuses on preventing and reducing back pain. The first six exercises focus on relaxation while the remaining focus on stretching and strengthening important muscles that support the spine.

1. While supine, with a pillow placed under the knees, tighten the abdominal muscles and flatten the lower back into the floor. Repeat 3 times.
2. In the same position, shrug shoulders by moving them toward the ears and then relax.
3. In the same position, allow the head to fall to the side like a pendulum. Do not force the head sideways but rather allow it to fall naturally.
4. In the same supine position, bend knees so that the soles of both feet are facing the floor. Slowly bring one knee upward toward the chest and return. Repeat with the other leg. Keep buttocks in contact with the floor at all times.
5. Lying on the side with a pillow placed under the head, slowly slide the upper leg toward the chest with the knee bent and then return to the starting position. Repeat with the opposite leg when lying on the other side.
6. Lying prone with the toes pointed inward, tighten the gluteal muscles and then relax.
7. Lying in the supine position, bring both knees to the chest and then return. Keep buttocks in contact with the floor.
8. Place hands and knees on the floor and support yourself "on all fours" like a cat. Hump your spine upward and lower your head like a stretching cat. Then reverse and arch your back, stick out your buttocks and lift your head high. Do everything slowly.
9. Lying on the back with knees raised and feet on the floor, take a breath and exhale slowly while lifting the head and shoulders. Arms at the side of the body should move toward the knees. Keep the lower back flat against the floor.
10. Kneel on the floor and keep the thighs perpendicular to the surface. Bend forward at waist and reach arms above head in front of the body on to the floor. Stretch chest muscles by drooping spine toward floor slowly.
11. While seated on a chair, bend forward at the waist and allow the head and arms to droop forward over the legs. Body should droop and hang; movement should not be forceful.

[2]Adapted from: *Y's Way to a Healthy Back* (1976). YMCA of the City of New York and National Council of YMCA's. 1976.

12. In this same loose drooped position, rotate hanging arms first to one side and then to the other.

13. In the supine position, alternately lift one leg toward the chest and then straighten the knee, moving the lower leg upward. Reverse and repeat with the other leg. Repeat two times.

14. With the feet supported and the knees bent and as close to the buttocks as possible, slowly curl upward to a sit-up position. Hands can be at the side, or for more vigor, placed behind the head with fingers crossed. (See Chapter 6 for a discussion of suggested variations in this exercise.)

Postural Enhancement Exercises[3]

The following exercises are designed to serve as a beginning set of exercises for enhancing postural asymmetries. Even though a postural problem may be visible only in one region of the body, the whole series of exercises should be done as a unit because very often asymmetries create compensations in other parts of the body. All these exercises should be done repeatedly with the number increasing progressively as needed.

1. Standing upright, shrug both shoulders upward, then pull shoulder blades together while still in the shrug position, and then return to the starting position. Repeat.

2. Kneel on the floor and crouch forward so that the head lies on the floor, supported by a pillow. Arms should be extended above the head. Lower the chest toward the knees and contract the abdominals for 3 seconds. Relax and repeat.

3. While seated on the floor with one leg extended ahead and the other with knee bent, tighten the leg muscles of the straight leg and lift it 6 inches off the floor for 3 seconds. Lower, relax and repeat.

4. Standing barefoot on the edge of a towel that is spread out before you on the floor, alternately contract the toes of each foot so as to pull the towel under the feet. Repeat.

5. Hang vertically from a bar, allowing the body to relax and weight be born by the arms. Slowly build up hanging time to 1 minute.

6. Balance a book on the head and slowly walk forward, sideways, backward, keeping the book in balance. Imagine trying to push weight upward by stretching the neck and shoulders.

---

[3]Adapted from Svoboda, M., Kauffman. L., Davis, R., Gilbert, G., Althoff, S., Robertson, L., Heyden, S. M., Lehman, A. E., and Schendel, J. S. (ed). (1985). *Health and Fitness for Life Laboratory Manual, 2nd Ed.* Scottsdale, AZ: Prospect Press.

4

Measuring Body Composition via Skinfold Fat (The Generalized Equations of Jackson and Pollock)

This technique involves the measurement of skinfold thickness at specific sites on the body and substituting the scores into an appropriate regression equation for predicting body density. The equations are different for each sex and include age as one of the variables. Once density is determined, another regression equation can be used to predict percent body fat. Research has shown that skinfold thickness can be used to make such predictions in the average individual, assuming that the measurements are taken by someone who is skillful with this technique. Even with a skillful technician, errors are estimated to range between 4–5.5% fat (see Chapter 7 for more on this). Research shows that without a skillful technician, errors can be considerably larger; therefore, if you elect to use this procedure, inquire about the background of the person measuring you. Note also that the limits of accuracy described above are most applicable for people who fall nearer the middle ranges of skinfold thickness. This means that for those who have extremely small or extremely large skinfold thicknesses, the errors can be larger than reported. Specific instructions that describe the sites and the general procedures follow:

1. Determine which three sites to use from the instructions given below. Figure 1, a–f, illustrates each of the sites and gives a close-up view of the technique for measuring skinfold thickness:

   Males sites: (a) chest, (b) abdomen, (c) thigh
   Females sites: (d) triceps, (e) suprailiac, (f) thigh

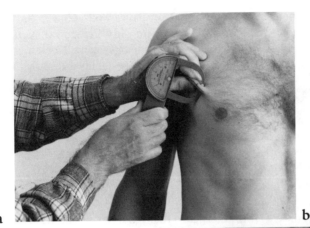

a

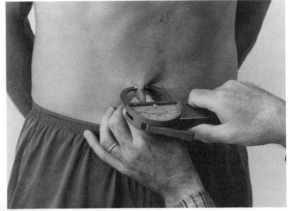

b

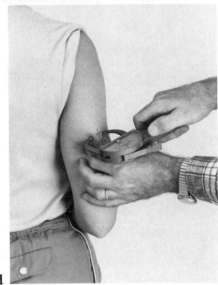

c

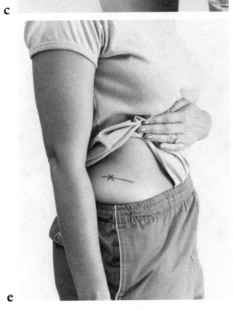

d

e

2. Sum the three measurements. Tables A and B on pages 362 and 363 have been developed to simplify your calculations and require only the sum of your three measurements and your age to the nearest year. Your answer will be an estimate of your percent fat. The formulas used to develop these tables are as follows:

Males: Density = $1.0994921 - (0.0009929)$ (sum) $+ (0.0000023)$ (sum)$^2 - 0.0001392$ (age)

Females: Density = $1.1093800 - (0.0008267$ (sum) $+ (0.0000016)$ (sum)$^2 - (0.0002574)$ (age)

where: sum = sum of your three skinfolds
age = age in years

Once density is known, the Siri formula is used to predict percent fat from density:

percent fat = $[(4.95/\text{density}) - 4.5][100]$

3. Having determined your percent fat, the components of body composition can be computed as follows:

Fat weight = $\dfrac{(\% \text{ fat})}{100}$ (body weight)

Fat-free weight = (body weight) − (fat weight)

Minimal weight = $\dfrac{\text{fat-free weight}}{1.0 - \dfrac{(\text{essential } \% \text{ fat})}{100}}$

Storage fat = (body weight) − (minimal weight)

Desired weight = $\dfrac{\text{fat-free weight}}{1.0 - \dfrac{(\text{desired } \% \text{ fat})}{100}}$

4. *Example:* Assume curious George, age 27 years and body weight 167 lbs., had his skinfold fat measured as follows:

chest = 17 mm   abdomen = 18 mm   thigh = 22 mm

percent fat = 16.5   (from Table B)

$$\text{Fat weight} = \frac{(\% \text{ fat})}{100} \text{ (body weight)}$$

$$= \frac{16.5}{100} \ (167 \text{ lbs}) = .165 \ (167) = 27.56 \text{ lbs}$$

Fat-free weight = (body weight) − (fat weight)

$$= 167 - 27.56 = 139.44 \text{ lbs}$$

$$\text{Minimal weight} = \frac{\text{fat-free weight}}{1.0 - \dfrac{(\text{essential \% fat})}{100}}$$

$$= \frac{139.44 \text{ lbs}}{1.0 - \dfrac{3}{100}} \quad = \quad \frac{139.44}{1.0 - .03} \quad = \quad \frac{139.44}{.97} \quad = \quad 143.75 \text{ lbs}$$

Storage fat = (body weight) − (minimal weight)

$$= 167 - 143.75 = 23.25 \text{ lbs}$$

$$\text{Desired weight} = \frac{\text{fat-free weight}}{1.0 - \dfrac{(\text{desired \% fat})}{100}}$$

(at 15% fat)

$$= \frac{139.44 \text{ lbs}}{1.0 - \dfrac{15}{100}} \quad = \quad \frac{139.44}{1.0 - .15} \quad = \quad \frac{139.44}{.85} \quad = \quad 164.05 \text{ lbs}$$

(at 10% fat)

$$= \frac{139.44 \text{ lbs}}{1.0 - \dfrac{10}{100}} \quad = \quad \frac{139.44}{1.0 - .10} \quad = \quad \frac{139.44}{.90} \quad = \quad 154.93$$

Therefore, assuming George were to lose only fat weight from his 23.25 lbs of total storage fat, his weight loss would be:

(at 15% fat)   167 − 164.05 = 2.95 lbs
(at 10% fat)   167 − 154.93 = 12.07 lbs

Table A. Percentage of body fat estimation from age and triceps, suprailium, and thigh skinfolds: WOMEN.*

SUM OF SKINFOLDS (MM)	AGE TO THE LAST YEAR								
	UNDER 22	23–27	28–32	33–37	38–42	43–47	48–52	53–57	OVER 58
23–25	9.7	9.9	10.2	10.4	10.7	10.9	11.2	11.4	11.7
26–28	11.0	11.2	11.5	11.7	12.0	12.3	12.5	12.7	13.0
29–31	12.3	12.5	12.8	13.0	13.3	13.5	13.8	14.0	14.3
32–34	13.6	13.8	14.0	14.3	14.5	14.8	15.0	15.3	15.5
35–37	14.8	15.0	15.3	15.5	15.8	16.0	16.3	16.5	16.8
38–40	16.0	16.3	16.5	16.7	17.0	17.2	17.5	17.7	18.0
41–43	17.2	17.4	17.7	17.9	18.2	18.4	18.7	18.9	19.2
44–46	18.3	18.6	18.8	19.1	19.3	19.6	19.8	20.1	20.3
47–49	19.5	19.7	20.0	20.2	20.5	20.7	21.0	21.2	21.5
50–52	20.6	20.8	21.1	21.3	21.6	21.8	22.1	22.3	22.6
53–55	21.7	21.9	22.1	22.4	22.6	22.9	23.1	23.4	23.6
56–58	22.7	23.0	23.2	23.4	23.7	23.9	24.2	24.4	24.7
59–61	23.7	24.0	24.2	24.5	24.7	25.0	25.2	25.5	25.7
62–64	24.7	25.0	25.2	25.5	25.7	26.0	26.7	26.4	26.7
65–67	25.7	25.9	26.2	26.4	26.7	26.9	27.2	27.4	27.7
68–70	26.6	26.9	27.1	27.4	27.6	27.9	28.1	28.4	28.6
71–73	27.5	27.8	28.0	28.3	28.5	28.8	28.0	29.3	29.5
74–76	28.4	28.7	28.9	29.2	29.4	29.7	29.9	30.2	30.4
77–79	29.3	29.5	29.8	30.0	30.3	30.5	30.8	31.0	31.3
80–82	30.1	30.4	30.6	30.9	31.1	31.4	31.6	31.9	32.1
83–85	30.9	31.2	31.4	31.7	31.9	32.2	32.4	32.7	32.9
86–88	31.7	32.0	32.2	32.5	32.7	32.9	33.2	33.4	33.7
89–91	32.5	32.7	33.0	33.2	33.5	33.7	33.9	34.2	34.4
92–94	33.2	33.4	33.7	33.9	34.2	34.4	34.7	34.9	35.2
95–97	33.9	34.1	34.4	34.6	34.9	35.1	35.4	35.6	35.9
98–100	34.6	34.8	35.1	35.3	35.5	35.8	36.0	36.3	36.5
101–103	35.3	35.4	35.7	35.9	36.2	36.4	36.7	36.9	37.2
104–106	35.8	36.1	36.3	36.6	36.8	37.1	37.3	37.5	37.8
107–109	36.4	36.7	36.9	37.1	37.4	37.6	37.9	38.1	38.4
110–112	37.0	37.2	37.5	37.7	38.0	38.2	38.5	38.7	38.9
113–115	37.5	37.8	38.0	38.2	38.5	38.7	39.0	39.2	39.5
116–118	38.0	38.3	38.5	38.8	39.0	39.3	39.5	39.7	40.0
119–121	38.5	38.7	39.0	39.2	39.5	39.7	40.0	40.2	40.5
122–124	39.0	39.2	39.4	39.7	39.9	40.2	40.4	40.7	40.9
125–127	39.4	39.6	39.9	40.1	40.4	40.6	40.9	41.1	41.4
128–130	39.8	40.0	40.3	40.5	40.8	41.0	41.3	41.5	41.8

*Percentage of fat calculated by the formula of Siri. Percentage of fat $= [(4.95/Db) - 4.5] \times 100$, where Db = body density.

From Pollock, M. L., Schmidt, D. H., and Jackson, A. S.: Measurement of cardiorespiratory fitness and body composition in the clinical setting. *Comprehensive Therapy,* Vol. 6, No. 9, pp. 12–27, 1980. Used with permission of The Laux Company, Inc., Ayer, MA.

Table B.   Percentage of body fat estimation from age and the sum of chest, abdominal, and thigh skinfolds: MEN.*

SUM OF SKINFOLDS (MM)	AGE TO THE LAST YEAR								
	UNDER 22	23–27	28–32	33–37	38–42	43–47	48–52	53–57	OVER 58
8–10	1.3	1.8	2.3	2.9	3.4	3.9	4.5	5.0	5.5
11–13	2.2	2.8	3.3	3.9	4.4	4.9	5.5	6.0	6.5
14–16	3.2	3.8	4.3	4.8	5.4	5.9	6.4	7.0	7.5
17–19	4.2	4.7	5.3	5.8	6.3	6.9	7.4	8.0	8.5
20–22	5.1	5.7	6.2	6.8	7.3	7.9	8.4	8.9	9.5
23–25	6.1	6.6	7.2	7.7	8.3	8.8	9.4	9.9	10.5
26–28	7.0	7.6	8.1	8.7	9.2	9.8	10.3	10.9	11.4
29–31	8.0	8.5	9.1	9.6	10.2	10.7	11.3	11.8	12.4
32–34	8.9	9.4	10.0	10.5	11.1	11.6	12.2	12.8	13.3
35–37	9.8	10.4	10.9	11.5	12.0	12.6	13.1	13.7	14.3
38–40	10.7	11.3	11.8	12.4	12.9	13.5	14.1	14.6	15.2
41–43	11.6	12.2	12.7	13.3	13.8	14.4	15.0	15.5	16.1
44–46	12.5	13.1	13.6	14.2	14.7	15.3	15.9	16.4	17.0
47–49	13.4	13.9	14.5	15.1	15.6	16.2	16.8	17.3	17.9
50–52	14.3	14.8	15.4	15.9	16.5	17.1	17.6	18.2	18.8
53–55	15.1	15.7	16.2	16.8	17.4	17.9	18.5	19.1	19.7
56–58	16.0	16.5	17.1	17.7	18.2	18.8	19.4	20.0	20.5
59–61	16.9	17.4	17.9	18.5	19.1	19.7	20.2	20.8	21.4
62–64	17.6	18.2	18.8	19.4	19.9	20.5	21.1	21.7	22.2
65–67	18.5	19.0	19.6	20.2	20.8	21.3	21.9	22.5	23.1
68–70	19.3	19.9	20.4	21.0	21.6	22.2	22.7	23.3	23.9
71–73	20.1	20.7	21.2	21.8	22.4	23.0	23.6	24.1	24.7
74–76	20.9	21.5	22.0	22.6	23.2	23.8	24.4	25.0	25.5
77–79	21.7	22.2	22.8	23.4	24.0	24.6	25.2	25.8	26.3
80–82	22.4	23.0	23.6	24.2	24.8	25.4	25.9	26.5	27.1
83–85	23.2	23.8	24.4	25.0	25.5	26.1	26.7	27.3	27.9
86–88	24.0	24.5	25.1	25.7	26.3	26.9	27.5	28.1	28.7
89–91	24.7	25.3	25.9	25.5	27.1	27.6	28.2	28.8	29.4
92–94	25.4	26.0	26.6	27.2	27.8	28.4	29.0	29.6	30.2
95–97	26.1	26.7	27.3	27.9	28.5	29.1	29.7	30.3	30.9
98–100	26.9	27.4	28.0	28.6	29.2	29.8	30.4	31.0	31.6
101–103	27.5	28.1	28.7	29.3	29.9	30.5	31.1	31.7	32.3
104–106	28.2	28.8	29.4	30.0	30.6	31.2	31.8	32.4	33.0
107–109	28.9	29.5	30.1	30.7	31.3	31.9	32.5	33.1	33.7
110–112	29.6	30.2	30.8	31.4	32.0	32.6	33.2	33.8	34.4
113–115	30.2	30.8	31.4	32.0	32.6	33.2	33.8	34.5	35.1
116–118	30.9	31.5	32.1	32.7	33.3	33.9	34.5	35.1	35.7
119–121	31.5	32.1	32.7	33.3	33.9	34.5	35.1	35.7	36.4
122–124	32.1	32.7	33.3	33.9	34.5	35.1	35.8	36.4	37.0
125–127	32.7	33.3	33.9	34.5	35.1	35.8	36.4	37.0	37.6

*Percentage of fat calculated by the formula of Siri. Percentage of fat = $[(4.95/Db) - 4.5] \times 100$, where Db = body density.

From Pollock, M. L., Schmidt, D. H., and Jackson, A. S.: Measurement of cardiorespiratory fitness and body composition in the clinical setting. *Comprehensive Therapy,* Vol. 6, No. 9, pp. 12–27, 1980. Used with permission of The Laux Company, Inc., Ayer, MA.

5

Table of Weights and Measures

1 ounce	=	28.3 grams					
1 pound	=	16 ounces	=	454 grams	=	.454 kilograms	
1 kilogram	=	1000 grams	=	2.2 pounds			
1 gram	=	1000 milligrams					

1 tablespoon	=	3 teaspoons					
1 teaspoon	=	5 milliliters					
1 cup	=	16 tablespoons	=	8 fluid ounces			
1 quart	=	2 pints	=	4 cups	=	.95 liters	
1 liter	=	1000 milliliters					
1 milliliter	=	.0338 ounces					

1 meter	=	100 centimeters	=	1000 millimeters	=	39.37 inches	
1 inch	=	2.54 centimeters					
1 yard	=	36 inches	=	.914 meters			
1 mile	=	1,609 meters	=	1,760 yards			

6

Caloric Expenditure (in calories per minute) for Selected Physical Activities.*

*Adapted from: McArdle, W. D., Katch, F. I., and Katch, V. L. (1986) *Exercise Physiology,* 2nd Ed., Philadelphia, Lea & Febiger (Appendix D); and Williams, M. H. (1983) *Nutrition for Fitness and Sport.* (Dubuque, Iowa, W. C. Brown (Appendix D).

The assistance of Albert G. Stefan, Jr., in helping to prepare this table is gratefully acknowledged.

ACTIVITY	CAL/MIN/LB	KG LB	43 94	45 100	48 106	51 112	54 118	56 124	59 130	62 136	65 142
Archery	.030		2.82	3.00	3.18	3.36	3.54	3.72	3.90	4.08	4.26
Badminton											
recreational singles	.036		3.38	3.60	3.82	4.03	4.25	4.46	4.68	4.90	5.11
social doubles	.027		2.54	2.70	2.86	3.02	3.19	3.35	3.51	3.67	3.83
competition	.059		5.55	5.90	6.25	6.61	6.96	7.32	7.67	8.02	8.38
Baseball											
player	.031		2.91	3.10	3.29	3.47	3.66	3.84	4.03	4.22	4.40
pitcher	.039		3.67	3.90	4.13	4.37	4.60	4.84	5.07	5.30	5.54
Basketball											
recreational	.049		4.61	4.90	5.19	5.49	5.78	6.08	6.37	6.66	6.96
competitive	.065		6.11	6.50	6.89	7.28	7.67	8.06	8.45	8.84	9.23
Bowling	.027		2.54	2.70	2.86	3.02	3.19	3.35	3.51	3.67	3.83
Boxing											
sparring	.063		5.92	6.30	6.68	7.06	7.43	7.81	8.19	8.57	8.95
in ring	.101		9.49	10.10	10.71	11.31	11.92	12.52	13.13	13.74	14.34
Canoeing											
leisure	.020		1.88	2.00	2.12	2.24	2.36	2.48	2.60	2.72	2.84
racing	.047		4.42	4.70	4.98	5.26	5.55	5.83	6.11	6.39	6.67
Calisthenics											
light	.034		3.20	3.40	3.60	3.81	4.01	4.22	4.42	4.62	4.83
vigorous	.097		9.12	9.70	10.28	10.86	11.45	12.03	12.61	13.19	13.77
Card Playing	.011		1.03	1.10	1.17	1.23	1.30	1.36	1.43	1.50	1.56
Carpentry	.024		2.26	2.40	2.54	2.69	2.83	2.98	3.12	3.26	3.41
Carpet Sweeping											
female	.020		1.88	2.00	2.12	2.24	2.36	2.48	2.60	2.72	2.84
male	.022		2.07	2.20	2.33	2.46	2.60	2.73	2.86	2.99	3.12
Chopping Wood											
fast	.136		12.78	13.60	14.42	15.23	16.05	16.86	17.68	18.50	19.31
slow	.039		3.67	3.90	4.13	4.37	4.60	4.84	5.07	5.30	5.54
Circuit Training											
Hydra-fitness	.060		5.64	6.00	6.36	6.72	7.08	7.44	7.80	8.16	8.52
Universal	.053		4.98	5.30	5.62	5.94	6.25	6.57	6.89	7.21	7.53
Nautilus	.042		3.95	4.20	4.45	4.70	4.96	5.21	5.46	5.71	5.96
free weights	.039		3.67	3.90	4.13	4.37	4.60	4.84	5.07	5.30	5.54
Cleaning											
female	.028		2.63	2.80	2.97	3.14	3.30	3.47	3.64	3.81	3.98
male	.026		2.44	2.60	2.76	2.91	3.07	3.22	3.38	3.54	3.69
Climbing Hills											
with 0 load	.055		5.17	5.50	5.83	6.16	6.49	6.82	7.15	7.48	7.81
with 5kg load	.059		5.55	5.90	6.25	6.61	6.96	7.32	7.67	8.02	8.38
with 10kg load	.064		6.02	6.40	6.78	7.17	7.55	7.94	8.32	8.70	9.09
with 20kg load	.067		6.30	6.70	7.10	7.50	7.91	8.31	8.71	9.11	9.51
Cooking											
female	.020		1.88	2.00	2.12	2.24	2.36	2.48	2.60	2.72	2.84
male	.022		2.07	2.20	2.33	2.46	2.60	2.73	2.86	2.99	3.12
Cycling											
leisure 5.5 mph	.029		2.73	2.90	3.07	3.25	3.42	3.60	3.77	3.94	4.12
leisure 9.4 mph	.045		4.23	4.50	4.77	5.04	5.31	5.58	5.85	6.12	6.39
racing	.077		7.24	7.70	8.16	8.62	9.09	9.55	10.01	10.47	10.93

67	70	73	75	78	81	84	86	89	92	95	97	100	103	105	108
148	154	160	166	172	178	184	190	196	202	208	214	220	226	232	238
4.44	4.62	4.80	4.98	5.16	5.34	5.52	5.70	5.88	6.06	6.24	6.42	6.60	6.78	6.96	7.14
5.33	5.54	5.76	5.98	6.19	6.41	6.62	6.84	7.06	7.27	7.49	7.70	7.92	8.14	8.35	8.57
4.00	4.16	4.32	4.48	4.64	4.81	4.97	5.13	5.29	5.45	5.62	5.78	5.94	6.10	6.26	6.43
8.73	9.09	9.44	9.79	10.15	10.50	10.86	11.21	11.56	11.92	12.27	12.63	12.98	13.33	13.69	14.04
4.59	4.77	4.96	5.15	5.33	5.52	5.70	5.89	6.08	6.26	6.45	6.63	6.82	7.01	7.19	7.38
5.77	6.01	6.24	6.47	6.71	6.94	7.18	7.41	7.64	7.88	8.11	8.35	8.58	8.81	9.05	9.28
7.25	7.55	7.84	8.13	8.43	8.72	9.02	9.31	9.60	9.90	10.19	10.49	10.78	11.07	11.37	11.66
9.62	10.01	10.40	10.79	11.18	11.57	11.96	12.35	12.74	13.13	13.52	13.91	14.30	14.69	15.08	15.47
4.00	4.16	4.32	4.48	4.64	4.81	4.97	5.13	5.29	5.45	5.62	5.78	5.94	6.10	6.26	6.43
9.32	9.70	10.08	10.46	10.84	11.21	11.59	11.97	12.35	12.73	13.10	13.48	13.86	14.24	14.62	14.99
14.95	15.55	16.16	16.77	17.37	17.98	18.58	19.19	19.80	20.40	21.01	21.61	22.22	22.83	23.43	24.04
2.96	3.08	3.20	3.32	3.44	3.56	3.68	3.80	3.92	4.04	4.16	4.28	4.40	4.52	4.64	4.76
6.96	7.24	7.52	7.80	8.08	8.37	8.65	8.93	9.21	9.49	9.78	10.06	10.34	10.62	10.90	11.19
5.03	5.24	5.44	5.64	5.85	6.05	6.26	6.46	6.66	6.87	7.07	7.28	7.48	7.68	7.89	8.09
14.36	14.94	15.52	16.10	16.68	17.27	17.85	18.43	19.01	19.59	20.18	20.76	21.34	21.92	22.50	23.09
1.63	1.69	1.76	1.83	1.89	1.96	2.02	2.09	2.16	2.22	2.29	2.35	2.42	2.49	2.55	2.62
3.55	3.70	3.84	3.98	4.13	4.27	4.42	4.56	4.70	4.85	4.99	5.14	5.28	5.42	5.57	5.71
2.96	3.08	3.20	3.32	3.44	3.56	3.68	3.80	3.92	4.04	4.16	4.28	4.40	4.52	4.64	4.76
3.26	3.39	3.52	3.65	3.78	3.92	4.05	4.18	4.31	4.44	4.58	4.71	4.84	4.97	5.10	5.24
20.13	20.94	21.76	22.58	23.39	24.21	25.02	25.84	26.66	27.47	28.29	29.10	29.92	30.74	31.55	32.37
5.77	6.01	6.24	6.47	6.71	6.94	7.18	7.41	7.64	7.88	8.11	8.35	8.58	8.81	9.05	9.28
8.88	9.24	9.60	9.96	10.32	10.68	11.04	11.40	11.76	12.12	12.48	12.84	13.20	13.56	13.92	14.28
7.84	8.16	8.48	8.80	9.12	9.43	9.75	10.07	10.39	10.71	11.02	11.34	11.66	11.98	12.30	12.61
6.22	6.47	6.72	6.97	7.22	7.48	7.73	7.98	8.23	8.48	8.74	8.99	9.24	9.49	9.74	10.00
5.77	6.01	6.24	6.47	6.71	6.94	7.18	7.41	7.64	7.88	8.11	8.35	8.58	8.81	9.05	9.28
4.14	4.31	4.48	4.65	4.82	4.98	5.15	5.32	5.49	5.66	5.82	5.99	6.16	6.33	6.50	6.66
3.85	4.00	4.16	4.32	4.47	4.63	4.78	4.94	5.10	5.25	5.41	5.56	5.72	5.88	6.03	6.19
8.14	8.47	8.80	9.13	9.46	9.79	10.12	10.45	10.78	11.11	11.44	11.77	12.10	12.43	12.76	13.09
8.73	9.09	9.44	9.79	10.15	10.50	10.86	11.21	11.56	11.92	12.27	12.63	12.98	13.33	13.69	14.04
9.47	9.86	10.24	10.62	11.01	11.39	11.78	12.16	12.54	12.93	13.31	13.70	14.08	14.46	14.85	15.23
9.92	10.32	10.72	11.12	11.52	11.93	12.33	12.73	13.13	13.53	13.94	14.34	14.74	15.14	15.54	15.95
2.96	3.08	3.20	3.32	3.44	3.56	3.68	3.80	3.92	4.04	4.16	4.28	4.40	4.52	4.64	4.76
3.26	3.39	3.52	3.65	3.78	3.92	4.05	4.18	4.31	4.44	4.58	4.71	4.84	4.97	5.10	5.24
4.29	4.47	4.64	4.81	4.99	5.16	5.34	5.51	5.68	5.86	6.03	6.21	6.38	6.55	6.73	6.90
6.66	6.93	7.20	7.47	7.74	8.01	8.28	8.55	8.82	9.09	9.36	9.63	9.90	10.17	10.44	10.71
11.40	11.86	12.32	12.78	13.24	13.71	14.17	14.63	15.09	15.55	16.02	16.48	16.94	17.40	17.86	18.33

ACTIVITY	CAL/MIN/LB	KG	43	45	48	51	54	56	59	62	65
		LB	94	100	106	112	118	124	130	136	142
Dancing (female)											
aerobic (medium)	.047		4.42	4.70	4.98	5.26	5.55	5.83	6.11	6.39	6.67
aerobic (intense)	.061		5.73	6.10	6.47	6.83	7.20	7.56	7.93	8.30	8.66
ballroom	.023		2.16	2.30	2.44	2.58	2.71	2.85	2.99	3.13	3.27
active (disco, square)	.045		4.23	4.50	4.77	5.04	5.31	5.58	5.85	6.12	6.39
Digging Trenches	.066		6.20	6.60	7.00	7.39	7.79	8.18	8.58	8.98	9.37
Eating (sitting)	.010		.94	1.00	1.06	1.12	1.18	1.24	1.30	1.36	1.42
Fencing											
moderately	.033		3.10	3.30	3.50	3.70	3.89	4.09	4.29	4.49	4.69
vigorously	.066		6.20	6.60	7.00	7.39	7.79	8.18	8.58	8.98	9.37
Field Hockey	.061		5.73	6.10	6.47	6.83	7.20	7.56	7.93	8.30	8.66
Fishing	.028		2.63	2.80	2.97	3.14	3.30	3.47	3.64	3.81	3.98
Football											
moderate	.033		3.10	3.30	3.50	3.70	3.89	4.09	4.29	4.49	4.69
touch, vigorous	.055		5.17	5.50	5.83	6.16	6.49	6.82	7.15	7.48	7.81
tackle	.060		5.64	6.00	6.36	6.72	7.08	7.44	7.80	8.16	8.52
Forestry											
chopping wood											
(fast)	.136		12.78	13.60	14.42	15.23	16.05	16.86	17.68	18.50	19.31
(slow)	.039		3.67	3.90	4.13	4.37	4.60	4.84	5.07	5.30	5.54
sawing by hand	.055		5.17	5.50	5.83	6.16	6.49	6.82	7.15	7.48	7.81
sawing (power)	.034		3.20	3.40	3.60	3.81	4.01	4.22	4.42	4.62	4.83
stacking firewood	.040		3.76	4.00	4.24	4.48	4.72	4.96	5.20	5.44	5.68
trimming trees	.059		5.55	5.90	6.25	6.61	6.96	7.32	7.67	8.02	8.38
Gardening											
digging	.057		5.36	5.70	6.04	6.38	6.73	7.07	7.41	7.75	8.09
hedging	.035		3.29	3.50	3.71	3.92	4.13	4.34	4.55	4.76	4.97
mowing	.051		4.79	5.10	5.41	5.71	6.02	6.32	6.63	6.94	7.24
raking	.025		2.35	2.50	2.65	2.80	2.95	3.10	3.25	3.40	3.55
weeding	.033		3.10	3.30	3.50	3.70	3.89	4.09	4.29	4.49	4.69
Golf											
2-some w/clubs	.036		3.38	3.60	3.82	4.03	4.25	4.46	4.68	4.90	5.11
4-some w/clubs	.027		2.54	2.70	2.86	3.02	3.19	3.35	3.51	3.67	3.83
golfcart	.019		1.79	1.90	2.01	2.13	2.24	2.36	2.47	2.58	2.70
Gymnastics	.030		2.82	3.00	3.18	3.36	3.54	3.72	3.90	4.08	4.26
Handball											
moderate	.065		6.11	6.50	6.89	7.28	7.67	8.06	8.45	8.84	9.23
competitive	.077		7.24	7.70	8.16	8.62	9.09	9.55	10.01	10.47	10.93
Hockey (ice)	.066		6.20	6.60	7.00	7.39	7.79	8.18	8.58	8.98	9.37
Horseback Riding											
walk	.019		1.79	1.90	2.01	2.13	2.24	2.36	2.47	2.58	2.70
sitting to trot	.027		2.54	2.70	2.86	3.02	3.19	3.35	3.51	3.67	3.83
posting to trot	.042		3.95	4.20	4.45	4.70	4.96	5.21	5.46	5.71	5.96
gallop	.057		5.36	5.70	6.04	6.38	6.73	7.07	7.41	7.75	8.09
Horseshoes	.025		2.35	2.50	2.65	2.80	2.95	3.10	3.25	3.40	3.55
Ironing	.015		1.41	1.50	1.59	1.68	1.77	1.86	1.95	2.04	2.13
Judo	.089		8.37	8.90	9.43	9.97	10.50	11.04	11.57	12.10	12.64

```
------------------------------------------------------------------------------------------
 67    70    73    75    78    81    84    86    89    92    95    97   100   103   105   108

148   154   160   166   172   178   184   190   196   202   208   214   220   226   232   238
------------------------------------------------------------------------------------------

6.96  7.24  7.52  7.80  8.08  8.37  8.65  8.93  9.21  9.49  9.78 10.06 10.34 10.62 10.90 11.19
9.03  9.39  9.76 10.13 10.49 10.86 11.22 11.59 11.96 12.32 12.69 13.05 13.42 13.79 14.15 14.52
3.40  3.54  3.68  3.82  3.96  4.09  4.23  4.37  4.51  4.65  4.78  4.92  5.06  5.20  5.34  5.47
6.66  6.93  7.20  7.47  7.74  8.01  8.28  8.55  8.82  9.09  9.36  9.63  9.90 10.17 10.44 10.71

9.77 10.16 10.56 10.96 11.35 11.75 12.14 12.54 12.94 13.33 13.73 14.12 14.52 14.92 15.31 15.71

1.48  1.54  1.60  1.66  1.72  1.78  1.84  1.90  1.96  2.02  2.08  2.14  2.20  2.26  2.32  2.38

4.88  5.08  5.28  5.48  5.68  5.87  6.07  6.27  6.47  6.67  6.86  7.06  7.26  7.46  7.66  7.85
9.77 10.16 10.56 10.96 11.35 11.75 12.14 12.54 12.94 13.33 13.73 14.12 14.52 14.92 15.31 15.71

9.03  9.39  9.76 10.13 10.49 10.86 11.22 11.59 11.96 12.32 12.69 13.05 13.42 13.79 14.15 14.52

4.14  4.31  4.48  4.65  4.82  4.98  5.15  5.32  5.49  5.66  5.82  5.99  6.16  6.33  6.50  6.66

4.88  5.08  5.28  5.48  5.68  5.87  6.07  6.27  6.47  6.67  6.86  7.06  7.26  7.46  7.66  7.85
8.14  8.47  8.80  9.13  9.46  9.79 10.12 10.45 10.78 11.11 11.44 11.77 12.10 12.43 12.76 13.09
8.88  9.24  9.60  9.96 10.32 10.68 11.04 11.40 11.76 12.12 12.48 12.84 13.20 13.56 13.92 14.28


20.13 20.94 21.76 22.58 23.39 24.21 25.02 25.84 26.66 27.47 28.29 29.10 29.92 30.74 31.55 32.37
5.77  6.01  6.24  6.47  6.71  6.94  7.18  7.41  7.64  7.88  8.11  8.35  8.58  8.81  9.05  9.28
8.14  8.47  8.80  9.13  9.46  9.79 10.12 10.45 10.78 11.11 11.44 11.77 12.10 12.43 12.76 13.09
5.03  5.24  5.44  5.64  5.85  6.05  6.26  6.46  6.66  6.87  7.07  7.28  7.48  7.68  7.89  8.09
5.92  6.16  6.40  6.64  6.88  7.12  7.36  7.60  7.84  8.08  8.32  8.56  8.80  9.04  9.28  9.52
8.73  9.09  9.44  9.79 10.15 10.50 10.86 11.21 11.56 11.92 12.27 12.63 12.98 13.33 13.69 14.04

8.44  8.78  9.12  9.46  9.80 10.15 10.49 10.83 11.17 11.51 11.86 12.20 12.54 12.88 13.22 13.57
5.18  5.39  5.60  5.81  6.02  6.23  6.44  6.65  6.86  7.07  7.28  7.49  7.70  7.91  8.12  8.33
7.55  7.85  8.16  8.47  8.77  9.08  9.38  9.69 10.00 10.30 10.61 10.91 11.22 11.53 11.83 12.14
3.70  3.85  4.00  4.15  4.30  4.45  4.60  4.75  4.90  5.05  5.20  5.35  5.50  5.65  5.80  5.95
4.88  5.08  5.28  5.48  5.68  5.87  6.07  6.27  6.47  6.67  6.86  7.06  7.26  7.46  7.66  7.85

5.33  5.54  5.76  5.98  6.19  6.41  6.62  6.84  7.06  7.27  7.49  7.70  7.92  8.14  8.35  8.57
4.00  4.16  4.32  4.48  4.64  4.81  4.97  5.13  5.29  5.45  5.62  5.78  5.94  6.10  6.26  6.43
2.81  2.93  3.04  3.15  3.27  3.38  3.50  3.61  3.72  3.84  3.95  4.07  4.18  4.29  4.41  4.52

4.44  4.62  4.80  4.98  5.16  5.34  5.52  5.70  5.88  6.06  6.24  6.42  6.60  6.78  6.96  7.14

9.62 10.01 10.40 10.79 11.18 11.57 11.96 12.35 12.74 13.13 13.52 13.91 14.30 14.69 15.08 15.47
11.40 11.86 12.32 12.78 13.24 13.71 14.17 14.63 15.09 15.55 16.02 16.48 16.94 17.40 17.86 18.33

9.77 10.16 10.56 10.96 11.35 11.75 12.14 12.54 12.94 13.33 13.73 14.12 14.52 14.92 15.31 15.71

2.81  2.93  3.04  3.15  3.27  3.38  3.50  3.61  3.72  3.84  3.95  4.07  4.18  4.29  4.41  4.52
4.00  4.16  4.32  4.48  4.64  4.81  4.97  5.13  5.29  5.45  5.62  5.78  5.94  6.10  6.26  6.43
6.22  6.47  6.72  6.97  7.22  7.48  7.73  7.98  8.23  8.48  8.74  8.99  9.24  9.49  9.74 10.00
8.44  8.78  9.12  9.46  9.80 10.15 10.49 10.83 11.17 11.51 11.86 12.20 12.54 12.88 13.22 13.57

3.70  3.85  4.00  4.15  4.30  4.45  4.60  4.75  4.90  5.05  5.20  5.35  5.50  5.65  5.80  5.95

2.22  2.31  2.40  2.49  2.58  2.67  2.76  2.85  2.94  3.03  3.12  3.21  3.30  3.39  3.48  3.57

13.17 13.71 14.24 14.77 15.31 15.84 16.38 16.91 17.44 17.98 18.51 19.05 19.58 20.11 20.65 21.18
```

ACTIVITY	CAL/MIN/LB	KG	43	45	48	51	54	56	59	62	65
		LB	94	100	106	112	118	124	130	136	142
Jumping Rope											
70/min	.074		6.96	7.40	7.84	8.29	8.73	9.18	9.62	10.06	10.51
80/min	.075		7.05	7.50	7.95	8.40	8.85	9.30	9.75	10.20	10.65
125/min	.080		7.52	8.00	8.48	8.96	9.44	9.92	10.40	10.88	11.36
145/min	.090		8.46	9.00	9.54	10.08	10.62	11.16	11.70	12.24	12.78
Karate	.085		7.99	8.50	9.01	9.52	10.03	10.54	11.05	11.56	12.07
Knitting/Sewing	.010		.94	1.00	1.06	1.12	1.18	1.24	1.30	1.36	1.42
Lying at Ease	.010		.94	1.00	1.06	1.12	1.18	1.24	1.30	1.36	1.42
Marching (rapid)	.065		6.11	6.50	6.89	7.28	7.67	8.06	8.45	8.84	9.23
Mopping	.027		2.54	2.70	2.86	3.02	3.19	3.35	3.51	3.67	3.83
Mountian Climbing	.065		6.11	6.50	6.89	7.28	7.67	8.06	8.45	8.84	9.23
Music											
accordian (sitting)	.015		1.41	1.50	1.59	1.68	1.77	1.86	1.95	2.04	2.13
cello (sitting)	.019		1.79	1.90	2.01	2.13	2.24	2.36	2.47	2.58	2.70
conducting	.018		1.69	1.80	1.91	2.02	2.12	2.23	2.34	2.45	2.56
drums (sitting)	.030		2.82	3.00	3.18	3.36	3.54	3.72	3.90	4.08	4.26
flute (sitting)	.016		1.50	1.60	1.70	1.79	1.89	1.98	2.08	2.18	2.27
horn (sitting)	.013		1.22	1.30	1.38	1.46	1.53	1.61	1.69	1.77	1.85
organ	.024		2.26	2.40	2.54	2.69	2.83	2.98	3.12	3.26	3.41
piano	.018		1.69	1.80	1.91	2.02	2.12	2.23	2.34	2.45	2.56
trumpet (standing)	.014		1.32	1.40	1.48	1.57	1.65	1.74	1.82	1.90	1.99
violin (sitting)	.020		1.88	2.00	2.12	2.24	2.36	2.48	2.60	2.72	2.84
woodwind (sitting)	.015		1.41	1.50	1.59	1.68	1.77	1.86	1.95	2.04	2.13
Paddleball	.057		5.36	5.70	6.04	6.38	6.73	7.07	7.41	7.75	8.09
Painting											
inside	.015		1.41	1.50	1.59	1.68	1.77	1.86	1.95	2.04	2.13
outside	.035		3.29	3.50	3.71	3.92	4.13	4.34	4.55	4.76	4.97
Pool (billiards)	.015		1.41	1.50	1.59	1.68	1.77	1.86	1.95	2.04	2.13
Racquetball											
moderate	.065		6.11	6.50	6.89	7.28	7.67	8.06	8.45	8.84	9.23
vigorous	.081		7.61	8.10	8.59	9.07	9.56	10.04	10.53	11.02	11.50
Rollerskating (9 mph)	.042		3.95	4.20	4.45	4.70	4.96	5.21	5.46	5.71	5.96
Running											
cross-country	.074		6.96	7.40	7.84	8.29	8.73	9.18	9.62	10.06	10.51
horizontal											
11:30 min/mi	.061		5.73	6.10	6.47	6.83	7.20	7.56	7.93	8.30	8.66
10 min/mi	.072		6.77	7.20	7.63	8.06	8.50	8.93	9.36	9.79	10.22
9 min/mi	.083		7.80	8.30	8.80	9.30	9.79	10.29	10.79	11.29	11.79
8 min/mi	.093		8.74	9.30	9.86	10.42	10.97	11.53	12.09	12.65	13.21
7 min/mi	.103		9.68	10.30	10.92	11.54	12.15	12.77	13.39	14.01	14.63
6 min/mi	.118		11.09	11.80	12.51	13.22	13.92	14.63	15.34	16.05	16.76
5:30 min/mi	.132		12.41	13.20	13.99	14.78	15.58	16.37	17.16	17.95	18.74
5 min/mi	.145		13.63	14.50	15.37	16.24	17.11	17.98	18.85	19.72	20.59
Sailing (small boat)	.027		2.54	2.70	2.86	3.02	3.19	3.35	3.51	3.67	3.83
Scrubbing Floors	.050		4.70	5.00	5.30	5.60	5.90	6.20	6.50	6.80	7.10
Shopping	.027		2.54	2.70	2.86	3.02	3.19	3.35	3.51	3.67	3.83
Sitting Quietly	.010		.94	1.00	1.06	1.12	1.18	1.24	1.30	1.36	1.42
Skating (ice)	.042		3.95	4.20	4.45	4.70	4.96	5.21	5.46	5.71	5.96

```
----------------------------------------------------------------------------------------------
 67    70    73    75    78    81    84    86    89    92    95    97   100   103   105   108

148   154   160   166   172   178   184   190   196   202   208   214   220   226   232   238
----------------------------------------------------------------------------------------------

10.95 11.40 11.84 12.28 12.73 13.17 13.62 14.06 14.50 14.95 15.39 15.84 16.28 16.72 17.17 17.61
11.10 11.55 12.00 12.45 12.90 13.35 13.80 14.25 14.70 15.15 15.60 16.05 16.50 16.95 17.40 17.85
11.84 12.32 12.80 13.28 13.76 14.24 14.72 15.20 15.68 16.16 16.64 17.12 17.60 18.08 18.56 19.04
13.32 13.86 14.40 14.94 15.48 16.02 16.56 17.10 17.64 18.18 18.72 19.26 19.80 20.34 20.88 21.42
12.58 13.09 13.60 14.11 14.62 15.13 15.64 16.15 16.66 17.17 17.68 18.19 18.70 19.21 19.72 20.23

 1.48  1.54  1.60  1.66  1.72  1.78  1.84  1.90  1.96  2.02  2.08  2.14  2.20  2.26  2.32  2.38

 1.48  1.54  1.60  1.66  1.72  1.78  1.84  1.90  1.96  2.02  2.08  2.14  2.20  2.26  2.32  2.38

 9.62 10.01 10.40 10.79 11.18 11.57 11.96 12.35 12.74 13.13 13.52 13.91 14.30 14.69 15.08 15.47

 4.00  4.16  4.32  4.48  4.64  4.81  4.97  5.13  5.29  5.45  5.62  5.78  5.94  6.10  6.26  6.43

 9.62 10.01 10.40 10.79 11.18 11.57 11.96 12.35 12.74 13.13 13.52 13.91 14.30 14.69 15.08 15.47

 2.22  2.31  2.40  2.49  2.58  2.67  2.76  2.85  2.94  3.03  3.12  3.21  3.30  3.39  3.48  3.57
 2.81  2.93  3.04  3.15  3.27  3.38  3.50  3.61  3.72  3.84  3.95  4.07  4.18  4.29  4.41  4.52
 2.66  2.77  2.88  2.99  3.10  3.20  3.31  3.42  3.53  3.64  3.74  3.85  3.96  4.07  4.18  4.28
 4.44  4.62  4.80  4.98  5.16  5.34  5.52  5.70  5.88  6.06  6.24  6.42  6.60  6.78  6.96  7.14
 2.37  2.46  2.56  2.66  2.75  2.85  2.94  3.04  3.14  3.23  3.33  3.42  3.52  3.62  3.71  3.81
 1.92  2.00  2.08  2.16  2.24  2.31  2.39  2.47  2.55  2.63  2.70  2.78  2.86  2.94  3.02  3.09
 3.55  3.70  3.84  3.98  4.13  4.27  4.42  4.56  4.70  4.85  4.99  5.14  5.28  5.42  5.57  5.71
 2.66  2.77  2.88  2.99  3.10  3.20  3.31  3.42  3.53  3.64  3.74  3.85  3.96  4.07  4.18  4.28
 2.07  2.16  2.24  2.32  2.41  2.49  2.58  2.66  2.74  2.83  2.91  3.00  3.08  3.16  3.25  3.33
 2.96  3.08  3.20  3.32  3.44  3.56  3.68  3.80  3.92  4.04  4.16  4.28  4.40  4.52  4.64  4.76
 2.22  2.31  2.40  2.49  2.58  2.67  2.76  2.85  2.94  3.03  3.12  3.21  3.30  3.39  3.48  3.57
 8.44  8.78  9.12  9.46  9.80 10.15 10.49 10.83 11.17 11.51 11.86 12.20 12.54 12.88 13.22 13.57

 2.22  2.31  2.40  2.49  2.58  2.67  2.76  2.85  2.94  3.03  3.12  3.21  3.30  3.39  3.48  3.57
 5.18  5.39  5.60  5.81  6.02  6.23  6.44  6.65  6.86  7.07  7.28  7.49  7.70  7.91  8.12  8.33
 2.22  2.31  2.40  2.49  2.58  2.67  2.76  2.85  2.94  3.03  3.12  3.21  3.30  3.39  3.48  3.57

 9.62 10.01 10.40 10.79 11.18 11.57 11.96 12.35 12.74 13.13 13.52 13.91 14.30 14.69 15.08 15.47
11.99 12.47 12.96 13.45 13.93 14.42 14.90 15.39 15.88 16.36 16.85 17.33 17.82 18.31 18.79 19.28
 6.22  6.47  6.72  6.97  7.22  7.48  7.73  7.98  8.23  8.48  8.74  8.99  9.24  9.49  9.74 10.00

10.95 11.40 11.84 12.28 12.73 13.17 13.62 14.06 14.50 14.95 15.39 15.84 16.28 16.72 17.17 17.61

 9.03  9.39  9.76 10.13 10.49 10.86 11.22 11.59 11.96 12.32 12.69 13.05 13.42 13.79 14.15 14.52
10.66 11.09 11.52 11.95 12.38 12.82 13.25 13.68 14.11 14.54 14.98 15.41 15.84 16.27 16.70 17.14
12.28 12.78 13.28 13.78 14.28 14.77 15.27 15.77 16.27 16.77 17.26 17.76 18.26 18.76 19.26 19.75
13.76 14.32 14.88 15.44 16.00 16.55 17.11 17.67 18.23 18.79 19.34 19.90 20.46 21.02 21.58 22.13
15.24 15.86 16.48 17.10 17.72 18.33 18.95 19.57 20.19 20.81 21.42 22.04 22.66 23.28 23.90 24.51
17.46 18.17 18.88 19.59 20.30 21.00 21.71 22.42 23.13 23.84 24.54 25.25 25.96 26.67 27.38 28.08
19.54 20.33 21.12 21.91 22.70 23.50 24.29 25.08 25.87 26.66 27.46 28.25 29.04 29.83 30.62 31.42
21.46 22.33 23.20 24.07 24.94 25.81 26.68 27.55 28.42 29.29 30.16 31.03 31.90 32.77 33.64 34.51
 4.00  4.16  4.32  4.48  4.64  4.81  4.97  5.13  5.29  5.45  5.62  5.78  5.94  6.10  6.26  6.43

 7.40  7.70  8.00  8.30  8.60  8.90  9.20  9.50  9.80 10.10 10.40 10.70 11.00 11.30 11.60 11.90

 4.00  4.16  4.32  4.48  4.64  4.81  4.97  5.13  5.29  5.45  5.62  5.78  5.94  6.10  6.26  6.43

 1.48  1.54  1.60  1.66  1.72  1.78  1.84  1.90  1.96  2.02  2.08  2.14  2.20  2.26  2.32  2.38

 6.22  6.47  6.72  6.97  7.22  7.48  7.73  7.98  8.23  8.48  8.74  8.99  9.24  9.49  9.74 10.00
```

ACTIVITY	CAL/MIN/LB	KG 43	45	48	51	54	56	59	62	65
		LB 94	100	106	112	118	124	130	136	142
Skiing (cross-country)										
24 min/mi	.050	4.70	5.00	5.30	5.60	5.90	6.20	6.50	6.80	7.10
15 min/mi	.065	6.11	6.50	6.89	7.28	7.67	8.06	8.45	8.84	9.23
12 min/mi	.077	7.24	7.70	8.16	8.62	9.09	9.55	10.01	10.47	10.93
uphill (fast)	.137	12.88	13.70	14.52	15.34	16.17	16.99	17.81	18.63	19.45
Skiing (downhill)	.065	6.11	6.50	6.89	7.28	7.67	8.06	8.45	8.84	9.23
Snowshoeing	.075	7.05	7.50	7.95	8.40	8.85	9.30	9.75	10.20	10.65
Soccer	.059	5.55	5.90	6.25	6.61	6.96	7.32	7.67	8.02	8.38
Squash										
moderate	.067	6.30	6.70	7.10	7.50	7.91	8.31	8.71	9.11	9.51
competitive	.077	7.24	7.70	8.16	8.62	9.09	9.55	10.01	10.47	10.93
Standing Quietly	.011	1.03	1.10	1.17	1.23	1.30	1.36	1.43	1.50	1.56
Studying (light work)	.027	2.54	2.70	2.86	3.02	3.19	3.35	3.51	3.67	3.83
Stock Clerking	.025	2.35	2.50	2.65	2.80	2.95	3.10	3.25	3.40	3.55
Swimming										
backstroke										
30 yards/min	.035	3.29	3.50	3.71	3.92	4.13	4.34	4.55	4.76	4.97
40 yards/min	.055	5.17	5.50	5.83	6.16	6.49	6.82	7.15	7.48	7.81
vigorous	.077	7.24	7.70	8.16	8.62	9.09	9.55	10.01	10.47	10.93
breaststroke										
20 yards/min	.031	2.91	3.10	3.29	3.47	3.66	3.84	4.03	4.22	4.40
40 yards/min	.063	5.92	6.30	6.68	7.06	7.43	7.81	8.19	8.57	8.95
vigorous	.074	6.96	7.40	7.84	8.29	8.73	9.18	9.62	10.06	10.51
crawl										
25 yards/min	.040	3.76	4.00	4.24	4.48	4.72	4.96	5.20	5.44	5.68
50 yards/min	.020	1.88	2.00	2.12	2.24	2.36	2.48	2.60	2.72	2.84
sidestroke	.055	5.17	5.50	5.83	6.16	6.49	6.82	7.15	7.48	7.81
Table Tennis	.031	2.91	3.10	3.29	3.47	3.66	3.84	4.03	4.22	4.40
Tennis										
singles, recreational	.050	4.70	5.00	5.30	5.60	5.90	6.20	6.50	6.80	7.10
doubles, recreational	.034	3.20	3.40	3.60	3.81	4.01	4.22	4.42	4.62	4.83
Typing										
electric	.012	1.13	1.20	1.27	1.34	1.42	1.49	1.56	1.63	1.70
manual	.014	1.32	1.40	1.48	1.57	1.65	1.74	1.82	1.90	1.99
Volleyball										
moderate	.029	2.73	2.90	3.07	3.25	3.42	3.60	3.77	3.94	4.12
vigorous	.065	6.11	6.50	6.89	7.28	7.67	8.06	8.45	8.84	9.23
Walking										
1.0 mph	.015	1.41	1.50	1.59	1.68	1.77	1.86	1.95	2.04	2.13
2.0 mph	.021	1.97	2.10	2.23	2.35	2.48	2.60	2.73	2.86	2.98
3.0 mph	.027	2.54	2.70	2.86	3.02	3.19	3.35	3.51	3.67	3.83
3.5 mph	.033	3.10	3.30	3.50	3.70	3.89	4.09	4.29	4.49	4.69
4.0 mph	.042	3.95	4.20	4.45	4.70	4.96	5.21	5.46	5.71	5.96
Water Skiing	.050	4.70	5.00	5.30	5.60	5.90	6.20	6.50	6.80	7.10
Weight Training	.052	4.89	5.20	5.51	5.82	6.14	6.45	6.76	7.07	7.38
Window-washing	.026	2.44	2.60	2.76	2.91	3.07	3.22	3.38	3.54	3.69
Wrestling	.085	7.99	8.50	9.01	9.52	10.03	10.54	11.05	11.56	12.07
Writing (sitting)	.013	1.22	1.30	1.38	1.46	1.53	1.61	1.69	1.77	1.85

67	70	73	75	78	81	84	86	89	92	95	97	100	103	105	108
148	154	160	166	172	178	184	190	196	202	208	214	220	226	232	238
7.40	7.70	8.00	8.30	8.60	8.90	9.20	9.50	9.80	10.10	10.40	10.70	11.00	11.30	11.60	11.90
9.62	10.01	10.40	10.79	11.18	11.57	11.96	12.35	12.74	13.13	13.52	13.91	14.30	14.69	15.08	15.47
11.40	11.86	12.32	12.78	13.24	13.71	14.17	14.63	15.09	15.55	16.02	16.48	16.94	17.40	17.86	18.33
20.28	21.10	21.92	22.74	23.56	24.39	25.21	26.03	26.85	27.67	28.50	29.32	30.14	30.96	31.78	32.61
9.62	10.01	10.40	10.79	11.18	11.57	11.96	12.35	12.74	13.13	13.52	13.91	14.30	14.69	15.08	15.47
11.10	11.55	12.00	12.45	12.90	13.35	13.80	14.25	14.70	15.15	15.60	16.05	16.50	16.95	17.40	17.85
8.73	9.09	9.44	9.79	10.15	10.50	10.86	11.21	11.56	11.92	12.27	12.63	12.98	13.33	13.69	14.04
9.92	10.32	10.72	11.12	11.52	11.93	12.33	12.73	13.13	13.53	13.94	14.34	14.74	15.14	15.54	15.95
11.40	11.86	12.32	12.78	13.24	13.71	14.17	14.63	15.09	15.55	16.02	16.48	16.94	17.40	17.86	18.33
1.63	1.69	1.76	1.83	1.89	1.96	2.02	2.09	2.16	2.22	2.29	2.35	2.42	2.49	2.55	2.62
4.00	4.16	4.32	4.48	4.64	4.81	4.97	5.13	5.29	5.45	5.62	5.78	5.94	6.10	6.26	6.43
3.70	3.85	4.00	4.15	4.30	4.45	4.60	4.75	4.90	5.05	5.20	5.35	5.50	5.65	5.80	5.95
5.18	5.39	5.60	5.81	6.02	6.23	6.44	6.65	6.86	7.07	7.28	7.49	7.70	7.91	8.12	8.33
8.14	8.47	8.80	9.13	9.46	9.79	10.12	10.45	10.78	11.11	11.44	11.77	12.10	12.43	12.76	13.09
11.40	11.86	12.32	12.78	13.24	13.71	14.17	14.63	15.09	15.55	16.02	16.48	16.94	17.40	17.86	18.33
4.59	4.77	4.96	5.15	5.33	5.52	5.70	5.89	6.08	6.26	6.45	6.63	6.82	7.01	7.19	7.38
9.32	9.70	10.08	10.46	10.84	11.21	11.59	11.97	12.35	12.73	13.10	13.48	13.86	14.24	14.62	14.99
10.95	11.40	11.84	12.28	12.73	13.17	13.62	14.06	14.50	14.95	15.39	15.84	16.28	16.72	17.17	17.61
5.92	6.16	6.40	6.64	6.88	7.12	7.36	7.60	7.84	8.08	8.32	8.56	8.80	9.04	9.28	9.52
2.96	3.08	3.20	3.32	3.44	3.56	3.68	3.80	3.92	4.04	4.16	4.28	4.40	4.52	4.64	4.76
8.14	8.47	8.80	9.13	9.46	9.79	10.12	10.45	10.78	11.11	11.44	11.77	12.10	12.43	12.76	13.09
4.59	4.77	4.96	5.15	5.33	5.52	5.70	5.89	6.08	6.26	6.45	6.63	6.82	7.01	7.19	7.38
7.40	7.70	8.00	8.30	8.60	8.90	9.20	9.50	9.80	10.10	10.40	10.70	11.00	11.30	11.60	11.90
5.03	5.24	5.44	5.64	5.85	6.05	6.26	6.46	6.66	6.87	7.07	7.28	7.48	7.68	7.89	8.09
1.78	1.85	1.92	1.99	2.06	2.14	2.21	2.28	2.35	2.42	2.50	2.57	2.64	2.71	2.78	2.86
2.07	2.16	2.24	2.32	2.41	2.49	2.58	2.66	2.74	2.83	2.91	3.00	3.08	3.16	3.25	3.33
4.29	4.47	4.64	4.81	4.99	5.16	5.34	5.51	5.68	5.86	6.03	6.21	6.38	6.55	6.73	6.90
9.62	10.01	10.40	10.79	11.18	11.57	11.96	12.35	12.74	13.13	13.52	13.91	14.30	14.69	15.08	15.47
2.22	2.31	2.40	2.49	2.58	2.67	2.76	2.85	2.94	3.03	3.12	3.21	3.30	3.39	3.48	3.57
3.11	3.23	3.36	3.49	3.61	3.74	3.86	3.99	4.12	4.24	4.37	4.49	4.62	4.75	4.87	5.00
4.00	4.16	4.32	4.48	4.64	4.81	4.97	5.13	5.29	5.45	5.62	5.78	5.94	6.10	6.26	6.43
4.88	5.08	5.28	5.48	5.68	5.87	6.07	6.27	6.47	6.67	6.86	7.06	7.26	7.46	7.66	7.85
6.22	6.47	6.72	6.97	7.22	7.48	7.73	7.98	8.23	8.48	8.74	8.99	9.24	9.49	9.74	10.00
7.40	7.70	8.00	8.30	8.60	8.90	9.20	9.50	9.80	10.10	10.40	10.70	11.00	11.30	11.60	11.90
7.70	8.01	8.32	8.63	8.94	9.26	9.57	9.88	10.19	10.50	10.82	11.13	11.44	11.75	12.06	12.38
3.85	4.00	4.16	4.32	4.47	4.63	4.78	4.94	5.10	5.25	5.41	5.56	5.72	5.88	6.03	6.19
12.58	13.09	13.60	14.11	14.62	15.13	15.64	16.15	16.66	17.17	17.68	18.19	18.70	19.21	19.72	20.23
1.92	2.00	2.08	2.16	2.24	2.31	2.39	2.47	2.55	2.63	2.70	2.78	2.86	2.94	3.02	3.09

7

Recommended Dietary Allowances (RDA), 1980*

AGE (YEARS)	WEIGHT (kg)	(lb)	HEIGHT (cm)	(in)	(g) PROTEIN	(RE) VITAMIN A	(µg) VITAMIN D	(mg) VITAMIN E	(mg) VITAMIN C	(mg) THIAMIN	(mg) RIBOFLAVIN	(mg equiv.) NIACIN	(mg) VITAMIN B_6	(µg) FOLACIN	(µg) VITAMIN B_{12}	(mg) CALCIUM	(mg) PHOSPHORUS	(mg) MAGNESIUM	(mg) IRON	(mg) ZINC	(µg) IODINE
INFANTS																					
0.0-0.5	6	13	60	24	kg × 2.2	420	10	3	35	0.3	0.4	6	0.3	30	0.5	360	240	50	10	3	40
0.5-1.0	9	20	71	28	kg × 2.0	400	10	4	35	0.5	0.6	8	0.6	45	1.5	540	360	70	15	5	50
CHILDREN																					
1-3	13	29	90	35	23	400	10	5	45	0.7	0.8	9	0.9	100	2.0	800	800	150	15	10	70
4-6	20	44	112	44	30	500	10	6	45	0.9	1.0	11	1.3	200	2.5	800	800	200	10	10	90
7-10	28	62	132	52	34	700	10	7	45	1.2	1.4	16	1.6	300	3.0	800	800	250	10	10	120
MALES																					
11-14	45	99	157	62	45	1,000	10	8	50	1.4	1.6	18	1.8	400	3.0	1,200	1,200	350	18	15	150
15-18	66	145	176	69	56	1,000	10	10	60	1.4	1.7	18	2.0	400	3.0	1,200	1,200	400	18	15	150
19-22	70	154	177	70	56	1,000	7.5	10	60	1.5	1.7	19	2.2	400	3.0	800	800	350	10	15	150
23-50	70	154	178	70	56	1,000	5	10	60	1.4	1.6	18	2.2	400	3.0	800	800	350	10	15	150
51+	70	154	178	70	56	1,000	5	10	60	1.2	1.4	16	2.2	400	3.0	800	800	350	10	15	150
FEMALES																					
11-14	46	101	157	62	46	800	10	8	50	1.1	1.3	15	1.8	400	3.0	1,200	1,200	300	18	15	150
15-18	55	120	163	64	46	800	10	8	60	1.1	1.3	14	2.0	400	3.0	1,200	1,200	300	18	15	150
19-22	55	120	163	64	44	800	7.5	8	60	1.1	1.3	14	2.0	400	3.0	800	800	300	18	15	150
23-50	55	120	163	64	44	800	5	8	60	1.0	1.2	13	2.0	400	3.0	800	800	300	18	15	150
51+	55	120	163	64	44	800	5	8	60	1.0	1.2	13	2.0	400	3.0	800	800	300	10	15	150
PREGNANT					+30	+200	+5	+2	+20	+0.4	+0.3	+2	+0.6	+400	+1.0	+400	+400	+150	**	+5	+25
LACTATING					+20	+400	+5	+3	+40	+0.5	+0.5	+5	+0.5	+100	+1.0	+400	+400	+150	**	+10	+50

*The allowances are intended to provide for individual variations among most normal, healthy people in the United States under usual environmental stresses. They were designed for the maintenance of good nutrition. Diets should be based on a variety of common foods in order to provide other nutrients for which human requirements have been less well defined.

**Supplemental iron is recommended.

Reproduced from *Recommended Dietary Allowances*, 9th ed. (1980), with the permission of the National Academy of Sciences, Washington, D.C.

8

Nutritive Value of Foods

Item No.	Foods, approximate measures, units, and weight (weight of edible portion only)			Water	Food energy	Pro-tein	Fat	Fatty acids		
								Satu-rated	Mono-unsatu-rated	Poly-unsatu-rated
	Beverages		Grams	Per-cent	Cal-ories	Grams	Grams	Grams	Grams	Grams
	Alcoholic:									
	Beer:									
1	Regular----------------------	12 fl oz--------	360	92	150	1	0	0.0	0.0	0.0
2	Light------------------------	12 fl oz--------	355	95	95	1	0	0.0	0.0	0.0
	Gin, rum, vodka, whiskey:									
3	80-proof--------------------	1-1/2 fl oz-----	42	67	95	0	0	0.0	0.0	0.0
4	86-proof--------------------	1-1/2 fl oz-----	42	64	105	0	0	0.0	0.0	0.0
5	90-proof--------------------	1-1/2 fl oz-----	42	62	110	0	0	0.0	0.0	0.0
	Wines:									
6	Dessert---------------------	3-1/2 fl oz-----	103	77	140	Tr	0	0.0	0.0	0.0
	Table:									
7	Red------------------------	3-1/2 fl oz-----	102	88	75	Tr	0	0.0	0.0	0.0
8	White----------------------	3-1/2 fl oz-----	102	87	80	Tr	0	0.0	0.0	0.0
	Carbonated:[2]									
9	Club soda--------------------	12 fl oz--------	355	100	0	0	0	0.0	0.0	0.0
	Cola type:									
10	Regular---------------------	12 fl oz--------	369	89	160	0	0	0.0	0.0	0.0
11	Diet, artificially sweetened	12 fl oz--------	355	100	Tr	0	0	0.0	0.0	0.0
12	Ginger ale--------------------	12 fl oz--------	366	91	125	0	0	0.0	0.0	0.0
13	Grape------------------------	12 fl oz--------	372	88	180	0	0	0.0	0.0	0.0
14	Lemon-lime-------------------	12 fl oz--------	372	89	155	0	0	0.0	0.0	0.0
15	Orange-----------------------	12 fl oz--------	372	88	180	0	0	0.0	0.0	0.0
16	Pepper type------------------	12 fl oz--------	369	89	160	0	0	0.0	0.0	0.0
17	Root beer--------------------	12 fl oz--------	370	89	165	0	0	0.0	0.0	0.0
	Cocoa and chocolate-flavored beverages. See Dairy Products (items 95-98).									
	Coffee:									
18	Brewed----------------------	6 fl oz--------	180	100	Tr	Tr	Tr	Tr	Tr	Tr
19	Instant, prepared (2 tsp powder plus 6 fl oz water)----------	6 fl oz--------	182	99	Tr	Tr	Tr	Tr	Tr	Tr
	Fruit drinks, noncarbonated:									
	Canned:									
20	Fruit punch drink------------	6 fl oz--------	190	88	85	Tr	0	0.0	0.0	0.0
21	Grape drink------------------	6 fl oz--------	187	86	100	Tr	0	0.0	0.0	0.0
22	Pineapple-grapefruit juice drink--------------------	6 fl oz--------	187	87	90	Tr	Tr	Tr	Tr	Tr
	Frozen:									
	Lemonade concentrate:									
23	Undiluted------------------	6-fl-oz can-----	219	49	425	Tr	Tr	Tr	Tr	Tr
24	Diluted with 4-1/3 parts water by volume---------	6 fl oz--------	185	89	80	Tr	Tr	Tr	Tr	Tr
	Limeade concentrate:									
25	Undiluted------------------	6-fl-oz can-----	218	50	410	Tr	Tr	Tr	Tr	Tr
26	Diluted with 4-1/3 parts water by volume---------	6 fl oz--------	185	89	75	Tr	Tr	Tr	Tr	Tr
	Fruit juices. See type under Fruits and Fruit Juices.									
	Milk beverages. See Dairy Products (items 92-105).									
	Tea:									
27	Brewed----------------------	8 fl oz--------	240	100	Tr	Tr	Tr	Tr	Tr	Tr
	Instant, powder, prepared:									
28	Unsweetened (1 tsp powder plus 8 fl oz water)--------	8 fl oz--------	241	100	Tr	Tr	Tr	Tr	Tr	Tr
29	Sweetened (3 tsp powder plus 8 fl oz water)-------------	8 fl oz--------	262	91	85	Tr	Tr	Tr	Tr	Tr

[1]Value not determined.
[2]Mineral content varies depending on water source.

Nutrients in Indicated Quantity

Cho-les-terol	Carbo-hydrate	Calcium	Phos-phorus	Iron	Potas-sium	Sodium	Vitamin A value (IU)	Vitamin A value (RE)	Thiamin	Ribo-flavin	Niacin	Ascorbic acid	Item No.
Milli-grams	Grams	Milli-grams	Milli-grams	Milli-grams	Milli-grams	Milli-grams	Inter-national units	Retinol equiva-lents	Milli-grams	Milli-grams	Milli-grams	Milli-grams	
0	13	14	50	0.1	115	18	0	0	0.02	0.09	1.8	0	1
0	5	14	43	0.1	64	11	0	0	0.03	0.11	1.4	0	2
0	Tr	Tr	Tr	Tr	1	Tr	0	0	Tr	Tr	Tr	0	3
0	Tr	Tr	Tr	Tr	1	Tr	0	0	Tr	Tr	Tr	0	4
0	Tr	Tr	Tr	Tr	1	Tr	0	0	Tr	Tr	Tr	0	5
0	8	8	9	0.2	95	9	([1])	([1])	0.01	0.02	0.2	0	6
0	3	8	18	0.4	113	5	([1])	([1])	0.00	0.03	0.1	0	7
0	3	9	14	0.3	83	5	([1])	([1])	0.00	0.01	0.1	0	8
0	0	18	0	Tr	0	78	0	0	0.00	0.00	0.0	0	9
0	41	11	52	0.2	7	18	0	0	0.00	0.00	0.0	0	10
0	Tr	14	39	0.2	7	[3]32	0	0	0.00	0.00	0.0	0	11
0	32	11	0	0.1	4	29	0	0	0.00	0.00	0.0	0	12
0	46	15	0	0.4	4	48	0	0	0.00	0.00	0.0	0	13
0	39	7	0	0.4	4	33	0	0	0.00	0.00	0.0	0	14
0	46	15	4	0.3	7	52	0	0	0.00	0.00	0.0	0	15
0	41	11	41	0.1	4	37	0	0	0.00	0.00	0.0	0	16
0	42	15	0	0.2	4	48	0	0	0.00	0.00	0.0	0	17
0	Tr	4	2	Tr	124	2	0	0	0.00	0.02	0.4	0	18
0	1	2	6	0.1	71	Tr	0	0	0.00	0.03	0.6	0	19
0	22	15	2	0.4	48	15	20	2	0.03	0.04	Tr	[4]61	20
0	26	2	2	0.3	9	11	Tr	Tr	0.01	0.01	Tr	[4]64	21
0	23	13	7	0.9	97	24	60	6	0.06	0.04	0.5	[4]110	22
0	112	9	13	0.4	153	4	40	4	0.04	0.07	0.7	66	23
0	21	2	2	0.1	30	1	10	1	0.01	0.02	0.2	13	24
0	108	11	13	0.2	129	Tr	Tr	Tr	0.02	0.02	0.2	26	25
0	20	2	2	Tr	24	Tr	Tr	Tr	Tr	Tr	Tr	4	26
0	Tr	0	2	Tr	36	1	0	0	0.00	0.03	Tr	0	27
0	1	1	4	Tr	61	1	0	0	0.00	0.02	0.1	0	28
0	22	1	3	Tr	49	Tr	0	0	0.00	0.04	0.1	0	29

[3]Blend of aspartame and saccharin; if only sodium saccharin is used, sodium is 75 mg; if only aspartame is used, ium is 23 mg.
[4]With added ascorbic acid.

Item No.	Foods, approximate measures, units, and weight (weight of edible portion only)		Water	Food energy	Pro-tein	Fat	Fatty acids		
							Satu-rated	Mono-unsatu-rated	Poly-unsatu-rated
	Dairy Products	Grams	Per-cent	Cal-ories	Grams	Grams	Grams	Grams	Grams
	Butter. See Fats and Oils (items 128-130).								
	Cheese:								
	Natural:								
30	Blue------------------------	1 oz------------	28	42	100	6	8	5.3	2.2	0.2
31	Camembert (3 wedges per 4-oz container)-----------------	1 wedge---------	38	52	115	8	9	5.8	2.7	0.3
	Cheddar:								
32	Cut pieces----------------	1 oz------------	28	37	115	7	9	6.0	2.7	0.3
33		1 in³-----------	17	37	70	4	6	3.6	1.6	0.2
34	Shredded------------------	1 cup----------	113	37	455	28	37	23.8	10.6	1.1
	Cottage (curd not pressed down):								
	Creamed (cottage cheese, 4% fat):								
35	Large curd--------------	1 cup----------	225	79	235	28	10	6.4	2.9	0.3
36	Small curd--------------	1 cup----------	210	79	215	26	9	6.0	2.7	0.3
37	With fruit-------------	1 cup----------	226	72	280	22	8	4.9	2.2	0.2
38	Lowfat (2%)--------------	1 cup----------	226	79	205	31	4	2.8	1.2	0.1
39	Uncreamed (cottage cheese dry curd, less than 1/2% fat)-------------------	1 cup----------	145	80	125	25	1	0.4	0.2	Tr
40	Cream------------------------	1 oz------------	28	54	100	2	10	6.2	2.8	0.4
41	Feta------------------------	1 oz------------	28	55	75	4	6	4.2	1.3	0.2
	Mozzarella, made with:								
42	Whole milk---------------	1 oz------------	28	54	80	6	6	3.7	1.9	0.2
43	Part skim milk (low moisture)----------------	1 oz------------	28	49	80	8	5	3.1	1.4	0.1
44	Muenster--------------------	1 oz------------	28	42	105	7	9	5.4	2.5	0.2
	Parmesan, grated:								
45	Cup, not pressed down------	1 cup----------	100	18	455	42	30	19.1	8.7	0.7
46	Tablespoon---------------	1 tbsp---------	5	18	25	2	2	1.0	0.4	Tr
47	Ounce-------------------	1 oz------------	28	18	130	12	9	5.4	2.5	0.2
48	Provolone-------------------	1 oz------------	28	41	100	7	8	4.8	2.1	0.2
	Ricotta, made with:								
49	Whole milk---------------	1 cup----------	246	72	430	28	32	20.4	8.9	0.9
50	Part skim milk-----------	1 cup----------	246	74	340	28	19	12.1	5.7	0.6
51	Swiss-----------------------	1 oz------------	28	37	105	8	8	5.0	2.1	0.3
	Pasteurized process cheese:								
52	American--------------------	1 oz------------	28	39	105	6	9	5.6	2.5	0.3
53	Swiss-----------------------	1 oz------------	28	42	95	7	7	4.5	2.0	0.2
54	Pasteurized process cheese food, American --------------	1 oz------------	28	43	95	6	7	4.4	2.0	0.2
55	Pasteurized process cheese spread, American------------	1 oz------------	28	48	80	5	6	3.8	1.8	0.2
	Cream, sweet:								
56	Half-and-half (cream and milk)	1 cup----------	242	81	315	7	28	17.3	8.0	1.0
57		1 tbsp---------	15	81	20	Tr	2	1.1	0.5	0.1
58	Light, coffee, or table--------	1 cup----------	240	74	470	6	46	28.8	13.4	1.7
59		1 tbsp---------	15	74	30	Tr	3	1.8	0.8	0.1
	Whipping, unwhipped (volume about double when whipped):								
60	Light----------------------	1 cup----------	239	64	700	5	74	46.2	21.7	2.1
61		1 tbsp---------	15	64	45	Tr	5	2.9	1.4	0.1
62	Heavy----------------------	1 cup----------	238	58	820	5	88	54.8	25.4	3.3
63		1 tbsp---------	15	58	50	Tr	6	3.5	1.6	0.2
64	Whipped topping, (pressurized)	1 cup----------	60	61	155	2	13	8.3	3.9	0.5
65		1 tbsp---------	3	61	10	Tr	1	0.4	0.2	Tr
66	Cream, sour-----------------	1 cup----------	230	71	495	7	48	30.0	13.9	1.8
67		1 tbsp---------	12	71	25	Tr	3	1.6	0.7	0.1

Nutrients in Indicated Quantity

Cho-les-terol	Carbo-hydrate	Calcium	Phos-phorus	Iron	Potas-sium	Sodium	Vitamin A value		Thiamin	Ribo-flavin	Niacin	Ascorbic acid	Item No.
							(IU)	(RE)					
Milli-grams	Grams	Milli-grams	Milli-grams	Milli-grams	Milli-grams	Milli-grams	Inter-national units	Retinol equiva-lents	Milli-grams	Milli-grams	Milli-grams	Milli-grams	
21	1	150	110	0.1	73	396	200	65	0.01	0.11	0.3	0	30
27	Tr	147	132	0.1	71	320	350	96	0.01	0.19	0.2	0	31
30	Tr	204	145	0.2	28	176	300	86	0.01	0.11	Tr	0	32
18	Tr	123	87	0.1	17	105	180	52	Tr	0.06	Tr	0	33
119	1	815	579	0.8	111	701	1,200	342	0.03	0.42	0.1	0	34
34	6	135	297	0.3	190	911	370	108	0.05	0.37	0.3	Tr	35
31	6	126	277	0.3	177	850	340	101	0.04	0.34	0.3	Tr	36
25	30	108	236	0.2	151	915	280	81	0.04	0.29	0.2	Tr	37
19	8	155	340	0.4	217	918	160	45	0.05	0.42	0.3	Tr	38
10	3	46	151	0.3	47	19	40	12	0.04	0.21	0.2	0	39
31	1	23	30	0.3	34	84	400	124	Tr	0.06	Tr	0	40
25	1	140	96	0.2	18	316	130	36	0.04	0.24	0.3	0	41
22	1	147	105	0.1	19	106	220	68	Tr	0.07	Tr	0	42
15	1	207	149	0.1	27	150	180	54	0.01	0.10	Tr	0	43
27	Tr	203	133	0.1	38	178	320	90	Tr	0.09	Tr	0	44
79	4	1,376	807	1.0	107	1,861	700	173	0.05	0.39	0.3	0	45
4	Tr	69	40	Tr	5	93	40	9	Tr	0.02	Tr	0	46
22	1	390	229	0.3	30	528	200	49	0.01	0.11	0.1	0	47
20	1	214	141	0.1	39	248	230	75	0.01	0.09	Tr	0	48
124	7	509	389	0.9	257	207	1,210	330	0.03	0.48	0.3	0	49
76	13	669	449	1.1	307	307	1,060	278	0.05	0.46	0.2	0	50
26	1	272	171	Tr	31	74	240	72	0.01	0.10	Tr	0	51
27	Tr	174	211	0.1	46	406	340	82	0.01	0.10	Tr	0	52
24	1	219	216	0.2	61	388	230	65	Tr	0.08	Tr	0	53
18	2	163	130	0.2	79	337	260	62	0.01	0.13	Tr	0	54
16	2	159	202	0.1	69	381	220	54	0.01	0.12	Tr	0	55
89	10	254	230	0.2	314	98	1,050	259	0.08	0.36	0.2	2	56
6	1	16	14	Tr	19	6	70	16	0.01	0.02	Tr	Tr	57
159	9	231	192	0.1	292	95	1,730	437	0.08	0.36	0.1	2	58
10	1	14	12	Tr	18	6	110	27	Tr	0.02	Tr	Tr	59
265	7	166	146	0.1	231	82	2,690	705	0.06	0.30	0.1	1	60
17	Tr	10	9	Tr	15	5	170	44	Tr	0.02	Tr	Tr	61
326	7	154	149	0.1	179	89	3,500	1,002	0.05	0.26	0.1	1	62
21	Tr	10	9	Tr	11	6	220	63	Tr	0.02	Tr	Tr	63
46	7	61	54	Tr	88	78	550	124	0.02	0.04	Tr	0	64
2	Tr	3	3	Tr	4	4	30	6	Tr	Tr	Tr	0	65
102	10	268	195	0.1	331	123	1,820	448	0.08	0.34	0.2	2	66
5	1	14	10	Tr	17	6	90	23	Tr	0.02	Tr	Tr	67

Item No.	Foods, approximate measures, units, and weight (weight of edible portion only)			Water	Food energy	Pro-tein	Fat	Fatty acids		
								Satu-rated	Mono-unsatu-rated	Poly-unsatu-rated
	Dairy Products—Con.		Grams	Per-cent	Cal-ories	Grams	Grams	Grams	Grams	Grams
	Cream products, imitation (made with vegetable fat):									
	Sweet:									
	Creamers:									
68	Liquid (frozen)------------	1 tbsp----------	15	77	20	Tr	1	1.4	Tr	Tr
69	Powdered------------------	1 tsp----------	2	2	10	Tr	1	0.7	Tr	Tr
	Whipped topping:									
70	Frozen--------------------	1 cup----------	75	50	240	1	19	16.3	1.2	0.4
71		1 tbsp----------	4	50	15	Tr	1	0.9	0.1	Tr
	Powdered, made with whole milk--------------------									
72		1 cup----------	80	67	150	3	10	8.5	0.7	0.2
73		1 tbsp----------	4	67	10	Tr	Tr	0.4	Tr	Tr
74	Pressurized--------------	1 cup----------	70	60	185	1	16	13.2	1.3	0.2
75		1 tbsp----------	4	60	10	Tr	1	0.8	0.1	Tr
76	Sour dressing (filled cream type product, nonbutterfat)--	1 cup----------	235	75	415	8	39	31.2	4.6	1.1
77		1 tbsp----------	12	75	20	Tr	2	1.6	0.2	0.1
	Ice cream. See Milk desserts, frozen (items 106-111).									
	Ice milk. See Milk desserts, frozen (items 112-114).									
	Milk:									
	Fluid:									
78	Whole (3.3% fat)-------------	1 cup----------	244	88	150	8	8	5.1	2.4	0.3
	Lowfat (2%):									
79	No milk solids added-------	1 cup----------	244	89	120	8	5	2.9	1.4	0.2
80	Milk solids added, label claim less than 10 g of protein per cup----------	1 cup----------	245	89	125	9	5	2.9	1.4	0.2
	Lowfat (1%):									
81	No milk solids added-------	1 cup----------	244	90	100	8	3	1.6	0.7	0.1
82	Milk solids added, label claim less than 10 g of protein per cup----------	1 cup----------	245	90	105	9	2	1.5	0.7	0.1
	Nonfat (skim):									
83	No milk solids added-------	1 cup----------	245	91	85	8	Tr	0.3	0.1	Tr
84	Milk solids added, label claim less than 10 g of protein per cup----------	1 cup----------	245	90	90	9	1	0.4	0.2	Tr
85	Buttermilk----------------	1 cup----------	245	90	100	8	2	1.3	0.6	0.1
	Canned:									
86	Condensed, sweetened---------	1 cup----------	306	27	980	24	27	16.8	7.4	1.0
	Evaporated:									
87	Whole milk----------------	1 cup----------	252	74	340	17	19	11.6	5.9	0.6
88	Skim milk-----------------	1 cup----------	255	79	200	19	1	0.3	0.2	Tr
	Dried:									
89	Buttermilk------------------	1 cup----------	120	3	465	41	7	4.3	2.0	0.3
	Nonfat, instantized:									
90	Envelope, 3.2 oz, net wt.[6]	1 envelope------	91	4	325	32	1	0.4	0.2	Tr
91	Cup----------------------	1 cup----------	68	4	245	24	Tr	0.3	0.1	Tr
	Milk beverages:									
	Chocolate milk (commercial):									
92	Regular-------------------	1 cup----------	250	82	210	8	8	5.3	2.5	0.3
93	Lowfat (2%)---------------	1 cup----------	250	84	180	8	5	3.1	1.5	0.2
94	Lowfat (1%)---------------	1 cup----------	250	85	160	8	3	1.5	0.8	0.1

[5]Vitamin A value is largely from beta-carotene used for coloring.
[6]Yields 1 qt of fluid milk when reconstituted according to package directions.

Nutrients in Indicated Quantity

Cholesterol	Carbohydrate	Calcium	Phosphorus	Iron	Potassium	Sodium	Vitamin A value		Thiamin	Riboflavin	Niacin	Ascorbic acid	Item No.
							(IU)	(RE)					
Milligrams	Grams	Milligrams	Milligrams	Milligrams	Milligrams	Milligrams	International units	Retinol equivalents	Milligrams	Milligrams	Milligrams	Milligrams	
0	2	1	10	Tr	29	12	[5]10	[5]1	0.00	0.00	0.0	0	68
0	1	Tr	8	Tr	16	4	Tr	Tr	0.00	Tr	0.0	0	69
0	17	5	6	0.1	14	19	[5]650	[5]65	0.00	0.00	0.0	0	70
0	1	Tr	Tr	Tr	1	1	[5]30	[5]3	0.00	0.00	0.0	0	71
8	13	72	69	Tr	121	53	[5]290	[5]39	0.02	0.09	Tr	1	72
Tr	1	4	3	Tr	6	3	[5]10	[5]2	Tr	Tr	Tr	Tr	73
0	11	4	13	Tr	13	43	[5]330	[5]33	0.00	0.00	0.0	0	74
0	1	Tr	1	Tr	1	2	[5]20	[5]2	0.00	0.00	0.0	0	75
13	11	266	205	0.1	380	113	20	5	0.09	0.38	0.2	2	76
1	1	14	10	Tr	19	6	Tr	Tr	Tr	0.02	Tr	Tr	77
33	11	291	228	0.1	370	120	310	76	0.09	0.40	0.2	2	78
18	12	297	232	0.1	377	122	500	139	0.10	0.40	0.2	2	79
18	12	313	245	0.1	397	128	500	140	0.10	0.42	0.2	2	80
10	12	300	235	0.1	381	123	500	144	0.10	0.41	0.2	2	81
10	12	313	245	0.1	397	128	500	145	0.10	0.42	0.2	2	82
4	12	302	247	0.1	406	126	500	149	0.09	0.34	0.2	2	83
5	12	316	255	0.1	418	130	500	149	0.10	0.43	0.2	2	84
9	12	285	219	0.1	371	257	80	20	0.08	0.38	0.1	2	85
104	166	868	775	0.6	1,136	389	1,000	248	0.28	1.27	0.6	8	86
74	25	657	510	0.5	764	267	610	136	0.12	0.80	0.5	5	87
9	29	738	497	0.7	845	293	1,000	298	0.11	0.79	0.4	3	88
83	59	1,421	1,119	0.4	1,910	621	260	65	0.47	1.89	1.1	7	89
17	47	1,120	896	0.3	1,552	499	[7]2,160	[7]646	0.38	1.59	0.8	5	90
12	35	837	670	0.2	1,160	373	[7]1,610	[7]483	0.28	1.19	0.6	4	91
31	26	280	251	0.6	417	149	300	73	0.09	0.41	0.3	2	92
17	26	284	254	0.6	422	151	500	143	0.09	0.41	0.3	2	93
7	26	287	256	0.6	425	152	500	148	0.10	0.42	0.3	2	94

[7]With added vitamin A.

Item No.	Foods, approximate measures, units, and weight (weight of edible portion only)		Grams	Water Per-cent	Food energy Cal-ories	Pro-tein Grams	Fat Grams	Fatty acids Satu-rated Grams	Mono-unsatu-rated Grams	Poly-unsatu-rated Grams
	Dairy Products—Con.									
	Milk beverages:									
	Cocoa and chocolate-flavored beverages:									
95	Powder containing nonfat dry milk	1 oz	28	1	100	3	1	0.6	0.3	Tr
96	Prepared (6 oz water plus 1 oz powder)	1 serving	206	86	100	3	1	0.6	0.3	Tr
97	Powder without nonfat dry milk	3/4 oz	21	1	75	1	1	0.3	0.2	Tr
98	Prepared (8 oz whole milk plus 3/4 oz powder)	1 serving	265	81	225	9	9	5.4	2.5	0.3
99	Eggnog (commercial)	1 cup	254	74	340	10	19	11.3	5.7	0.9
	Malted milk: Chocolate:									
100	Powder	3/4 oz	21	2	85	1	1	0.5	0.3	0.1
101	Prepared (8 oz whole milk plus 3/4 oz powder)	1 serving	265	81	235	9	9	5.5	2.7	0.4
	Natural:									
102	Powder	3/4 oz	21	3	85	3	2	0.9	0.5	0.3
103	Prepared (8 oz whole milk plus 3/4 oz powder)	1 serving	265	81	235	11	10	6.0	2.9	0.6
	Shakes, thick:									
104	Chocolate	10-oz container	283	72	335	9	8	4.8	2.2	0.3
105	Vanilla	10-oz container	283	74	315	11	9	5.3	2.5	0.3
	Milk desserts, frozen: Ice cream, vanilla: Regular (about 11% fat):									
106	Hardened	1/2 gal	1,064	61	2,155	38	115	71.3	33.1	4.3
107		1 cup	133	61	270	5	14	8.9	4.1	0.5
108		3 fl oz	50	61	100	2	5	3.4	1.6	0.2
109	Soft serve (frozen custard)	1 cup	173	60	375	7	23	13.5	6.7	1.0
110	Rich (about 16% fat), hardened	1/2 gal	1,188	59	2,805	33	190	118.3	54.9	7.1
111		1 cup	148	59	350	4	24	14.7	6.8	0.9
	Ice milk, vanilla:									
112	Hardened (about 4% fat)	1/2 gal	1,048	69	1,470	41	45	28.1	13.0	1.7
113		1 cup	131	69	185	5	6	3.5	1.6	0.2
114	Soft serve (about 3% fat)	1 cup	175	70	225	8	5	2.9	1.3	0.2
115	Sherbet (about 2% fat)	1/2 gal	1,542	66	2,160	17	31	19.0	8.8	1.1
116		1 cup	193	66	270	2	4	2.4	1.1	0.1
	Yogurt: With added milk solids: Made with lowfat milk:									
117	Fruit-flavored[8]	8-oz container	227	74	230	10	2	1.6	0.7	0.1
118	Plain	8-oz container	227	85	145	12	4	2.3	1.0	0.1
119	Made with nonfat milk	8-oz container	227	85	125	13	Tr	0.3	0.1	Tr
	Without added milk solids:									
120	Made with whole milk	8-oz container	227	88	140	8	7	4.8	2.0	0.2
	Eggs									
	Eggs, large (24 oz per dozen): Raw:									
121	Whole, without shell	1 egg	50	75	80	6	6	1.7	2.2	0.7
122	White	1 white	33	88	15	3	Tr	0.0	0.0	0.0
123	Yolk	1 yolk	17	49	65	3	6	1.7	2.2	0.7
	Cooked:									
124	Fried in butter	1 egg	46	68	95	6	7	2.7	2.7	0.8
125	Hard-cooked, shell removed	1 egg	50	75	80	6	6	1.7	2.2	0.7
126	Poached	1 egg	50	74	80	6	6	1.7	2.2	0.7
127	Scrambled (milk added) in butter. Also omelet	1 egg	64	73	110	7	8	3.2	2.9	0.8

[8]Carbohydrate content varies widely because of amount of sugar added and amount and solids content of added flavoring. Consult the label if more precise values for carbohydrate and calories are needed.

							Vitamin A value						
Nutrients in Indicated Quantity													
Cho-les-terol	Carbo-hydrate	Calcium	Phos-phorus	Iron	Potas-sium	Sodium	(IU)	(RE)	Thiamin	Ribo-flavin	Niacin	Ascorbic acid	Item No.
Milli-grams	Grams	Milli-grams	Milli-grams	Milli-grams	Milli-grams	Milli-grams	Inter-national units	Retinol equiva-lents	Milli-grams	Milli-grams	Milli-grams	Milli-grams	
1	22	90	88	0.3	223	139	Tr	Tr	0.03	0.17	0.2	Tr	95
1	22	90	88	0.3	223	139	Tr	Tr	0.03	0.17	0.2	Tr	96
0	19	7	26	0.7	136	56	Tr	Tr	Tr	0.03	0.1	Tr	97
33	30	298	254	0.9	508	176	310	76	0.10	0.43	0.3	3	98
149	34	330	278	0.5	420	138	890	203	0.09	0.48	0.3	4	99
1	18	13	37	0.4	130	49	20	5	0.04	0.04	0.4	0	100
34	29	304	265	0.5	500	168	330	80	0.14	0.43	0.7	2	101
4	15	56	79	0.2	159	96	70	17	0.11	0.14	1.1	0	102
37	27	347	307	0.3	529	215	380	93	0.20	0.54	1.3	2	103
30	60	374	357	0.9	634	314	240	59	0.13	0.63	0.4	0	104
33	50	413	326	0.3	517	270	320	79	0.08	0.55	0.4	0	105
476	254	1,406	1,075	1.0	2,052	929	4,340	1,064	0.42	2.63	1.1	6	106
59	32	176	134	0.1	257	116	540	133	0.05	0.33	0.1	1	107
22	12	66	51	Tr	96	44	200	50	0.02	0.12	0.1	Tr	108
153	38	236	199	0.4	338	153	790	199	0.08	0.45	0.2	1	109
703	256	1,213	927	0.8	1,771	868	7,200	1,758	0.36	2.27	0.9	5	110
88	32	151	115	0.1	221	108	900	219	0.04	0.28	0.1	1	111
146	232	1,409	1,035	1.5	2,117	836	1,710	419	0.61	2.78	0.9	6	112
18	29	176	129	0.2	265	105	210	52	0.08	0.35	0.1	1	113
13	38	274	202	0.3	412	163	175	44	0.12	0.54	0.2	1	114
113	469	827	594	2.5	1,585	706	1,480	308	0.26	0.71	1.0	31	115
14	59	103	74	0.3	198	88	190	39	0.03	0.09	0.1	4	116
10	43	345	271	0.2	442	133	100	25	0.08	0.40	0.2	1	117
14	16	415	326	0.2	531	159	150	36	0.10	0.49	0.3	2	118
4	17	452	355	0.2	579	174	20	5	0.11	0.53	0.3	2	119
29	11	274	215	0.1	351	105	280	68	0.07	0.32	0.2	1	120
274	1	28	90	1.0	65	69	260	78	0.04	0.15	Tr	0	121
0	Tr	4	4	Tr	45	50	0	0	Tr	0.09	Tr	0	122
272	Tr	26	86	0.9	15	8	310	94	0.04	0.07	Tr	0	123
278	1	29	91	1.1	66	162	320	94	0.04	0.14	Tr	0	124
274	1	28	90	1.0	65	69	260	78	0.04	0.14	Tr	0	125
273	1	28	90	1.0	65	146	260	78	0.03	0.13	Tr	0	126
282	2	54	109	1.0	97	176	350	102	0.04	0.18	Tr	Tr	127

Item No.	Foods, approximate measures, units, and weight (weight of edible portion only)			Water	Food energy	Pro-tein	Fat	Fatty acids		
								Satu-rated	Mono-unsatu-rated	Poly-unsatu-rated
	Fats and Oils		Grams	Per-cent	Cal-ories	Grams	Grams	Grams	Grams	Grams
	Butter (4 sticks per lb):									
128	Stick--------------------------	1/2 cup---------	113	16	810	1	92	57.1	26.4	3.4
129	Tablespoon (1/8 stick)---------	1 tbsp----------	14	16	100	Tr	11	7.1	3.3	0.4
130	Pat (1 in square, 1/3 in high; 90 per lb)-------------	1 pat----------	5	16	35	Tr	4	2.5	1.2	0.2
131	Fats, cooking (vegetable shortenings)-------------------	1 cup-----------	205	0	1,810	0	205	51.3	91.2	53.5
132		1 tbsp----------	13	0	115	0	13	3.3	5.8	3.4
133	Lard--------------------------	1 cup-----------	205	0	1,850	0	205	80.4	92.5	23.0
134		1 tbsp----------	13	0	115	0	13	5.1	5.9	1.5
	Margarine:									
135	Imitation (about 40% fat), soft	8-oz container--	227	58	785	1	88	17.5	35.6	31.3
136		1 tbsp----------	14	58	50	Tr	5	1.1	2.2	1.9
	Regular (about 80% fat): Hard (4 sticks per lb):									
137	Stick----------------------	1/2 cup---------	113	16	810	1	91	17.9	40.5	28.7
138	Tablespoon (1/8 stick)-----	1 tbsp----------	14	16	100	Tr	11	2.2	5.0	3.6
139	Pat (1 in square, 1/3 in high; 90 per lb)---------	1 pat----------	5	16	35	Tr	4	0.8	1.8	1.3
140	Soft----------------------	8-oz container--	227	16	1,625	2	183	31.3	64.7	78.5
141		1 tbsp----------	14	16	100	Tr	11	1.9	4.0	4.8
	Spread (about 60% fat): Hard (4 sticks per lb):									
142	Stick----------------------	1/2 cup---------	113	37	610	1	69	15.9	29.4	20.5
143	Tablespoon (1/8 stick)-----	1 tbsp----------	14	37	75	Tr	9	2.0	3.6	2.5
144	Pat (1 in square, 1/3 in high; 90 per lb)---------	1 pat----------	5	37	25	Tr	3	0.7	1.3	0.9
145	Soft----------------------	8-oz container--	227	37	1,225	1	138	29.1	71.5	31.3
146		1 tbsp----------	14	37	75	Tr	9	1.8	4.4	1.9
	Oils, salad or cooking:									
147	Corn-------------------------	1 cup-----------	218	0	1,925	0	218	27.7	52.8	128.0
148		1 tbsp----------	14	0	125	0	14	1.8	3.4	8.2
149	Olive-------------------------	1 cup-----------	216	0	1,910	0	216	29.2	159.2	18.1
150		1 tbsp----------	14	0	125	0	14	1.9	10.3	1.2
151	Peanut-----------------------	1 cup-----------	216	0	1,910	0	216	36.5	99.8	69.1
152		1 tbsp----------	14	0	125	0	14	2.4	6.5	4.5
153	Safflower--------------------	1 cup-----------	218	0	1,925	0	218	19.8	26.4	162.4
154		1 tbsp----------	14	0	125	0	14	1.3	1.7	10.4
155	Soybean oil, hydrogenated (partially hardened)---------	1 cup-----------	218	0	1,925	0	218	32.5	93.7	82.0
156		1 tbsp----------	14	0	125	0	14	2.1	6.0	5.3
157	Soybean-cottonseed oil blend, hydrogenated----------------	1 cup-----------	218	0	1,925	0	218	39.2	64.3	104.9
158		1 tbsp----------	14	0	125	0	14	2.5	4.1	6.7
159	Sunflower--------------------	1 cup-----------	218	0	1,925	0	218	22.5	42.5	143.2
160		1 tbsp----------	14	0	125	0	14	1.4	2.7	9.2
	Salad dressings: Commercial:									
161	Blue cheese------------------	1 tbsp----------	15	32	75	1	8	1.5	1.8	4.2
	French:									
162	Regular---------------------	1 tbsp----------	16	35	85	Tr	9	1.4	4.0	3.5
163	Low calorie----------------	1 tbsp----------	16	75	25	Tr	2	0.2	0.3	1.0
	Italian:									
164	Regular---------------------	1 tbsp----------	15	34	80	Tr	9	1.3	3.7	3.2
165	Low calorie----------------	1 tbsp----------	15	86	5	Tr	Tr	Tr	Tr	Tr
	Mayonnaise:									
166	Regular---------------------	1 tbsp----------	14	15	100	Tr	11	1.7	3.2	5.8
167	Imitation------------------	1 tbsp----------	15	63	35	Tr	3	0.5	0.7	1.6
168	Mayonnaise type-------------	1 tbsp----------	15	40	60	Tr	5	0.7	1.4	2.7
169	Tartar sauce----------------	1 tbsp----------	14	34	75	Tr	8	1.2	2.6	3.9
	Thousand island:									
170	Regular---------------------	1 tbsp----------	16	46	60	Tr	6	1.0	1.3	3.2
171	Low calorie----------------	1 tbsp----------	15	69	25	Tr	2	0.2	0.4	0.9

[9]For salted butter; unsalted butter contains 12 mg sodium per stick, 2 mg per tbsp, or 1 mg per pat.
[10]Values for vitamin A are year-round average.

Nutrients in Indicated Quantity

Cho-les-terol	Carbo-hydrate	Calcium	Phos-phorus	Iron	Potas-sium	Sodium	Vitamin A value (IU)	Vitamin A value (RE)	Thiamin	Ribo-flavin	Niacin	Ascorbic acid	Item No.
Milli-grams	Grams	Milli-grams	Milli-grams	Milli-grams	Milli-grams	Milli-grams	Inter-national units	Retinol equiva-lents	Milli-grams	Milli-grams	Milli-grams	Milli-grams	
247	Tr	27	26	0.2	29	[9]933	[10]3,460	[10]852	0.01	0.04	Tr	0	128
31	Tr	3	3	Tr	4	[9]116	[10]430	[10]106	Tr	Tr	Tr	0	129
11	Tr	1	1	Tr	1	[9]41	[10]150	[10]38	Tr	Tr	Tr	0	130
0	0	0	0	0.0	0	0	0	0	0.00	0.00	0.0	0	131
0	0	0	0	0.0	0	0	0	0	0.00	0.00	0.0	0	132
195	0	0	0	0.0	0	0	0	0	0.00	0.00	0.0	0	133
12	0	0	0	0.0	0	0	0	0	0.00	0.00	0.0	0	134
0	1	40	31	0.0	57	[11]2,178	[12]7,510	[12]2,254	0.01	0.05	Tr	Tr	135
0	Tr	2	2	0.0	4	[11]134	[12]460	[12]139	Tr	Tr	Tr	Tr	136
0	1	34	26	0.1	48	[11]1,066	[12]3,740	[12]1,122	0.01	0.04	Tr	Tr	137
0	Tr	4	3	Tr	6	[11]132	[12]460	[12]139	Tr	0.01	Tr	Tr	138
0	Tr	1	1	Tr	2	[11]47	[12]170	[12]50	Tr	Tr	Tr	Tr	139
0	1	60	46	0.0	86	[11]2,449	[12]7,510	[12]2,254	0.02	0.07	Tr	Tr	140
0	Tr	4	3	0.0	5	[11]151	[12]460	[12]139	Tr	Tr	Tr	Tr	141
0	0	24	18	0.0	34	[11]1,123	[12]3,740	[12]1,122	0.01	0.03	Tr	Tr	142
0	0	3	2	0.0	4	[11]139	[12]460	[12]139	Tr	Tr	Tr	Tr	143
0	0	1	1	0.0	1	[11]50	[12]170	[12]50	Tr	Tr	Tr	Tr	144
0	0	47	37	0.0	68	[11]2,256	[12]7,510	[12]2,254	0.02	0.06	Tr	Tr	145
0	0	3	2	0.0	4	[11]139	[12]460	[12]139	Tr	Tr	Tr	Tr	146
0	0	0	0	0.0	0	0	0	0	0.00	0.00	0.0	0	147
0	0	0	0	0.0	0	0	0	0	0.00	0.00	0.0	0	148
0	0	0	0	0.0	0	0	0	0	0.00	0.00	0.0	0	149
0	0	0	0	0.0	0	0	0	0	0.00	0.00	0.0	0	150
0	0	0	0	0.0	0	0	0	0	0.00	0.00	0.0	0	151
0	0	0	0	0.0	0	0	0	0	0.00	0.00	0.0	0	152
0	0	0	0	0.0	0	0	0	0	0.00	0.00	0.0	0	153
0	0	0	0	0.0	0	0	0	0	0.00	0.00	0.0	0	154
0	0	0	0	0.0	0	0	0	0	0.00	0.00	0.0	0	155
0	0	0	0	0.0	0	0	0	0	0.00	0.00	0.0	0	156
0	0	0	0	0.0	0	0	0	0	0.00	0.00	0.0	0	157
0	0	0	0	0.0	0	0	0	0	0.00	0.00	0.0	0	158
0	0	0	0	0.0	0	0	0	0	0.00	0.00	0.0	0	159
0	0	0	0	0.0	0	0	0	0	0.00	0.00	0.0	0	160
3	1	12	11	Tr	6	164	30	10	Tr	0.02	Tr	Tr	161
0	1	2	1	Tr	2	188	Tr	Tr	Tr	Tr	Tr	Tr	162
0	2	6	5	Tr	3	306	Tr	Tr	Tr	Tr	Tr	Tr	163
0	1	1	1	Tr	5	162	30	3	Tr	Tr	Tr	Tr	164
0	2	1	1	Tr	4	136	Tr	Tr	Tr	Tr	Tr	Tr	165
8	Tr	3	4	0.1	5	80	40	12	0.00	0.00	Tr	0	166
4	2	Tr	Tr	0.0	2	75	0	0	0.00	0.00	0.0	0	167
4	4	2	4	Tr	1	107	30	13	Tr	Tr	Tr	0	168
4	1	3	4	0.1	11	182	30	9	Tr	Tr	0.0	Tr	169
4	2	2	3	0.1	18	112	50	15	Tr	Tr	Tr	0	170
2	2	2	3	0.1	17	150	50	14	Tr	Tr	Tr	0	171

For salted margarine.
Based on average vitamin A content of fortified margarine. Federal specifications for fortified margarine require minimum of 15,000 IU per pound.

Item No.	Foods, approximate measures, units, and weight (weight of edible portion only)		Grams	Water Percent	Food energy Calories	Protein Grams	Fat Grams	Saturated Grams	Monounsaturated Grams	Polyunsaturated Grams
	Fats and Oils—Con.									
	Salad dressings:									
	Prepared from home recipe:									
172	Cooked type[13]	1 tbsp	16	69	25	1	2	0.5	0.6	0.3
173	Vinegar and oil	1 tbsp	16	47	70	0	8	1.5	2.4	3.9
	Fish and Shellfish									
	Clams:									
174	Raw, meat only	3 oz	85	82	65	11	1	0.3	0.3	0.3
175	Canned, drained solids	3 oz	85	77	85	13	2	0.5	0.5	0.4
176	Crabmeat, canned	1 cup	135	77	135	23	3	0.5	0.8	1.4
177	Fish sticks, frozen, reheated, (stick, 4 by 1 by 1/2 in)	1 fish stick	28	52	70	6	3	0.8	1.4	0.8
	Flounder or Sole, baked, with lemon juice:									
178	With butter	3 oz	85	73	120	16	6	3.2	1.5	0.5
179	With margarine	3 oz	85	73	120	16	6	1.2	2.3	1.9
180	Without added fat	3 oz	85	78	80	17	1	0.3	0.2	0.4
181	Haddock, breaded, fried[14]	3 oz	85	61	175	17	9	2.4	3.9	2.4
182	Halibut, broiled, with butter and lemon juice	3 oz	85	67	140	20	6	3.3	1.6	0.7
183	Herring, pickled	3 oz	85	59	190	17	13	4.3	4.6	3.1
184	Ocean perch, breaded, fried[14]	1 fillet	85	59	185	16	11	2.6	4.6	2.8
	Oysters:									
185	Raw, meat only (13-19 medium Selects)	1 cup	240	85	160	20	4	1.4	0.5	1.4
186	Breaded, fried[14]	1 oyster	45	65	90	5	5	1.4	2.1	1.4
	Salmon:									
187	Canned (pink), solids and liquid	3 oz	85	71	120	17	5	0.9	1.5	2.1
188	Baked (red)	3 oz	85	67	140	21	5	1.2	2.4	1.4
189	Smoked	3 oz	85	59	150	18	8	2.6	·3.9	0.7
190	Sardines, Atlantic, canned in oil, drained solids	3 oz	85	62	175	20	9	2.1	3.7	2.9
191	Scallops, breaded, frozen, reheated	6 scallops	90	59	195	15	10	2.5	4.1	2.5
	Shrimp:									
192	Canned, drained solids	3 oz	85	70	100	21	1	0.2	0.2	0.4
193	French fried (7 medium)[16]	3 oz	85	55	200	16	10	2.5	4.1	2.6
194	Trout, broiled, with butter and lemon juice	3 oz	85	63	175	21	9	4.1	2.9	1.6
	Tuna, canned, drained solids:									
195	Oil pack, chunk light	3 oz	85	61	165	24	7	1.4	1.9	3.1
196	Water pack, solid white	3 oz	85	63	135	30	1	0.3	0.2	0.3
197	Tuna salad[17]	1 cup	205	63	375	33	19	3.3	4.9	9.2
	Fruits and Fruit Juices									
	Apples:									
	Raw:									
	Unpeeled, without cores:									
198	2-3/4-in diam. (about 3 per lb with cores)	1 apple	138	84	80	Tr	Tr	0.1	Tr	0.1
199	3-1/4-in diam. (about 2 per lb with cores)	1 apple	212	84	125	Tr	1	0.1	Tr	0.2
200	Peeled, sliced	1 cup	110	84	65	Tr	Tr	0.1	Tr	0.1
201	Dried, sulfured	10 rings	64	32	155	1	Tr	Tr	Tr	0.1
202	Apple juice, bottled or canned[19]	1 cup	248	88	115	Tr	Tr	Tr	Tr	0.1
	Applesauce, canned:									
203	Sweetened	1 cup	255	80	195	Tr	Tr	0.1	Tr	0.1
204	Unsweetened	1 cup	244	88	105	Tr	Tr	Tr	Tr	Tr

[13] Fatty acid values apply to product made with regular margarine.
[14] Dipped in egg, milk, and breadcrumbs; fried in vegetable shortening.
[15] If bones are discarded, value for calcium will be greatly reduced.
[16] Dipped in egg, breadcrumbs, and flour; fried in vegetable shortening.

Cho-les-terol	Carbo-hydrate	Calcium	Phos-phorus	Iron	Potas-sium	Sodium	Vitamin A value		Thiamin	Ribo-flavin	Niacin	Ascorbic acid	Item No.
							(IU)	(RE)					
Milli-grams	Grams	Milli-grams	Milli-grams	Milli-grams	Milli-grams	Milli-grams	Inter-national units	Retinol equiva-lents	Milli-grams	Milli-grams	Milli-grams	Milli-grams	
9	2	13	14	0.1	19	117	70	20	0.01	0.02	Tr	Tr	172
0	Tr	0	0	0.0	1	Tr	0	0	0.00	0.00	0.0	0	173
43	2	59	138	2.6	154	102	90	26	0.09	0.15	1.1	9	174
54	2	47	116	3.5	119	102	90	26	0.01	0.09	0.9	3	175
135	1	61	246	1.1	149	1,350	50	14	0.11	0.11	2.6	0	176
26	4	11	58	0.3	94	53	20	5	0.03	0.05	0.6	0	177
68	Tr	13	187	0.3	272	145	210	54	0.05	0.08	1.6	1	178
55	Tr	14	187	0.3	273	151	230	69	0.05	0.08	1.6	1	179
59	Tr	13	197	0.3	286	101	30	10	0.05	0.08	1.7	1	180
75	7	34	183	1.0	270	123	70	20	0.06	0.10	2.9	0	181
62	Tr	14	206	0.7	441	103	610	174	0.06	0.07	7.7	1	182
85	0	29	128	0.9	85	850	110	33	0.04	0.18	2.8	0	183
66	7	31	191	1.2	241	138	70	20	0.10	0.11	2.0	0	184
120	8	226	343	15.6	290	175	740	223	0.34	0.43	6.0	24	185
35	5	49	73	3.0	64	70	150	44	0.07	0.10	1.3	4	186
34	0	[15]167	243	0.7	307	443	60	18	0.03	0.15	6.8	0	187
60	0	26	269	0.5	305	55	290	87	0.18	0.14	5.5	0	188
51	0	12	208	0.8	327	1,700	260	77	0.17	0.17	6.8	0	189
85	0	[15]371	424	2.6	349	425	190	56	0.03	0.17	4.6	0	190
70	10	39	203	2.0	369	298	70	21	0.11	0.11	1.6	0	191
128	1	98	224	1.4	104	1,955	50	15	0.01	0.03	1.5	0	192
168	11	61	154	2.0	189	384	90	26	0.06	0.09	2.8	0	193
71	Tr	26	259	1.0	297	122	230	60	0.07	0.07	2.3	1	194
55	0	7	199	1.6	298	303	70	20	0.04	0.09	10.1	0	195
48	0	17	202	0.6	255	468	110	32	0.03	0.10	13.4	0	196
80	19	31	281	2.5	531	877	230	53	0.06	0.14	13.3	6	197
0	21	10	10	0.2	159	Tr	70	7	0.02	0.02	0.1	8	198
0	32	15	15	0.4	244	Tr	110	11	0.04	0.03	0.2	12	199
0	16	4	8	0.1	124	Tr	50	5	0.02	0.01	0.1	4	200
0	42	9	24	0.9	288	[18]56	0	0	0.00	0.10	0.6	[20]2	201
0	29	17	17	0.9	295	7	Tr	Tr	0.05	0.04	0.2	[20]2	202
0	51	10	18	0.9	156	8	30	3	0.03	0.07	0.5	[20]4	203
0	28	7	17	0.3	183	5	70	7	0.03	0.06	0.5	[20]3	204

[17] Made with drained chunk light tuna, celery, onion, pickle relish, and mayonnaise-type salad dressing.
[18] Sodium bisulfite used to preserve color; unsulfited product would contain less sodium.
[19] Also applies to pasteurized apple cider.
[20] Without added ascorbic acid. For value with added ascorbic acid, refer to label.

Item No.	Foods, approximate measures, units, and weight (weight of edible portion only)		Water	Food energy	Pro-tein	Fat	Fatty acids		
							Satu-rated	Mono-unsatu-rated	Poly-unsatu-rated
		Grams	Per-cent	Cal-ories	Grams	Grams	Grams	Grams	Grams

Fruits and Fruit Juices—Con.

	Apricots:								
205	Raw, without pits (about 12 per lb with pits)----------------	3 apricots------	106	86	50	1	Tr	Tr	0.2	0.1
	Canned (fruit and liquid):								
206	Heavy syrup pack------------	1 cup----------	258	78	215	1	Tr	Tr	0.1	Tr
207		3 halves--------	85	78	70	Tr	Tr	Tr	Tr	Tr
208	Juice pack-----------------	1 cup----------	248	87	120	2	Tr	Tr	Tr	Tr
209		3 halves--------	84	87	40	1	Tr	Tr	Tr	Tr
	Dried:								
210	Uncooked (28 large or 37 medium halves per cup)-----	1 cup----------	130	31	310	5	1	Tr	0.3	0.1
211	Cooked, unsweetened, fruit and liquid-----------------	1 cup----------	250	76	210	3	Tr	Tr	0.2	0.1
212	Apricot nectar, canned----------	1 cup----------	251	85	140	1	Tr	Tr	0.1	Tr
	Avocados, raw, whole, without skin and seed:								
213	California (about 2 per lb with skin and seed)---------------	1 avocado-------	173	73	305	4	30	4.5	19.4	3.5
214	Florida (about 1 per lb with skin and seed)---------------	1 avocado-------	304	80	340	5	27	5.3	14.8	4.5
	Bananas, raw, without peel:								
215	Whole (about 2-1/2 per lb with peel)---------------	1 banana--------	114	74	105	1	1	0.2	Tr	0.1
216	Sliced---------------------	1 cup----------	150	74	140	2	1	0.3	0.1	0.1
217	Blackberries, raw---------------	1 cup----------	144	86	75	1	1	0.2	0.1	0.1
	Blueberries:								
218	Raw-----------------------	1 cup----------	145	85	80	1	1	Tr	0.1	0.3
219	Frozen, sweetened-------------	10-oz container	284	77	230	1	Tr	Tr	0.1	0.2
220		1 cup----------	230	77	185	1	Tr	Tr	Tr	0.1
	Cantaloup. See Melons (item 251).								
	Cherries:								
221	Sour, red, pitted, canned, water pack------------------	1 cup----------	244	90	90	2	Tr	0.1	0.1	0.1
222	Sweet, raw, without pits and stems---------------------	10 cherries-----	68	81	50	1	1	0.1	0.2	0.2
223	Cranberry juice cocktail, bottled, sweetened----------	1 cup----------	253	85	145	Tr	Tr	Tr	Tr	0.1
224	Cranberry sauce, sweetened, canned, strained--------------	1 cup----------	277	61	420	1	Tr	Tr	0.1	0.2
	Dates:								
225	Whole, without pits-----------	10 dates-------	83	23	230	2	Tr	0.1	0.1	Tr
226	Chopped---------------------	1 cup----------	178	23	490	4	1	0.3	0.2	Tr
227	Figs, dried--------------------	10 figs--------	187	28	475	6	2	0.4	0.5	1.0
	Fruit cocktail, canned, fruit and liquid:								
228	Heavy syrup pack--------------	1 cup----------	255	80	185	1	Tr	Tr	Tr	0.1
229	Juice pack-------------------	1 cup----------	248	87	115	1	Tr	Tr	Tr	Tr
	Grapefruit:								
230	Raw, without peel, membrane and seeds (3-3/4-in diam., 1 lb 1 oz, whole, with refuse)----	1/2 grapefruit--	120	91	40	1	Tr	Tr	Tr	Tr
231	Canned, sections with syrup----	1 cup----------	254	84	150	1	Tr	Tr	Tr	0.1
	Grapefruit juice:								
232	Raw--------------------------	1 cup----------	247	90	95	1	Tr	Tr	Tr	0.1
	Canned:								
233	Unsweetened-----------------	1 cup----------	247	90	95	1	Tr	Tr	Tr	0.1
234	Sweetened-------------------	1 cup----------	250	87	115	1	Tr	Tr	Tr	0.1
	Frozen concentrate, unsweetened								
235	Undiluted-------------------	6-fl-oz can-----	207	62	300	4	1	0.1	0.1	0.2
236	Diluted with 3 parts water by volume-------------------	1 cup----------	247	89	100	1	Tr	Tr	Tr	0.1

[20] Without added ascorbic acid. For value with added ascorbic acid, refer to label.
[21] With added ascorbic acid.

Nutrients in Indicated Quantity

Cholesterol	Carbohydrate	Calcium	Phosphorus	Iron	Potassium	Sodium	Vitamin A value		Thiamin	Riboflavin	Niacin	Ascorbic acid	Item No.
							(IU)	(RE)					
Milligrams	Grams	Milligrams	Milligrams	Milligrams	Milligrams	Milligrams	International units	Retinol equivalents	Milligrams	Milligrams	Milligrams	Milligrams	
0	12	15	20	0.6	314	1	2,770	277	0.03	0.04	0.6	11	205
0	55	23	31	0.8	361	10	3,170	317	0.05	0.06	1.0	8	206
0	18	8	10	0.3	119	3	1,050	105	0.02	0.02	0.3	3	207
0	31	30	50	0.7	409	10	4,190	419	0.04	0.05	0.9	12	208
0	10	10	17	0.3	139	3	1,420	142	0.02	0.02	0.3	4	209
0	80	59	152	6.1	1,791	13	9,410	941	0.01	0.20	3.9	3	210
0	55	40	103	4.2	1,222	8	5,910	591	0.02	0.08	2.4	4	211
0	36	18	23	1.0	286	8	3,300	330	0.02	0.04	0.7	[20]2	212
0	12	19	73	2.0	1,097	21	1,060	106	0.19	0.21	3.3	14	213
0	27	33	119	1.6	1,484	15	1,860	186	0.33	0.37	5.8	24	214
0	27	7	23	0.4	451	1	90	9	0.05	0.11	0.6	10	215
0	35	9	30	0.5	594	2	120	12	0.07	0.15	0.8	14	216
0	18	46	30	0.8	282	Tr	240	24	0.04	0.06	0.6	30	217
0	20	9	15	0.2	129	9	150	15	0.07	0.07	0.5	19	218
0	62	17	20	1.1	170	3	120	12	0.06	0.15	0.7	3	219
0	50	14	16	0.9	138	2	100	10	0.05	0.12	0.6	2	220
0	22	27	24	3.3	239	17	1,840	184	0.04	0.10	0.4	5	221
0	11	10	13	0.3	152	Tr	150	15	0.03	0.04	0.3	5	222
0	38	8	3	0.4	61	10	10	1	0.01	0.04	0.1	[21]108	223
0	108	11	17	0.6	72	80	60	6	0.04	0.06	0.3	6	224
0	61	27	33	1.0	541	2	40	4	0.07	0.08	1.8	0	225
0	131	57	71	2.0	1,161	5	90	9	0.16	0.18	3.9	0	226
0	122	269	127	4.2	1,331	21	250	25	0.13	0.16	1.3	1	227
0	48	15	28	0.7	224	15	520	52	0.05	0.05	1.0	5	228
0	29	20	35	0.5	236	10	760	76	0.03	0.04	1.0	7	229
0	10	14	10	0.1	167	Tr	[22]10	[22]1	0.04	0.02	0.3	41	230
0	39	36	25	1.0	328	5	Tr	Tr	0.10	0.05	0.6	54	231
0	23	22	37	0.5	400	2	20	2	0.10	0.05	0.5	94	232
0	22	17	27	0.5	378	2	20	2	0.10	0.05	0.6	72	233
0	28	20	28	0.9	405	5	20	2	0.10	0.06	0.8	67	234
0	72	56	101	1.0	1,002	6	60	6	0.30	0.16	1.6	248	235
0	24	20	35	0.3	336	2	20	2	0.10	0.05	0.5	83	236

[22]For white grapefruit; pink grapefruit have about 310 IU or 31 RE.

Item No.	Foods, approximate measures, units, and weight (weight of edible portion only)			Water	Food energy	Pro-tein	Fat	Fatty acids		
								Satu-rated	Mono-unsatu-rated	Poly-unsatu-rated
			Grams	Per-cent	Cal-ories	Grams	Grams	Grams	Grams	Grams
	Fruits and Fruit Juices—Con.									
	Grapes, European type (adherent skin), raw:									
237	Thompson Seedless---------------	10 grapes-------	50	81	35	Tr	Tr	0.1	Tr	0.1
238	Tokay and Emperor, seeded types	10 grapes-------	57	81	40	Tr	Tr	0.1	Tr	0.1
	Grape juice:									
239	Canned or bottled--------------	1 cup-----------	253	84	155	1	Tr	0.1	Tr	0.1
	Frozen concentrate, sweetened:									
240	Undiluted--------------------	6-fl-oz can-----	216	54	385	1	1	0.2	Tr	0.2
241	Diluted with 3 parts water by volume-----------------	1 cup-----------	250	87	125	Tr	Tr	0.1	Tr	0.1
242	Kiwifruit, raw, without skin (about 5 per lb with skin)-----	1 kiwifruit-----	76	83	45	1	Tr	Tr	0.1	0.1
243	Lemons, raw, without peel and seeds (about 4 per lb with peel and seeds)---------------------	1 lemon---------	58	89	15	1	Tr	Tr	Tr	0.1
	Lemon juice:									
244	Raw-------------------------	1 cup-----------	244	91	60	1	Tr	Tr	Tr	Tr
245	Canned or bottled, unsweetened	1 cup-----------	244	92	50	1	1	0.1	Tr	0.2
246		1 tbsp----------	15	92	5	Tr	Tr	Tr	Tr	Tr
247	Frozen, single-strength, unsweetened------------------	6-fl-oz can-----	244	92	55	1	1	0.1	Tr	0.2
	Lime juice:									
248	Raw-------------------------	1 cup-----------	246	90	65	1	Tr	Tr	Tr	0.1
249	Canned, unsweetened-----------	1 cup-----------	246	93	50	1	1	0.1	0.1	0.2
250	Mangos, raw, without skin and seed (about 1-1/2 per lb with skin and seed)------------------	1 mango---------	207	82	135	1	1	0.1	0.2	0.1
	Melons, raw, without rind and cavity contents:									
251	Cantaloup, orange-fleshed (5-in diam., 2-1/3 lb, whole, with rind and cavity contents)----	1/2 melon-------	267	90	95	2	1	0.1	0:1	0.3
252	Honeydew (6-1/2-in diam., 5-1/4 lb, whole, with rind and cav-ity contents)--------------	1/10 melon------	129	90	45	1	Tr	Tr	Tr	0.1
253	Nectarines, raw, without pits (about 3 per lb with pits)-----	1 nectarine-----	136	86	65	1	1	0.1	0.2	0.3
	Oranges, raw:									
254	Whole, without peel and seeds (2-5/8-in diam., about 2-1/2 per lb, with peel and seeds)	1 orange--------	131	87	60	1	Tr	Tr	Tr	Tr
255	Sections without membranes-----	1 cup-----------	180	87	85	2	Tr	Tr	Tr	Tr
	Orange juice:									
256	Raw, all varieties------------	1 cup-----------	248	88	110	2	Tr	0.1	0.1	0.1
257	Canned, unsweetened-----------	1 cup-----------	249	89	105	1	Tr	Tr	0.1	0.1
258	Chilled------------------------	1 cup-----------	249	88	110	2	1	0.1	0.1	0.2
	Frozen concentrate:									
259	Undiluted--------------------	6-fl-oz can-----	213	58	340	5	Tr	0.1	0.1	0.1
260	Diluted with 3 parts water by volume-----------------	1 cup-----------	249	88	110	2	Tr	Tr	Tr	Tr
261	Orange and grapefruit juice, canned-----------------------	1 cup-----------	247	89	105	1	Tr	Tr	Tr	Tr
262	Papayas, raw, 1/2-in cubes-------	1 cup-----------	140	86	65	1	Tr	0.1	0.1	Tr
	Peaches: Raw:									
263	Whole, 2-1/2-in diam., peeled, pitted (about 4 per lb with peels and pits)----	1 peach---------	87	88	35	1	Tr	Tr	Tr	Tr
264	Sliced-----------------------	1 cup-----------	170	88	75	1	Tr	Tr	0.1	0.1
	Canned, fruit and liquid:									
265	Heavy syrup pack-------------	1 cup-----------	256	79	190	1	Tr	Tr	0.1	0.1
266		1 half----------	81	79	60	Tr	Tr	Tr	Tr	Tr
267	Juice pack-------------------	1 cup-----------	248	87	110	2	Tr	Tr	Tr	Tr
268		1 half----------	77	87	35	Tr	Tr	Tr	Tr	Tr

[20]Without added ascorbic acid. For value with added ascorbic acid, refer to label.
[21]With added ascorbic acid.

							Vitamin A value						

Nutrients in Indicated Quantity

Cho-les-terol	Carbo-hydrate	Calcium	Phos-phorus	Iron	Potas-sium	Sodium	Vitamin A value		Thiamin	Ribo-flavin	Niacin	Ascorbic acid	Item No.
							(IU)	(RE)					
Milli-grams	Grams	Milli-grams	Milli-grams	Milli-grams	Milli-grams	Milli-grams	Inter-national units	Retinol equiva-lents	Milli-grams	Milli-grams	Milli-grams	Milli-grams	
0	9	6	7	0.1	93	1	40	4	0.05	0.03	0.2	5	237
0	10	6	7	0.1	105	1	40	4	0.05	0.03	0.2	6	238
0	38	23	28	0.6	334	8	20	2	0.07	0.09	0.7	[20]Tr	239
0	96	28	32	0.8	160	15	60	6	0.11	0.20	0.9	[21]179	240
0	32	10	10	0.3	53	5	20	2	0.04	0.07	0.3	[21]60	241
0	11	20	30	0.3	252	4	130	13	0.02	0.04	0.4	74	242
0	5	15	9	0.3	80	1	20	2	0.02	0.01	0.1	31	243
0	21	17	15	0.1	303	2	50	5	0.07	0.02	0.2	112	244
0	16	27	22	0.3	249	[23]51	40	4	0.10	0.02	0.5	61	245
0	1	2	1	Tr	15	[23]3	Tr	Tr	0.01	Tr	Tr	4	246
0	16	20	20	0.3	217	2	30	3	0.14	0.03	0.3	77	247
0	22	22	17	0.1	268	2	20	2	0.05	0.02	0.2	72	248
0	16	30	25	0.6	185	[23]39	40	4	0.08	0.01	0.4	16	249
0	35	21	23	0.3	323	4	8,060	806	0.12	0.12	1.2	57	250
0	22	29	45	0.6	825	24	8,610	861	0.10	0.06	1.5	113	251
0	12	8	13	0.1	350	13	50	5	0.10	0.02	0.8	32	252
0	16	7	22	0.2	288	Tr	1,000	100	0.02	0.06	1.3	7	253
0	15	52	18	0.1	237	Tr	270	27	0.11	0.05	0.4	70	254
0	21	72	25	0.2	326	Tr	370	37	0.16	0.07	0.5	96	255
0	26	27	42	0.5	496	2	500	50	0.22	0.07	1.0	124	256
0	25	20	35	1.1	436	5	440	44	0.15	0.07	0.8	86	257
0	25	25	27	0.4	473	2	190	19	0.28	0.05	0.7	82	258
0	81	68	121	0.7	1,436	6	590	59	0.60	0.14	1.5	294	259
0	27	22	40	0.2	473	2	190	19	0.20	0.04	0.5	97	260
0	25	20	35	1.1	390	7	290	29	0.14	0.07	0.8	72	261
0	17	35	12	0.3	247	9	400	40	0.04	0.04	0.5	92	262
0	10	4	10	0.1	171	Tr	470	47	0.01	0.04	0.9	6	263
0	19	9	20	0.2	335	Tr	910	91	0.03	0.07	1.7	11	264
0	51	8	28	0.7	236	15	850	85	0.03	0.06	1.6	7	265
0	16	2	9	0.2	75	5	270	27	0.01	0.02	0.5	2	266
0	29	15	42	0.7	317	10	940	94	0.02	0.04	1.4	9	267
0	9	5	13	0.2	99	3	290	29	0.01	0.01	0.4	3	268

[23]Sodium benzoate and sodium bisulfite added as preservatives.

Item No.	Foods, approximate measures, units, and weight (weight of edible portion only)			Water	Food energy	Protein	Fat	Fatty acids		
								Saturated	Monounsaturated	Polyunsaturated
			Grams	Percent	Calories	Grams	Grams	Grams	Grams	Grams

Fruits and Fruit Juices—Con.

	Peaches:									
	Dried:									
269	Uncooked----------------------	1 cup------------	160	32	380	6	1	0.1	0.4	0.6
270	Cooked, unsweetened, fruit and liquid-----------------	1 cup-----------	258	78	200	3	1	0.1	0.2	0.3
271	Frozen, sliced, sweetened------	10-oz container	284	75	265	2	Tr	Tr	0.1	0.2
272		1 cup-----------	250	75	235	2	Tr	Tr	0.1	0.2
	Pears:									
	Raw, with skin, cored:									
273	Bartlett, 2-1/2-in diam. (about 2-1/2 per lb with cores and stems)-----------	1 pear----------	166	84	100	1	1	Tr	0.1	0.2
274	Bosc, 2-1/2-in diam. (about 3 per lb with cores and stems)---------------------	1 pear----------	141	84	85	1	1	Tr	0.1	0.1
275	D'Anjou, 3-in diam. (about 2 per lb with cores and stems)---------------------	1 pear----------	200	84	120	1	1	Tr	0.2	0.2
	Canned, fruit and liquid:									
276	Heavy syrup pack-------------	1 cup-----------	255	80	190	1	Tr	Tr	0.1	0.1
277		1 half----------	79	80	60	Tr	Tr	Tr	Tr	Tr
278	Juice pack-------------------	1 cup-----------	248	86	125	1	Tr	Tr	Tr	Tr
279		1 half----------	77	86	40	Tr	Tr	Tr	Tr	Tr
	Pineapple:									
280	Raw, diced---------------------	1 cup-----------	155	87	75	1	1	Tr	0.1	0.2
	Canned, fruit and liquid:									
	Heavy syrup pack:									
281	Crushed, chunks, tidbits---	1 cup-----------	255	79	200	1	Tr	Tr	Tr	0.1
282	Slices--------------------	1 slice---------	58	79	45	Tr	Tr	Tr	Tr	Tr
	Juice pack:									
283	Chunks or tidbits----------	1 cup-----------	250	84	150	1	Tr	Tr	·Tr	0.1
284	Slices---------------------	1 slice---------	58	84	35	Tr	Tr	Tr	Tr	Tr
285	Pineapple juice, unsweetened, canned-------------------------	1 cup-----------	250	86	140	1	Tr	Tr	Tr	0.1
	Plantains, without peel:									
286	Raw---------------------------	1 plantain------	179	65	220	2	1	0.3	0.1	0.1
287	Cooked, boiled, sliced---------	1 cup-----------	154	67	180	1	Tr	0.1	Tr	0.1
	Plums, without pits:									
	Raw:									
288	2-1/8-in diam. (about 6-1/2 per lb with pits)----------	1 plum----------	66	85	35	1	Tr	Tr	0.3	0.1
289	1-1/2-in diam. (about 15 per lb with pits)-------------	1 plum----------	28	85	15	Tr	Tr	Tr	0.1	Tr
	Canned, purple, fruit and liquid:									
290	Heavy syrup pack-------------	1 cup-----------	258	76	230	1	Tr	Tr	0.2	0.1
291		3 plums---------	133	76	120	Tr	Tr	Tr	0.1	Tr
292	Juice pack-------------------	1 cup-----------	252	84	145	1	Tr	Tr	Tr	Tr
293		3 plums---------	95	84	55	Tr	Tr	Tr	Tr	Tr
	Prunes, dried:									
294	Uncooked----------------------	4 extra large or 5 large prunes	49	32	115	1	Tr	Tr	0.2	0.1
295	Cooked, unsweetened, fruit and liquid-----------------	1 cup-----------	212	70	225	2	Tr	Tr	0.3	0.1
296	Prune juice, canned or bottled---	1 cup-----------	256	81	180	2	Tr	Tr	0.1	Tr
	Raisins, seedless:									
297	Cup, not pressed down----------	1 cup-----------	145	15	435	5	1	0.2	Tr	0.2
298	Packet, 1/2 oz (1-1/2 tbsp)----	1 packet--------	14	15	40	Tr	Tr	Tr	Tr	Tr
	Raspberries:									
299	Raw---------------------------	1 cup-----------	123	87	60	1	1	Tr	0.1	0.4
300	Frozen, sweetened-------------	10-oz container	284	73	295	2	Tr	Tr	Tr	0.3
301		1 cup-----------	250	73	255	2	Tr	Tr	Tr	0.2

[21] With added ascorbic acid.

Nutrients in Indicated Quantity

Cho-les-terol	Carbo-hydrate	Calcium	Phos-phorus	Iron	Potas-sium	Sodium	Vitamin A value		Thiamin	Ribo-flavin	Niacin	Ascorbic acid	Item No.
							(IU)	(RE)					
Milli-grams	Grams	Milli-grams	Milli-grams	Milli-grams	Milli-grams	Milli-grams	Inter-national units	Retinol equiva-lents	Milli-grams	Milli-grams	Milli-grams	Milli-grams	
0	98	45	190	6.5	1,594	11	3,460	346	Tr	0.34	7.0	8	269
0	51	23	98	3.4	826	5	510	51	0.01	0.05	3.9	[21]10	270
0	68	9	31	1.1	369	17	810	81	0.04	0.10	1.9	[21]268	271
0	60	8	28	0.9	325	15	710	71	0.03	0.09	1.6	[21]236	272
0	25	18	18	0.4	208	Tr	30	3	0.03	0.07	0.2	7	273
0	21	16	16	0.4	176	Tr	30	3	0.03	0.06	0.1	6	274
0	30	22	22	0.5	250	Tr	40	4	0.04	0.08	0.2	8	275
0	49	13	18	0.6	166	13	10	1	0.03	0.06	0.6	3	276
0	15	4	6	0.2	51	4	Tr	Tr	0.01	0.02	0.2	1	277
0	32	22	30	0.7	238	10	10	1	0.03	0.03	0.5	4	278
0	10	7	9	0.2	74	3	Tr	Tr	0.01	0.01	0.2	1	279
0	19	11	11	0.6	175	2	40	4	0.14	0.06	0.7	24	280
0	52	36	18	1.0	265	3	40	4	0.23	0.06	0.7	19	281
0	12	8	4	0.2	60	1	10	1	0.05	0.01	0.2	4	282
0	39	35	15	0.7	305	3	100	10	0.24	0.05	0.7	24	283
0	9	8	3	0.2	71	1	20	2	0.06	0.01	0.2	6	284
0	34	43	20	0.7	335	3	10	1	0.14	0.06	0.6	27	285
0	57	5	61	1.1	893	7	2,020	202	0.09	0.10	1.2	33	286
0	48	3	43	0.9	716	8	1,400	140	0.07	0.08	1.2	17	287
0	9	3	7	0.1	114	Tr	210	21	0.03	0.06	0.3	6	288
0	4	1	3	Tr	48	Tr	90	9	0.01	0.03	0.1	3	289
0	60	23	34	2.2	235	49	670	67	0.04	0.10	0.8	1	290
0	31	12	17	1.1	121	25	340	34	0.02	0.05	0.4	1	291
0	38	25	38	0.9	388	3	2,540	254	0.06	0.15	1.2	7	292
0	14	10	14	0.3	146	1	960	96	0.02	0.06	0.4	3	293
0	31	25	39	1.2	365	2	970	97	0.04	0.08	1.0	2	294
0	60	49	74	2.4	708	4	650	65	0.05	0.21	1.5	6	295
0	45	31	64	3.0	707	10	10	1	0.04	0.18	2.0	10	296
0	115	71	141	3.0	1,089	17	10	1	0.23	0.13	1.2	5	297
0	11	7	14	0.3	105	2	Tr	Tr	0.02	0.01	0.1	Tr	298
0	14	27	15	0.7	187	Tr	160	16	0.04	0.11	1.1	31	299
0	74	43	48	1.8	324	3	170	17	0.05	0.13	0.7	47	300
0	65	38	43	1.6	285	3	150	15	0.05	0.11	0.6	41	301

Item No.	Foods, approximate measures, units, and weight (weight of edible portion only)			Water	Food energy	Pro-tein	Fat	Fatty acids		
								Satu-rated	Mono-unsatu-rated	Poly-unsatu-rated
			Grams	Per-cent	Cal-ories	Grams	Grams	Grams	Grams	Grams
	Fruits and Fruit Juices—Con.									
302	Rhubarb, cooked, added sugar-----	1 cup-----------	240	68	280	1	Tr	Tr	Tr	0.1
	Strawberries:									
303	Raw, capped, whole-------------	1 cup-----------	149	92	45	1	1	Tr	0.1	0.3
304	Frozen, sweetened, sliced------	10-oz container	284	73	275	2	Tr	Tr	0.1	0.2
305		1 cup-----------	255	73	245	1	Tr	Tr	Tr	0.2
	Tangerines:									
306	Raw, without peel and seeds (2-3/8-in diam., about 4 per lb, with peel and seeds)-----	1 tangerine-----	84	88	35	1	Tr	Tr	Tr	Tr
307	Canned, light syrup, fruit and liquid----------------------	1 cup-----------	252	83	155	1	Tr	Tr	Tr	0.1
308	Tangerine juice, canned, sweet-ened------------------------	1 cup-----------	249	87	125	1	Tr	Tr	Tr	0.1
	Watermelon, raw, without rind and seeds:									
309	Piece (4 by 8 in wedge with rind and seeds; 1/16 of 32-2/3-lb melon, 10 by 16 in)	1 piece---------	482	92	155	3	2	0.3	0.2	1.0
310	Diced-------------------------	1 cup-----------	160	92	50	1	1	0.1	0.1	0.3
	Grain Products									
311	Bagels, plain or water, enriched, 3-1/2-in diam.[24] ----------------	1 bagel---------	68	29	200	7	2	0.3	0.5	0.7
312	Barley, pearled, light, uncooked	1 cup-----------	200	11	700	16	2	0.3	0.2	0.9
	Biscuits, baking powder, 2-in diam. (enriched flour, vege-table shortening):									
313	From home recipe---------------	1 biscuit-------	28	28	100	2	5	1.2	2.0	1.3
314	From mix-----------------------	1 biscuit-------	28	29	95	2	3	0.8	1.4	0.9
315	From refrigerated dough--------	1 biscuit-------	20	30	65	1	2	0.6	0.9	0.6
	Breadcrumbs, enriched:									
316	Dry, grated-------------------	1 cup-----------	100	7	390	13	5	1.5	1.6	1.0
	Soft. See White bread (item 351).									
	Breads:									
317	Boston brown bread, canned, slice, 3-1/4 in by 1/2 in[25]--	1 slice---------	45	45	95	2	1	0.3	0.1	0.1
	Cracked-wheat bread (3/4 en-riched wheat flour, 1/4 cracked wheat flour):[25]									
318	Loaf, 1 lb-------------------	1 loaf----------	454	35	1,190	42	16	3.1	4.3	5.7
319	Slice (18 per loaf)----------	1 slice---------	25	35	65	2	1	0.2	0.2	0.3
320	Toasted-------------------	1 slice---------	21	26	65	2	1	0.2	0.2	0.3
	French or vienna bread, en-riched:[25]									
321	Loaf, 1 lb-------------------	1 loaf----------	454	34	1,270	43	18	3.8	5.7	5.9
	Slice:									
322	French, 5 by 2-1/2 by 1 in	1 slice---------	35	34	100	3	1	0.3	0.4	0.5
323	Vienna, 4-3/4 by 4 by 1/2 in----------------------	1 slice---------	25	34	70	2	1	0.2	0.3	0.3
	Italian bread, enriched:									
324	Loaf, 1 lb-------------------	1 loaf----------	454	32	1,255	41	4	0.6	0.3	1.6
325	Slice, 4-1/2 by 3-1/4 by 3/4 in----------------------	1 slice---------	30	32	85	3	Tr	Tr	Tr	0.1
	Mixed grain bread, enriched:[25]									
326	Loaf, 1 lb-------------------	1 loaf----------	454	37	1,165	45	17	3.2	4.1	6.5
327	Slice (18 per loaf)----------	1 slice---------	25	37	65	2	1	0.2	0.2	0.4
328	Toasted-------------------	1 slice---------	23	27	65	2	1	0.2	0.2	0.4

[24] Egg bagels have 44 mg cholesterol and 22 IU or 7 RE vitamin A per bagel.
[25] Made with vegetable shortening.

Nutrients in Indicated Quantity

Cho-les-terol	Carbo-hydrate	Calcium	Phos-phorus	Iron	Potas-sium	Sodium	Vitamin A value (IU)	Vitamin A value (RE)	Thiamin	Ribo-flavin	Niacin	Ascorbic acid	Item No.
Milli-grams	Grams	Milli-grams	Milli-grams	Milli-grams	Milli-grams	Milli-grams	Inter-national units	Retinol equiva-lents	Milli-grams	Milli-grams	Milli-grams	Milli-grams	
0	75	348	19	0.5	230	2	170	17	0.04	0.06	0.5	8	302
0	10	21	28	0.6	247	1	40	4	0.03	0.10	0.3	84	303
0	74	31	37	1.7	278	9	70	7	0.05	0.14	1.1	118	304
0	66	28	33	1.5	250	8	60	6	0.04	0.13	1.0	106	305
0	9	12	8	0.1	132	1	770	77	0.09	0.02	0.1	26	306
0	41	18	25	0.9	197	15	2,120	212	0.13	0.11	1.1	50	307
0	30	45	35	0.5	443	2	1,050	105	0.15	0.05	0.2	55	308
0	35	39	43	0.8	559	10	1,760	176	0.39	0.10	1.0	46	309
0	11	13	14	0.3	186	3	590	59	0.13	0.03	0.3	15	310
0	38	29	46	1.8	50	245	0	0	0.26	0.20	2.4	0	311
0	158	32	378	4.2	320	6	0	0	0.24	0.10	6.2	0	312
Tr	13	47	36	0.7	32	195	10	3	0.08	0.08	0.8	Tr	313
Tr	14	58	128	0.7	56	262	20	4	0.12	0.11	0.8	Tr	314
1	10	4	79	0.5	18	249	0	0	0.08	0.05	0.7	0	315
5	73	122	141	4.1	152	736	0	0	0.35	0.35	4.8	0	316
3	21	41	72	0.9	131	113	[26]0	[26]0	0.06	0.04	0.7	0	317
0	227	295	581	12.1	608	1,966	Tr	Tr	1.73	1.73	15.3	Tr	318
0	12	16	32	0.7	34	106	Tr	Tr	0.10	0.09	0.8	Tr	319
0	12	16	32	0.7	34	106	Tr	Tr	0.07	0.09	0.8	Tr	320
0	230	499	386	14.0	409	2,633	Tr	Tr	2.09	1.59	18.2	Tr	321
0	18	39	30	1.1	32	203	Tr	Tr	0.16	0.12	1.4	Tr	322
0	13	28	21	0.8	23	145	Tr	Tr	0.12	0.09	1.0	Tr	323
0	256	77	350	12.7	336	2,656	0	0	1.80	1.10	15.0	0	324
0	17	5	23	0.8	22	176	0	0	0.12	0.07	1.0	0	325
0	212	472	962	14.8	990	1,870	Tr	Tr	1.77	1.73	18.9	Tr	326
0	12	27	55	0.8	56	106	Tr	Tr	0.10	0.10	1.1	Tr	327
0	12	27	55	0.8	56	106	Tr	Tr	0.08	0.10	1.1	Tr	328

Made with white cornmeal. If made with yellow cornmeal, value is 32 IU or 3 RE.

Item No.	Foods, approximate measures, units, and weight (weight of edible portion only)			Water	Food energy	Protein	Fat	Fatty acids		
								Saturated	Mono-unsaturated	Poly-unsaturated
	Grain Products—Con.		Grams	Percent	Calories	Grams	Grams	Grams	Grams	Grams
	Breads:									
	Oatmeal bread, enriched:[25]									
329	Loaf, 1 lb-------------------	1 loaf----------	454	37	1,145	38	20	3.7	7.1	8.2
330	Slice (18 per loaf)----------	1 slice---------	25	37	65	2	1	0.2	0.4	0.5
331	Toasted--------------------	1 slice---------	23	30	65	2	1	0.2	0.4	0.5
332	Pita bread, enriched, white, 6-1/2-in diam.--------------	1 pita----------	60	31	165	6	1	0.1	0.1	0.4
	Pumpernickel (2/3 rye flour, 1/3 enriched wheat flour):[25]									
333	Loaf, 1 lb-------------------	1 loaf----------	454	37	1,160	42	16	2.6	3.6	6.4
334	Slice, 5 by 4 by 3/8 in------	1 slice---------	32	37	80	3	1	0.2	0.3	0.5
335	Toasted--------------------	1 slice---------	29	28	80	3	1	0.2	0.3	0.5
	Raisin bread, enriched:[25]									
336	Loaf, 1 lb-------------------	1 loaf----------	454	33	1,260	37	18	4.1	6.5	6.7
337	Slice (18 per loaf)----------	1 slice---------	25	33	65	2	1	0.2	0.3	0.4
338	Toasted--------------------	1 slice---------	21	24	65	2	1	0.2	0.3	0.4
	Rye bread, light (2/3 enriched wheat flour, 1/3 rye flour):[25]									
339	Loaf, 1 lb-------------------	1 loaf----------	454	37	1,190	38	17	3.3	5.2	5.5
340	Slice, 4-3/4 by 3-3/4 by 7/16 in------------------	1 slice---------	25	37	65	2	1	0.2	0.3	0.3
341	Toasted--------------------	1 slice---------	22	28	65	2	1	0.2	0.3	0.3
	Wheat bread, enriched:[25]									
342	Loaf, 1 lb-------------------	1 loaf----------	454	37	1,160	43	19	3.9	7.3	4.5
343	Slice (18 per loaf)----------	1 slice---------	25	37	65	2	1	0.2	0.4	0.3
344	Toasted--------------------	1 slice---------	23	28	65	3	1	0.2	0.4	0.3
	White bread, enriched:[25]									
345	Loaf, 1 lb-------------------	1 loaf----------	454	37	1,210	38	18	5.6	6.5	4.2
346	Slice (18 per loaf)--------	1 slice---------	25	37	65	2	1	0.3	0.4	0.2
347	Toasted------------------	1 slice---------	22	28	65	2	1	0.3	0.4	0.2
348	Slice (22 per loaf)--------	1 slice---------	20	37	55	2	1	0.2	0.3	0.2
349	Toasted------------------	1 slice---------	17	28	55	2	1	0.2	0.3	0.2
350	Cubes---------------------	1 cup----------	30	37	80	2	1	0.4	0.4	0.3
351	Crumbs, soft---------------	1 cup----------	45	37	120	4	2	0.6	0.6	0.4
	Whole-wheat bread:[25]									
352	Loaf, 1 lb-------------------	1 loaf----------	454	38	1,110	44	20	5.8	6.8	5.2
353	Slice (16 per loaf)----------	1 slice---------	28	38	70	3	1	0.4	0.4	0.3
354	Toasted--------------------	1 slice---------	25	29	70	3	1	0.4	0.4	0.3
	Bread stuffing (from enriched bread), prepared from mix:									
355	Dry type-------------------	1 cup----------	140	33	500	9	31	6.1	13.3	9.6
356	Moist type-----------------	1 cup----------	203	61	420	9	26	5.3	11.3	8.0
	Breakfast cereals:									
	Hot type, cooked:									
	Corn (hominy) grits:									
357	Regular and quick, enriched	1 cup----------	242	85	145	3	Tr	Tr	0.1	0.2
358	Instant, plain------------	1 pkt----------	137	85	80	2	Tr	Tr	Tr	0.1
	Cream of Wheat®:									
359	Regular, quick, instant----	1 cup----------	244	86	140	4	Tr	0.1	Tr	0.2
360	Mix'n Eat, plain----------	1 pkt----------	142	82	100	3	Tr	Tr	Tr	0.1
361	Malt-O-Meal® -------------	1 cup----------	240	88	120	4	Tr	Tr	Tr	0.1
	Oatmeal or rolled oats:									
362	Regular, quick, instant, nonfortified------------	1 cup----------	234	85	145	6	2	0.4	0.8	1.0
	Instant, fortified:									
363	Plain-------------------	1 pkt----------	177	86	105	4	2	0.3	0.6	0.7
364	Flavored----------------	1 pkt----------	164	76	160	5	2	0.3	0.7	0.8

[25] Made with vegetable shortening.
[27] Nutrient added.
[28] Cooked without salt. If salt is added according to label recommendations, sodium content is 540 mg.
[29] For white corn grits. Cooked yellow grits contain 145 IU or 14 RE.
[30] Value based on label declaration for added nutrients.

Nutrients in Indicated Quantity

Cho-les-terol	Carbo-hydrate	Calcium	Phos-phorus	Iron	Potas-sium	Sodium	Vitamin A value (IU)	Vitamin A value (RE)	Thiamin	Ribo-flavin	Niacin	Ascorbic acid	Item No.
Milli-grams	Grams	Milli-grams	Milli-grams	Milli-grams	Milli-grams	Milli-grams	Inter-national units	Retinol equiva-lents	Milli-grams	Milli-grams	Milli-grams	Milli-grams	
0	212	267	563	12.0	707	2,231	0	0	2.09	1.20	15.4	0	329
0	12	15	31	0.7	39	124	0	0	0.12	0.07	0.9	0	330
0	12	15	31	0.7	39	124	0	0	0.09	0.07	0.9	0	331
0	33	49	60	1.4	71	339	0	0	0.27	0.12	2.2	0	332
0	218	322	990	12.4	1,966	2,461	0	0	1.54	2.36	15.0	0	333
0	16	23	71	0.9	141	177	0	0	0.11	0.17	1.1	0	334
0	16	23	71	0.9	141	177	0	0	0.09	0.17	1.1	0	335
0	239	463	395	14.1	1,058	1,657	Tr	Tr	1.50	2.81	18.6	Tr	336
0	13	25	22	0.8	59	92	Tr	Tr	0.08	0.15	1.0	Tr	337
0	13	25	22	0.8	59	92	Tr	Tr	0.06	0.15	1.0	Tr	338
0	218	363	658	12.3	926	3,164	0	0	1.86	1.45	15.0	0	339
0	12	20	36	0.7	51	175	0	0	0.10	0.08	0.8	0	340
0	12	20	36	0.7	51	175	0	0	0.08	0.08	0.8	0	341
0	213	572	835	15.8	627	2,447	Tr	Tr	2.09	1.45	20.5	Tr	342
0	12	32	47	0.9	35	138	Tr	Tr	0.12	0.08	1.2	Tr	343
0	12	32	47	0.9	35	138	Tr	Tr	0.10	0.08	1.2	Tr	344
0	222	572	490	12.9	508	2,334	Tr	Tr	2.13	1.41	17.0	Tr	345
0	12	32	27	0.7	28	129	Tr	Tr	0.12	0.08	0.9	Tr	346
0	12	32	27	0.7	28	129	Tr	Tr	0.09	0.08	0.9	Tr	347
0	10	25	21	0.6	22	101	Tr	Tr	0.09	0.06	0.7	Tr	348
0	10	25	21	0.6	22	101	Tr	Tr	0.07	0.06	0.7	Tr	349
0	15	38	32	0.9	34	154	Tr	Tr	0.14	0.09	1.1	Tr	350
0	22	57	49	1.3	50	231	Tr	Tr	0.21	0.14	1.7	Tr	351
0	206	327	1,180	15.5	799	2,887	Tr	Tr	1.59	0.95	17.4	Tr	352
0	13	20	74	1.0	50	180	Tr	Tr	0.10	0.06	1.1	Tr	353
0	13	20	74	1.0	50	180	Tr	Tr	0.08	0.06	1.1	Tr	354
0	50	92	136	2.2	126	1,254	910	273	0.17	0.20	2.5	0	355
67	40	81	134	2.0	118	1,023	850	256	0.10	0.18	1.6	0	356
0	31	0	29	[27]1.5	53	[28]0	[29]0	[29]0	[27]0.24	[27]0.15	[27]2.0	0	357
0	18	7	16	[27]1.0	29	343	0	0	[27]0.18	[27]0.08	[27]1.3	0	358
0	29	[30]54	[31]43	[30]10.9	46	[31,32]5	0	0	[30]0.24	[30]0.07	[30]1.5	0	359
0	21	[30]20	[30]20	[30]8.1	38	241	[30]1,250	[30]376	[30]0.43	[30]0.28	[30]5.0	0	360
0	26	5	[30]24	[30]9.6	31	[33]2	0	0	[30]0.48	[30]0.24	[30]5.8	0	361
0	25	19	178	1.6	131	[34]2	40	4	0.26	0.05	0.3	0	362
0	18	[27]163	133	[27]6.3	99	[27]285	[27]1,510	[27]453	[27]0.53	[27]0.28	[27]5.5	0	363
0	31	[27]168	148	[27]6.7	137	[27]254	[27]1,530	[27]460	[27]0.53	[27]0.38	[27]5.9	Tr	364

For regular and instant cereal. For quick cereal, phosphorus is 102 mg and sodium is 142 mg.
Cooked without salt. If salt is added according to label recommendations, sodium content is 390 mg.
Cooked without salt. If salt is added according to label recommendations, sodium content is 324 mg.
Cooked without salt. If salt is added according to label recommendations, sodium content is 374 mg.

Item No.	Foods, approximate measures, units, and weight (weight of edible portion only)		Grams	Water	Food energy	Protein	Fat	Fatty acids Saturated	Fatty acids Monounsaturated	Fatty acids Polyunsaturated
			Grams	Percent	Calories	Grams	Grams	Grams	Grams	Grams
	Grain Products—Con.									
	Breakfast cereals:									
	Ready to eat:									
365	All-Bran® (about 1/3 cup)----	1 oz------------	28	3	70	4	1	0.1	0.1	0.3
366	Cap'n Crunch® (about 3/4 cup)	1 oz------------	28	3	120	1	3	1.7	0.3	0.4
367	Cheerios® (about 1-1/4 cup)--	1 oz------------	28	5	110	4	2	0.3	0.6	0.7
	Corn Flakes (about 1-1/4 cup):									
368	Kellogg's® ----------------	1 oz------------	28	3	110	2	Tr	Tr	Tr	Tr
369	Toasties® -----------------	1 oz------------	28	3	110	2	Tr	Tr	Tr	Tr
	40% Bran Flakes:									
370	Kellogg's® (about 3/4 cup)	1 oz------------	28	3	90	4	1	0.1	0.1	0.3
371	Post® (about 2/3 cup)------	1 oz------------	28	3	90	3	Tr	0.1	0.1	0.2
372	Froot Loops® (about 1 cup)---	1 oz------------	28	3	110	2	1	0.2	0.1	0.1
373	Golden Grahams® (about 3/4 cup)------------------	1 oz------------	28	2	110	2	1	0.7	0.1	0.2
374	Grape-Nuts® (about 1/4 cup)--	1 oz------------	28	3	100	3	Tr	Tr	Tr	0.1
375	Honey Nut Cheerios® (about 3/4 cup)------------------	1 oz------------	28	3	105	3	1	0.1	0.3	0.3
376	Lucky Charms® (about 1 cup)--	1 oz------------	28	3	110	3	1	0.2	0.4	0.4
377	Nature Valley® Granola (about 1/3 cup)-------------------	1 oz------------	28	4	125	3	5	3.3	0.7	0.7
378	100% Natural Cereal (about 1/4 cup)-------------------	1 oz------------	28	2	135	3	6	4.1	1.2	0.5
379	Product 19® (about 3/4 cup)--	1 oz------------	28	3	110	3	Tr	Tr	Tr	0.1
	Raisin Bran:									
380	Kellogg's® (about 3/4 cup)	1 oz------------	28	8	90	3	1	0.1	0.1	0.3
381	Post® (about 1/2 cup)------	1 oz------------	28	9	85	3	1	0.1	0.1	0.3
382	Rice Krispies® (about 1 cup)	1 oz------------	28	2	110	2	Tr	Tr	Tr	0.1
383	Shredded Wheat (about 2/3 cup)-------------------	1 oz------------	28	5	100	3	1	0.1	0.1	0.3
384	Special K® (about 1-1/3 cup)	1 oz------------	28	2	110	6	Tr	Tr	Tr	Tr
385	Super Sugar Crisp® (about 7/8 cup)-----------------------	1 oz------------	28	2	105	2	Tr	Tr	Tr	0.1
386	Sugar Frosted Flakes, Kellogg's® (about 3/4 cup)	1 oz------------	28	3	110	1	Tr	Tr	Tr	Tr
387	Sugar Smacks® (about 3/4 cup)	1 oz------------	28	3	105	2	1	0.1	0.1	0.2
388	Total® (about 1 cup)---------	1 oz------------	28	4	100	3	1	0.1	0.1	0.3
389	Trix® (about 1 cup)----------	1 oz------------	28	3	110	2	Tr	0.2	0.1	0.1
390	Wheaties® (about 1 cup)------	1 oz------------	28	5	100	3	Tr	0.1	Tr	0.2
391	Buckwheat flour, light, sifted---	1 cup----------	98	12	340	6	1	0.2	0.4	0.4
392	Bulgur, uncooked-----------------	1 cup----------	170	10	600	19	3	1.2	0.3	1.2
	Cakes prepared from cake mixes with enriched flour:[35]									
	Angelfood:									
393	Whole cake, 9-3/4-in diam. tube cake------------------	1 cake----------	635	38	1,510	38	2	0.4	0.2	1.0
394	Piece, 1/12 of cake----------	1 piece--------	53	38	125	3	Tr	Tr	Tr	0.1
	Coffeecake, crumb:									
395	Whole cake, 7-3/4 by 5-5/8 by 1-1/4 in---------------	1 cake----------	430	30	1,385	27	41	11.8	16.7	9.6
396	Piece, 1/6 of cake-----------	1 piece--------	72	30	230	5	7	2.0	2.8	1.6
	Devil's food with chocolate frosting:									
397	Whole, 2-layer cake, 8- or 9-in diam.-----------------	1 cake----------	1,107	24	3,755	49	136	55.6	51.4	19.7
398	Piece, 1/16 of cake----------	1 piece--------	69	24	235	3	8	3.5	3.2	1.2
399	Cupcake, 2-1/2-in diam.------	1 cupcake-------	35	24	120	2	4	1.8	1.6	0.6
	Gingerbread:									
400	Whole cake, 8 in square------	1 cake----------	570	37	1,575	18	39	9.6	16.4	10.5
401	Piece, 1/9 of cake-----------	1 piece--------	63	37	175	2	4	1.1	1.8	1.2

[27] Nutrient added.
[30] Value based on label declaration for added nutrients.

Nutrients in Indicated Quantity

Cho-les-terol	Carbo-hydrate	Calcium	Phos-phorus	Iron	Potas-sium	Sodium	Vitamin A value (IU)	Vitamin A value (RE)	Thiamin	Ribo-flavin	Niacin	Ascorbic acid	Item No.
Milli-grams	Grams	Milli-grams	Milli-grams	Milli-grams	Milli-grams	Milli-grams	Inter-national units	Retinol equiva-lents	Milli-grams	Milli-grams	Milli-grams	Milli-grams	
0	21	23	264	[30]4.5	350	320	[30]1,250	[30]375	[30]0.37	[30]0.43	[30]5.0	[30]15	365
0	23	5	36	[27]7.5	37	213	[30]40	[30]4	[27]0.50	[27]0.55	[27]6.6	[30]0	366
0	20	48	134	[30]4.5	101	307	[30]1,250	[30]375	[30]0.37	[30]0.43	[30]5.0	[30]15	367
0	24	1	18	[30]1.8	26	351	[30]1,250	[30]375	[30]0.37	[30]0.43	[30]5.0	[30]15	368
0	24	1	12	[27]0.7	33	297	[30]1,250	[30]375	[30]0.37	[30]0.43	[30]5.0	0	369
0	22	14	139	[30]8.1	180	264	[30]1,250	[30]375	[30]0.37	[30]0.43	[30]5.0	0	370
0	22	12	179	[30]4.5	151	260	[30]1,250	[30]375	[30]0.37	[30]0.43	[30]5.0	0	371
0	25	3	24	[30]4.5	26	145	[30]1,250	[30]375	[30]0.37	[30]0.43	[30]5.0	[30]15	372
Tr	24	17	41	[30]4.5	63	346	[30]1,250	[30]375	[30]0.37	[30]0.43	[30]5.0	[30]15	373
0	23	11	71	1.2	95	197	[30]1,250	[30]375	[30]0.37	[30]0.43	[30]5.0	0	374
0	23	20	105	[30]4.5	99	257	[30]1,250	[30]375	[30]0.37	[30]0.43	[30]5.0	[30]15	375
0	23	32	79	[30]4.5	59	201	[30]1,250	[30]375	[30]0.37	[30]0.43	[30]5.0	[30]15	376
0	19	18	89	0.9	98	58	20	2	0.10	0.05	0.2	0	377
Tr	18	49	104	0.8	140	12	20	2	0.09	0.15	0.6	0	378
0	24	3	40	[30]18.0	44	325	[30]5,000	[30]1,501	[30]1.50	[30]1.70	[30]20.0	[30]60	379
0	21	10	105	[30]3.5	147	207	[30]960	[30]288	[30]0.28	[30]0.34	[30]3.9	0	380
0	21	13	119	[30]4.5	175	185	[30]1,250	[30]375	[30]0.37	[30]0.43	[30]5.0	0	381
0	25	4	34	[30]1.8	29	340	[30]1,250	[30]375	[30]0.37	[30]0.43	[30]5.0	[30]15	382
0	23	11	100	1.2	102	3	0	0	0.07	0.08	1.5	0	383
Tr	21	8	55	[30]4.5	49	265	[30]1,250	[30]375	[30]0.37	[30]0.43	[30]5.0	[30]15	384
0	26	6	52	[30]1.8	105	25	[30]1,250	[30]375	[30]0.37	[30]0.43	[30]5.0	0	385
0	26	1	21	[30]1.8	18	230	[30]1,250	[30]375	[30]0.37	[30]0.43	[30]5.0	[30]15	386
0	25	3	31	[30]1.8	42	75	[30]1,250	[30]375	[30]0.37	[30]0.43	[30]5.0	[30]15	387
0	22	48	118	[30]18.0	106	352	[30]5,000	[30]1,501	[30]1.50	[30]1.70	[30]20.0	[30]60	388
0	25	6	19	[30]4.5	27	181	[30]1,250	[30]375	[30]0.37	[30]0.43	[30]5.0	[30]15	389
0	23	43	98	[30]4.5	106	354	[30]1,250	[30]375	[30]0.37	[30]0.43	[30]5.0	[30]15	390
0	78	11	86	1.0	314	2	0	0	0.08	0.04	0.4	0	391
0	129	49	575	9.5	389	7	0	0	0.48	0.24	7.7	0	392
0	342	527	1,086	2.7	845	3,226	0	0	0.32	1.27	1.6	0	393
0	29	44	91	0.2	71	269	0	0	0.03	0.11	0.1	0	394
279	225	262	748	7.3	469	1,853	690	194	0.82	0.90	7.7	1	395
47	38	44	125	1.2	78	310	120	32	0.14	0.15	1.3	Tr	396
598	645	653	1,162	22.1	1,439	2,900	1,660	498	1.11	1.66	10.0	1	397
37	40	41	72	1.4	90	181	100	31	0.07	0.10	0.6	Tr	398
19	20	21	37	0.7	46	92	50	16	0.04	0.05	0.3	Tr	399
6	291	513	570	10.8	1,562	1,733	0	0	0.86	1.03	7.4	1	400
1	32	57	63	1.2	173	192	0	0	0.09	0.11	0.8	Tr	401

[5] Excepting angelfood cake, cakes were made from mixes containing vegetable shortening and frostings were made with margarine.

Item No.	Foods, approximate measures, units, and weight (weight of edible portion only)		Grams	Water Percent	Food energy Calories	Protein Grams	Fat Grams	Saturated Grams	Mono-unsaturated Grams	Poly-unsaturated Grams
	Grain Products—Con.									
	Cakes prepared from cake mixes with enriched flour:[35]									
	Yellow with chocolate frosting:									
402	Whole, 2-layer cake, 8- or 9-in diam.	1 cake	1,108	26	3,735	45	125	47.8	48.8	21.8
403	Piece, 1/16 of cake	1 piece	69	26	235	3	8	3.0	3.0	1.4
	Cakes prepared from home recipes using enriched flour:									
	Carrot, with cream cheese frosting:[36]									
404	Whole cake, 10-in diam. tube cake	1 cake	1,536	23	6,175	63	328	66.0	135.2	107.5
405	Piece, 1/16 of cake	1 piece	96	23	385	4	21	4.1	8.4	6.7
	Fruitcake, dark:[36]									
406	Whole cake, 7-1/2-in diam., 2-1/4-in high tube cake	1 cake	1,361	18	5,185	74	228	47.6	113.0	51.7
407	Piece, 1/32 of cake, 2/3-in arc	1 piece	43	18	165	2	7	1.5	3.6	1.6
	Plain sheet cake:[37]									
	Without frosting:									
408	Whole cake, 9-in square	1 cake	777	25	2,830	35	108	29.5	45.1	25.6
409	Piece, 1/9 of cake	1 piece	86	25	315	4	12	3.3	5.0	2.8
	With uncooked white frosting:									
410	Whole cake, 9-in square	1 cake	1,096	21	4,020	37	129	41.6	50.4	26.3
411	Piece, 1/9 of cake	1 piece	121	21	445	4	14	4.6	5.6	2.9
	Pound:[38]									
412	Loaf, 8-1/2 by 3-1/2 by 3-1/4 in	1 loaf	514	22	2,025	33	94	21.1	40.9	26.7
413	Slice, 1/17 of loaf	1 slice	30	22	120	2	5	1.2	2.4	1.6
	Cakes, commercial, made with enriched flour:									
	Pound:									
414	Loaf, 8-1/2 by 3-1/2 by 3 in	1 loaf	500	24	1,935	26	94	52.0	30.0	4.0
415	Slice, 1/17 of loaf	1 slice	29	24	110	2	5	3.0	1.7	0.2
	Snack cakes:									
416	Devil's food with creme filling (2 small cakes per pkg)	1 small cake	28	20	105	1	4	1.7	1.5	0.6
417	Sponge with creme filling (2 small cakes per pkg)	1 small cake	42	19	155	1	5	2.3	2.1	0.5
	White with white frosting:									
418	Whole, 2-layer cake, 8- or 9-in diam.	1 cake	1,140	24	4,170	43	148	33.1	61.6	42.2
419	Piece, 1/16 of cake	1 piece	71	24	260	3	9	2.1	3.8	2.6
	Yellow with chocolate frosting:									
420	Whole, 2-layer cake, 8- or 9-in diam.	1 cake	1,108	23	3,895	40	175	92.0	58.7	10.0
421	Piece, 1/16 of cake	1 piece	69	23	245	2	11	5.7	3.7	0.6
	Cheesecake:									
422	Whole cake, 9-in diam.	1 cake	1,110	46	3,350	60	213	119.9	65.5	14.4
423	Piece, 1/12 of cake	1 piece	92	46	280	5	18	9.9	5.4	1.2
	Cookies made with enriched flour:									
	Brownies with nuts:									
424	Commercial, with frosting, 1-1/2 by 1-3/4 by 7/8 in	1 brownie	25	13	100	1	4	1.6	2.0	0.6
425	From home recipe, 1-3/4 by 1-3/4 by 7/8 in[36]	1 brownie	20	10	95	1	6	1.4	2.8	1.2
	Chocolate chip:									
426	Commercial, 2-1/4-in diam., 3/8 in thick	4 cookies	42	4	180	2	9	2.9	3.1	2.6

[35] Excepting angelfood cake, cakes were made from mixes containing vegetable shortening and frostings were made with margarine.
[36] Made with vegetable oil.

Nutrients in Indicated Quantity

Cho-les-terol	Carbo-hydrate	Calcium	Phos-phorus	Iron	Potas-sium	Sodium	Vitamin A value (IU)	Vitamin A value (RE)	Thiamin	Ribo-flavin	Niacin	Ascorbic acid	Item No.
Milli-grams	Grams	Milli-grams	Milli-grams	Milli-grams	Milli-grams	Milli-grams	Inter-national units	Retinol equiva-lents	Milli-grams	Milli-grams	Milli-grams	Milli-grams	
576	638	1,008	2,017	15.5	1,208	2,515	1,550	465	1.22	1.66	11.1	1	402
36	40	63	126	1.0	75	157	100	29	0.08	0.10	0.7	Tr	403
183	775	707	998	21.0	1,720	4,470	2,240	246	1.83	1.97	14.7	23	404
74	48	44	62	1.3	108	279	140	15	0.11	0.12	0.9	1	405
640	783	1,293	1,592	37.6	6,138	2,123	1,720	422	2.41	2.55	17.0	504	406
20	25	41	50	1.2	194	67	50	13	0.08	0.08	0.5	16	407
552	434	497	793	11.7	614	2,331	1,320	373	1.24	1.40	10.1	2	408
61	48	55	88	1.3	68	258	150	41	0.14	0.15	1.1	Tr	409
636	694	548	822	11.0	669	2,488	2,190	647	1.21	1.42	9.9	2	410
70	77	61	91	1.2	74	275	240	71	0.13	0.16	1.1	Tr	411
555	265	339	473	9.3	483	1,645	3,470	1,033	0.93	1.08	7.8	1	412
32	15	20	28	0.5	28	96	200	60	0.05	0.06	0.5	Tr	413
100	257	146	517	8.0	443	1,857	2,820	715	0.96	1.12	8.1	0	414
64	15	8	30	0.5	26	108	160	41	0.06	0.06	0.5	0	415
15	17	21	26	1.0	34	105	20	4	0.06	0.09	0.7	0	416
7	27	14	44	0.6	37	155	30	9	0.07	0.06	0.6	0	417
46	670	536	1,585	15.5	832	2,827	640	194	3.19	2.05	27.6	0	418
3	42	33	99	1.0	52	176	40	12	0.20	0.13	1.7	0	419
609	620	366	1,884	19.9	1,972	3,080	1,850	488	0.78	2.22	10.0	0	420
38	39	23	117	1.2	123	192	120	30	0.05	0.14	0.6	0	421
2053	317	622	977	5.3	1,088	2,464	2,820	833	0.33	1.44	5.1	56	422
170	26	52	81	0.4	90	204	230	69	0.03	0.12	0.4	5	423
14	16	13	26	0.6	50	59	70	18	0.08	0.07	0.3	Tr	424
18	11	9	26	0.4	35	51	20	6	0.05	0.05	0.3	Tr	425
5	28	13	41	0.8	68	140	50	15	0.10	0.23	1.0	Tr	426

Cake made with vegetable shortening; frosting with margarine.
Made with margarine.

Item No.	Foods, approximate measures, units, and weight (weight of edible portion only)		Grams	Water Percent	Food energy Calories	Protein Grams	Fat Grams	Fatty acids		
								Saturated Grams	Monounsaturated Grams	Polyunsaturated Grams
	Grain Products—Con.									
	Cookies made with enriched flour:									
	Chocolate chip:									
427	From home recipe, 2-1/3-in diam.[25]	4 cookies	40	3	185	2	11	3.9	4.3	2.0
428	From refrigerated dough, 2-1/4-in diam., 3/8 in thick	4 cookies	48	5	225	2	11	4.0	4.4	2.0
429	Fig bars, square, 1-5/8 by 1-5/8 by 3/8 in or rectangular, 1-1/2 by 1-3/4 by 1/2 in	4 cookies	56	12	210	2	4	1.0	1.5	1.0
430	Oatmeal with raisins, 2-5/8-in diam., 1/4 in thick	4 cookies	52	4	245	3	10	2.5	4.5	2.8
431	Peanut butter cookie, from home recipe, 2-5/8-in diam.[25]	4 cookies	48	3	245	4	14	4.0	5.8	2.8
432	Sandwich type (chocolate or vanilla), 1-3/4-in diam., 3/8 in thick	4 cookies	40	2	195	2	8	2.0	3.6	2.2
	Shortbread:									
433	Commercial	4 small cookies	32	6	155	2	8	2.9	3.0	1.1
434	From home recipe[38]	2 large cookies	28	3	145	2	8	1.3	2.7	3.4
435	Sugar cookie, from refrigerated dough, 2-1/2-in diam., 1/4 in thick	4 cookies	48	4	235	2	12	2.3	5.0	3.6
436	Vanilla wafers, 1-3/4-in diam., 1/4 in thick	10 cookies	40	4	185	2	7	1.8	3.0	1.8
437	Corn chips	1-oz package	28	1	155	2	9	1.4	2.4	3.7
	Cornmeal:									
438	Whole-ground, unbolted, dry form	1 cup	122	12	435	11	5	0.5	1.1	2.5
439	Bolted (nearly whole-grain), dry form	1 cup	122	12	440	11	4	0.5	0.9	2.2
	Degermed, enriched:									
440	Dry form	1 cup	138	12	500	11	2	0.2	0.4	0.9
441	Cooked	1 cup	240	88	120	3	Tr	Tr	0.1	0.2
	Crackers:[39]									
	Cheese:									
442	Plain, 1 in square	10 crackers	10	4	50	1	3	0.9	1.2	0.3
443	Sandwich type (peanut butter)	1 sandwich	8	3	40	1	2	0.4	0.8	0.3
444	Graham, plain, 2-1/2 in square	2 crackers	14	5	60	1	1	0.4	0.6	0.4
445	Melba toast, plain	1 piece	5	4	20	1	Tr	0.1	0.1	0.1
446	Rye wafers, whole-grain, 1-7/8 by 3-1/2 in	2 wafers	14	5	55	1	1	0.3	0.4	0.3
447	Saltines[40]	4 crackers	12	4	50	1	1	0.5	0.4	0.2
448	Snack-type, standard	1 round cracker	3	3	15	Tr	1	0.2	0.4	0.1
449	Wheat, thin	4 crackers	8	3	35	1	1	0.5	0.5	0.4
450	Whole-wheat wafers	2 crackers	8	4	35	1	2	0.5	0.6	0.4
451	Croissants, made with enriched flour, 4-1/2 by 4 by 1-3/4 in	1 croissant	57	22	235	5	12	3.5	6.7	1.4
	Danish pastry, made with enriched flour:									
	Plain without fruit or nuts:									
452	Packaged ring, 12 oz	1 ring	340	27	1,305	21	71	21.8	28.6	15.6
453	Round piece, about 4-1/4-in diam., 1 in high	1 pastry	57	27	220	4	12	3.6	4.8	2.6
454	Ounce	1 oz	28	27	110	2	6	1.8	2.4	1.3
455	Fruit, round piece	1 pastry	65	30	235	4	13	3.9	5.2	2.9
	Doughnuts, made with enriched flour:									
456	Cake type, plain, 3-1/4-in diam., 1 in high	1 doughnut	50	21	210	3	12	2.8	5.0	3.0
457	Yeast-leavened, glazed, 3-3/4-in diam., 1-1/4 in high	1 doughnut	60	27	235	4	13	5.2	5.5	0.9
458	English muffins, plain, enriched	1 muffin	57	42	140	5	1	0.3	0.2	0.3
459	Toasted	1 muffin	50	29	140	5	1	0.3	0.2	0.3

[25]Made with vegetable shortening.
[38]Made with margarine.

Nutrients in Indicated Quantity

Cho-les-terol	Carbo-hydrate	Calcium	Phos-phorus	Iron	Potas-sium	Sodium	Vitamin A value		Thiamin	Ribo-flavin	Niacin	Ascorbic acid	Item No.
							(IU)	(RE)					
Milli-grams	Grams	Milli-grams	Milli-grams	Milli-grams	Milli-grams	Milli-grams	Inter-national units	Retinol equiva-lents	Milli-grams	Milli-grams	Milli-grams	Milli-grams	
18	26	13	34	1.0	82	82	20	5	0.06	0.06	0.6	0	427
22	32	13	34	1.0	62	173	30	8	0.06	0.10	0.9	0	428
27	42	40	34	1.4	162	180	60	6	0.08	0.07	0.7	Tr	429
2	36	18	58	1.1	90	148	40	12	0.09	0.08	1.0	0	430
22	28	21	60	1.1	110	142	20	5	0.07	0.07	1.9	0	431
0	29	12	40	1.4	66	189	0	0	0.09	0.07	0.8	0	432
27	20	13	39	0.8	38	123	30	8	0.10	0.09	0.9	0	433
0	17	6	31	0.6	18	125	300	89	0.08	0.06	0.7	Tr	434
29	31	50	91	0.9	33	261	40	11	0.09	0.06	1.1	0	435
25	29	16	36	0.8	50	150	50	14	0.07	0.10	1.0	0	436
0	16	35	52	0.5	52	233	110	11	0.04	0.05	0.4	1	437
0	90	24	312	2.2	346	1	620	62	0.46	0.13	2.4	0	438
0	91	21	272	2.2	303	1	590	59	0.37	0.10	2.3	0	439
0	108	8	137	5.9	166	1	610	61	0.61	0.36	4.8	0	440
0	26	2	34	1.4	38	0	140	14	0.14	0.10	1.2	0	441
6	6	11	17	0.3	17	112	20	5	0.05	0.04	0.4	0	442
1	5	7	25	0.3	17	90	Tr	Tr	0.04	0.03	0.6	0	443
0	11	6	20	0.4	36	86	0	0	0.02	0.03	0.6	0	444
0	4	6	10	0.1	11	44	0	0	0.01	0.01	0.1	0	445
0	10	7	44	0.5	65	115	0	0	0.06	0.03	0.5	0	446
4	9	3	12	0.5	17	165	0	0	0.06	0.05	0.6	0	447
0	2	3	6	0.1	4	30	Tr	Tr	0.01	0.01	0.1	0	448
0	5	3	15	0.3	17	69	Tr	Tr	0.04	0.03	0.4	0	449
0	5	3	22	0.2	31	59	0	0	0.02	0.03	0.4	0	450
13	27	20	64	2.1	68	452	50	13	0.17	0.13	1.3	0	451
292	152	360	347	6.5	316	1,302	360	99	0.95	1.02	8.5	Tr	452
49	26	60	58	1.1	53	218	60	17	0.16	0.17	1.4	Tr	453
24	13	30	29	0.5	26	109	30	8	0.08	0.09	0.7	Tr	454
56	28	17	80	1.3	57	233	40	11	0.16	0.14	1.4	Tr	455
20	24	22	111	1.0	58	192	20	5	0.12	0.12	1.1	Tr	456
21	26	17	55	1.4	64	222	Tr	Tr	0.28	0.12	1.8	0	457
0	27	96	67	1.7	331	378	0	0	0.26	0.19	2.2	0	458
0	27	96	67	1.7	331	378	0	0	0.23	0.19	2.2	0	459

Crackers made with enriched flour except for rye wafers and whole-wheat wafers.
Made with lard.

Item No.	Foods, approximate measures, units, and weight (weight of edible portion only)		Grams	Water Per-cent	Food energy Cal-ories	Pro-tein Grams	Fat Grams	Fatty acids Satu-rated Grams	Mono-unsatu-rated Grams	Poly-unsatu-rated Grams
	Grain Products—Con.									
460	French toast, from home recipe---	1 slice--------	65	53	155	6	7	1.6	2.0	1.6
	Macaroni, enriched, cooked (cut lengths, elbows, shells):									
461	Firm stage (hot)-------------	1 cup-----------	130	64	190	7	1	0.1	0.1	0.3
	Tender stage:									
462	Cold------------------------	1 cup-----------	105	72	115	4	Tr	0.1	0.1	0.2
463	Hot-------------------------	1 cup-----------	140	72	155	5	1	0.1	0.1	0.2
	Muffins made with enriched flour, 2-1/2-in diam., 1-1/2 in high:									
	From home recipe:									
464	Blueberry [25]--------------	1 muffin--------	45	37	135	3	5	1.5	2.1	1.2
465	Bran [36]-------------------	1 muffin--------	45	35	125	3	6	1.4	1.6	2.3
466	Corn (enriched, degermed cornmeal and flour) [25] -----	1 muffin--------	45	33	145	3	5	1.5	2.2	1.4
	From commercial mix (egg and water added):									
467	Blueberry-------------------	1 muffin--------	45	33	140	3	5	1.4	2.0	1.2
468	Bran------------------------	1 muffin--------	45	28	140	3	4	1.3	1.6	1.0
469	Corn------------------------	1 muffin--------	45	30	145	3	6	1.7	2.3	1.4
470	Noodles (egg noodles), enriched, cooked------------------------	1 cup-----------	160	70	200	7	2	0.5	0.6	0.6
471	Noodles, chow mein, canned------	1 cup-----------	45	11	220	6	11	2.1	7.3	0.4
	Pancakes, 4-in diam.:									
472	Buckwheat, from mix (with buckwheat and enriched flours), egg and milk added-----------	1 pancake-------	27	58	55	2	2	0.9	0.9	0.5
	Plain:									
473	From home recipe using enriched flour-------------	1 pancake-------	27	50	60	2	2	0.5	0.8	0.5
474	From mix (with enriched flour), egg, milk, and oil added--------------------	1 pancake-------	27	54	60	2	2	0.5	0.9	0.5
	Piecrust, made with enriched flour and vegetable shortening, baked:									
475	From home recipe, 9-in diam.---	1 pie shell-----	180	15	900	11	60	14.8	25.9	15.7
476	From mix, 9-in diam.-----------	Piecrust for 2-crust pie-----	320	19	1,485	20	93	22.7	41.0	25.0
	Pies, piecrust made with enriched flour, vegetable shortening, 9-in diam.:									
	Apple:									
477	Whole-----------------------	1 pie-----------	945	48	2,420	21	105	27.4	44.4	26.5
478	Piece, 1/6 of pie-----------	1 piece---------	158	48	405	3	18	4.6	7.4	4.4
	Blueberry:									
479	Whole-----------------------	1 pie-----------	945	51	2,285	23	102	25.5	44.4	27.4
480	Piece, 1/6 of pie-----------	1 piece---------	158	51	380	4	17	4.3	7.4	4.6
	Cherry:									
481	Whole-----------------------	1 pie-----------	945	47	2,465	25	107	28.4	46.3	27.4
482	Piece, 1/6 of pie-----------	1 piece---------	158	47	410	4	18	4.7	7.7	4.6
	Creme:									
483	Whole-----------------------	1 pie-----------	910	43	2,710	20	139	90.1	23.7	6.4
484	Piece, 1/6 of pie-----------	1 piece---------	152	43	455	3	23	15.0	4.0	1.1
	Custard:									
485	Whole-----------------------	1 pie-----------	910	58	1,985	56	101	33.7	40.0	19.1
486	Piece, 1/6 of pie-----------	1 piece---------	152	58	330	9	17	5.6	6.7	3.2
	Lemon meringue:									
487	Whole-----------------------	1 pie-----------	840	47	2,140	31	86	26.0	34.4	17.6
488	Piece, 1/6 of pie-----------	1 piece---------	140	47	355	5	14	4.3	5.7	2.9
	Peach:									
489	Whole-----------------------	1 pie-----------	945	48	2,410	24	101	24.6	43.5	26.5
490	Piece, 1/6 of pie-----------	1 piece---------	158	48	405	4	17	4.1	7.3	4.4

[25] Made with vegetable shortening.

							Vitamin A value						
Cho-les-terol	Carbo-hydrate	Calcium	Phos-phorus	Iron	Potas-sium	Sodium	(IU)	(RE)	Thiamin	Ribo-flavin	Niacin	Ascorbic acid	Item No.
Milli-grams	Grams	Milli-grams	Milli-grams	Milli-grams	Milli-grams	Milli-grams	Inter-national units	Retinol equiva-lents	Milli-grams	Milli-grams	Milli-grams	Milli-grams	
112	17	72	85	1.3	86	257	110	32	0.12	0.16	1.0	Tr	460
0	39	14	85	2.1	103	1	0	0	0.23	0.13	1.8	0	461
0	24	8	53	1.3	64	1	0	0	0.15	0.08	1.2	0	462
0	32	11	70	1.7	85	1	0	0	0.20	0.11	1.5	0	463
19	20	54	46	0.9	47	198	40	9	0.10	0.11	0.9	1	464
24	19	60	125	1.4	99	189	230	30	0.11	0.13	1.3	3	465
23	21	66	59	0.9	57	169	80	15	0.11	0.11	0.9	Tr	466
45	22	15	90	0.9	54	225	50	11	0.10	0.17	1.1	Tr	467
28	24	27	182	1.7	50	385	100	14	0.08	0.12	1.9	0	468
42	22	30	128	1.3	31	291	90	16	0.09	0.09	0.8	Tr	469
50	37	16	94	2.6	70	3	110	34	0.22	0.13	1.9	0	470
5	26	14	41	0.4	33	450	0	0	0.05	0.03	0.6	0	471
20	6	59	91	0.4	66	125	60	17	0.04	0.05	0.2	Tr	472
16	9	27	38	0.5	33	115	30	10	0.06	0.07	0.5	Tr	473
16	8	36	71	0.7	43	160	30	7	0.09	0.12	0.8	Tr	474
0	79	25	90	4.5	90	1,100	0	0	0.54	0.40	5.0	0	475
0	141	131	272	9.3	179	2,602	0	0	1.06	0.80	9.9	0	476
0	360	76	208	9.5	756	2,844	280	28	1.04	0.76	9.5	9	477
0	60	13	35	1.6	126	476	50	5	0.17	0.13	1.6	2	478
0	330	104	217	12.3	945	2,533	850	85	1.04	0.85	10.4	38	479
0	55	17	36	2.1	158	423	140	14	0.17	0.14	1.7	6	480
0	363	132	236	9.5	992	2,873	4,160	416	1.13	0.85	9.5	0	481
0	61	22	40	1.6	166	480	700	70	0.19	0.14	1.6	0	482
46	351	273	919	6.8	796	2,207	1,250	391	0.36	0.89	6.4	0	483
8	59	46	154	1.1	133	369	210	65	0.06	0.15	1.1	0	484
1010	213	874	1,028	9.1	1,247	2,612	2,090	573	0.82	1.91	5.5	0	485
169	36	146	172	1.5	208	436	350	96	0.14	0.32	0.9	0	486
857	317	118	412	8.4	420	2,369	1,430	395	0.59	0.84	5.0	25	487
143	53	20	69	1.4	70	395	240	66	0.10	0.14	0.8	4	488
0	361	95	274	11.3	1,408	2,533	6,900	690	1.04	0.95	14.2	28	489
0	60	16	46	1.9	235	423	1,150	115	0.17	0.16	2.4	5	490

Made with vegetable oil.

Item No.	Foods, approximate measures, units, and weight (weight of edible portion only)			Water	Food energy	Pro-tein	Fat	Fatty acids		
								Satu-rated	Mono-unsatu-rated	Poly-unsatu-rated
			Grams	Per-cent	Cal-ories	Grams	Grams	Grams	Grams	Grams
	Grain Products—Con.									
	Pies, piecrust made with enriched flour, vegetable shortening, 9-inch diam.:									
	Pecan:									
491	Whole	1 pie	825	20	3,450	42	189	28.1	101.5	47.0
492	Piece, 1/6 of pie	1 piece	138	20	575	7	32	4.7	17.0	7.9
	Pumpkin:									
493	Whole	1 pie	910	59	1,920	36	102	38.2	40.0	18.2
494	Piece, 1/6 of pie	1 piece	152	59	320	6	17	6.4	6.7	3.0
	Pies, fried:									
495	Apple	1 pie	85	43	255	2	14	5.8	6.6	0.6
496	Cherry	1 pie	85	42	250	2	14	5.8	6.7	0.6
	Popcorn, popped:									
497	Air-popped, unsalted	1 cup	8	4	30	1	Tr	Tr	0.1	0.2
498	Popped in vegetable oil, salted	1 cup	11	3	55	1	3	0.5	1.4	1.2
499	Sugar syrup coated	1 cup	35	4	135	2	1	0.1	0.3	0.6
	Pretzels, made with enriched flour:									
500	Stick, 2-1/4 in long	10 pretzels	3	3	10	Tr	Tr	Tr	Tr	Tr
501	Twisted, dutch, 2-3/4 by 2-5/8 in	1 pretzel	16	3	65	2	1	0.1	0.2	0.2
502	Twisted, thin, 3-1/4 by 2-1/4 by 1/4 in	10 pretzels	60	3	240	6	2	0.4	0.8	0.6
	Rice:									
503	Brown, cooked, served hot	1 cup	195	70	230	5	1	0.3	0.3	0.4
	White, enriched:									
	Commercial varieties, all types:									
504	Raw	1 cup	185	12	670	12	1	0.2	0.2	0.3
505	Cooked, served hot	1 cup	205	73	225	4	Tr	0.1	0.1	0.1
506	Instant, ready-to-serve, hot	1 cup	165	73	180	4	0	0.1	0.1	0.1
	Parboiled:									
507	Raw	1 cup	185	10	685	14	1	0.1	0.1	0.2
508	Cooked, served hot	1 cup	175	73	185	4	Tr	Tr	Tr	0.1
	Rolls, enriched:									
	Commercial:									
509	Dinner, 2-1/2-in diam., 2 in high	1 roll	28	32	85	2	2	0.5	0.8	0.6
510	Frankfurter and hamburger (8 per 11-1/2-oz pkg.)	1 roll	40	34	115	3	2	0.5	0.8	0.6
511	Hard, 3-3/4-in diam., 2 in high	1 roll	50	25	155	5	2	0.4	0.5	0.6
512	Hoagie or submarine, 11-1/2 by 3 by 2-1/2 in	1 roll	135	31	400	11	8	1.8	3.0	2.2
	From home recipe:									
513	Dinner, 2-1/2-in diam., 2 in high	1 roll	35	26	120	3	3	0.8	1.2	0.9
	Spaghetti, enriched, cooked:									
514	Firm stage, "al dente," served hot	1 cup	130	64	190	7	1	0.1	0.1	0.3
515	Tender stage, served hot	1 cup	140	73	155	5	1	0.1	0.1	0.2
516	Toaster pastries	1 pastry	54	13	210	2	6	1.7	3.6	0.4
517	Tortillas, corn	1 tortilla	30	45	65	2	1	0.1	0.3	0.6
	Waffles, made with enriched flour, 7-in diam.:									
518	From home recipe	1 waffle	75	37	245	7	13	4.0	4.9	2.6
519	From mix, egg and milk added	1 waffle	75	42	205	7	8	2.7	2.9	1.5
	Wheat flours:									
	All-purpose or family flour, enriched:									
520	Sifted, spooned	1 cup	115	12	420	12	1	0.2	0.1	0.5
521	Unsifted, spooned	1 cup	125	12	455	13	1	0.2	0.1	0.5
522	Cake or pastry flour, enriched, sifted, spooned	1 cup	96	12	350	7	1	0.1	0.1	0.3
523	Self-rising, enriched, unsifted, spooned	1 cup	125	12	440	12	1	0.2	0.1	0.5
524	Whole-wheat, from hard wheats, stirred	1 cup	120	12	400	16	2	0.3	0.3	1.1

							Vitamin A value						
Cho-les-terol	Carbo-hydrate	Calcium	Phos-phorus	Iron	Potas-sium	Sodium	(IU)	(RE)	Thiamin	Ribo-flavin	Niacin	Ascorbic acid	Item No.
Milli-grams	Grams	Milli-grams	Milli-grams	Milli-grams	Milli-grams	Milli-grams	Inter-national units	Retinol equiva-lents	Milli-grams	Milli-grams	Milli-grams	Milli-grams	
569	423	388	850	27.2	1,015	1,823	1,320	322	1.82	0.99	6.6	0	491
95	71	65	142	4.6	170	305	220	54	0.30	0.17	1.1	0	492
655	223	464	628	8.2	1,456	1,947	22,480	2,493	0.82	1.27	7.3	0	493
109	37	78	105	1.4	243	325	3,750	416	0.14	0.21	1.2	0	494
14	31	12	34	0.9	42	326	30	3	0.09	0.06	1.0	1	495
13	32	11	41	0.7	61	371	190	19	0.06	0.06	0.6	1	496
0	6	1	22	0.2	20	Tr	10	1	0.03	0.01	0.2	0	497
0	6	3	31	0.3	19	86	20	2	0.01	0.02	0.1	0	498
0	30	2	47	0.5	90	Tr	30	3	0.13	0.02	0.4	0	499
0	2	1	3	0.1	3	48	0	0	0.01	0.01	0.1	0	500
0	13	4	15	0.3	16	258	0	0	0.05	0.04	0.7	0	501
0	48	16	55	1.2	61	966	0	0	0.19	0.15	2.6	0	502
0	50	23	142	1.0	137	0	0	0	0.18	0.04	2.7	0	503
0	149	44	174	5.4	170	9	0	0	0.81	0.06	6.5	0	504
0	50	21	57	1.8	57	0	0	0	0.23	0.02	2.1	0	505
0	40	5	31	1.3	0	0	0	0	0.21	0.02	1.7	0	506
0	150	111	370	5.4	278	17	0	0	0.81	0.07	6.5	0	507
0	41	33	100	1.4	75	0	0	0	0.19	0.02	2.1	0	508
Tr	14	33	44	0.8	36	155	Tr	Tr	0.14	0.09	1.1	Tr	509
Tr	20	54	44	1.2	56	241	Tr	Tr	0.20	0.13	1.6	Tr	510
Tr	30	24	46	1.4	49	313	0	0	0.20	0.12	1.7	0	511
Tr	72	100	115	3.8	128	683	0	0	0.54	0.33	4.5	0	512
12	20	16	36	1.1	41	98	30	8	0.12	0.12	1.2	0	513
0	39	14	85	2.0	103	1	0	0	0.23	0.13	1.8	0	514
0	32	11	70	1.7	85	1	0	0	0.20	0.11	1.5	0	515
0	38	104	104	2.2	91	248	520	52	0.17	0.18	2.3	4	516
0	13	42	55	0.6	43	1	80	8	0.05	0.03	0.4	0	517
102	26	154	135	1.5	129	445	140	39	0.18	0.24	1.5	Tr	518
59	27	179	257	1.2	146	515	170	49	0.14	0.23	0.9	Tr	519
0	88	18	100	5.1	109	2	0	0	0.73	0.46	6.1	0	520
0	95	20	109	5.5	119	3	0	0	0.80	0.50	6.6	0	521
0	76	16	70	4.2	91	2	0	0	0.58	0.38	5.1	0	522
0	93	331	583	5.5	113	1,349	0	0	0.80	0.50	6.6	0	523
0	85	49	446	5.2	444	4	0	0	0.66	0.14	5.2	0	524

Item No.	Foods, approximate measures, units, and weight (weight of edible portion only)		Grams	Water Per-cent	Food energy Cal-ories	Pro-tein Grams	Fat Grams	Fatty acids		
								Satu-rated Grams	Mono-unsatu-rated Grams	Poly-unsatu-rated Grams
	Legumes, Nuts, and Seeds									
	Almonds, shelled:									
525	Slivered, packed---------------	1 cup-----------	135	4	795	27	70	6.7	45.8	14.8
526	Whole-------------------------	1 oz-----------	28	4	165	6	15	1.4	9.6	3.1
	Beans, dry:									
	Cooked, drained:									
527	Black-------------------------	1 cup-----------	171	66	225	15	1	0.1	0.1	0.5
528	Great Northern----------------	1 cup-----------	180	69	210	14	1	0.1	0.1	0.6
529	Lima--------------------------	1 cup-----------	190	64	260	16	1	0.2	0.1	0.5
530	Pea (navy)--------------------	1 cup-----------	190	69	225	15	1	0.1	0.1	0.7
531	Pinto-------------------------	1 cup-----------	180	65	265	15	1	0.1	0.1	0.5
	Canned, solids and liquid:									
	White with:									
532	Frankfurters (sliced)------	1 cup-----------	255	71	365	19	18	7.4	8.8	0.7
533	Pork and tomato sauce------	1 cup-----------	255	71	310	16	7	2.4	2.7	0.7
534	Pork and sweet sauce------	1 cup-----------	255	66	385	16	12	4.3	4.9	1.2
535	Red kidney-------------------	1 cup-----------	255	76	230	15	1	0.1	0.1	0.6
536	Black-eyed peas, dry, cooked (with residual cooking liquid)	1 cup-----------	250	80	190	13	1	0.2	Tr	0.3
537	Brazil nuts, shelled-------------	1 oz-----------	28	3	185	4	19	4.6	6.5	6.8
538	Carob flour--------------------	1 cup-----------	140	3	255	6	Tr	Tr	0.1	0.1
	Cashew nuts, salted:									
539	Dry roasted-------------------	1 cup-----------	137	2	785	21	63	12.5	37.4	10.7
540		1 oz-----------	28	2	165	4	13	2.6	7.7	2.2
541	Roasted in oil----------------	1 cup-----------	130	4	750	21	63	12.4	36.9	10.6
542		1 oz-----------	28	4	165	5	14	2.7	8.1	2.3
543	Chestnuts, European (Italian), roasted, shelled--------------	1 cup-----------	143	40	350	5	3	0.6	1.1	1.2
544	Chickpeas, cooked, drained-------	1 cup-----------	163	60	270	15	4	0.4	0.9	1.9
	Coconut:									
	Raw:									
545	Piece, about 2 by 2 by 1/2 in	1 piece---------	45	47	160	1	15	13.4	0.6	0.2
546	Shredded or grated----------	1 cup-----------	80	47	285	3	27	23.8	1.1	0.3
547	Dried, sweetened, shredded-----	1 cup-----------	93	13	470	3	33	29.3	1.4	0.4
548	Filberts (hazelnuts), chopped----	1 cup-----------	115	5	725	15	72	5.3	56.5	6.9
549		1 oz-----------	28	5	180	4	18	1.3	13.9	1.7
550	Lentils, dry, cooked-------------	1 cup-----------	200	72	215	16	1	0.1	0.2	0.5
551	Macadamia nuts, roasted in oil, salted------------------------	1 cup-----------	134	2	960	10	103	15.4	80.9	1.8
552		1 oz-----------	28	2	205	2	22	3.2	17.1	0.4
	Mixed nuts, with peanuts, salted:									
553	Dry roasted-------------------	1 oz-----------	28	2	170	5	15	2.0	8.9	3.1
554	Roasted in oil----------------	1 oz-----------	28	2	175	5	16	2.5	9.0	3.8
555	Peanuts, roasted in oil, salted--	1 cup-----------	145	2	840	39	71	9.9	35.5	22.6
556		1 oz-----------	28	2	165	8	14	1.9	6.9	4.4
557	Peanut butter-------------------	1 tbsp---------	16	1	95	5	8	1.4	4.0	2.5
558	Peas, split, dry, cooked---------	1 cup-----------	200	70	230	16	1	0.1	0.1	0.3
559	Pecans, halves------------------	1 cup-----------	108	5	720	8	73	5.9	45.5	18.1
560		1 oz-----------	28	5	190	2	19	1.5	12.0	4.7
561	Pine nuts (pinyons), shelled-----	1 oz-----------	28	6	160	3	17	2.7	6.5	7.3
562	Pistachio nuts, dried, shelled---	1 oz-----------	28	4	165	6	14	1.7	9.3	2.1
563	Pumpkin and squash kernels, dry, hulled--------------------------	1 oz-----------	28	7	155	7	13	2.5	4.0	5.9
564	Refried beans, canned-----------	1 cup-----------	290	72	295	18	3	0.4	0.6	1.4
565	Sesame seeds, dry, hulled--------	1 tbsp---------	8	5	45	2	4	0.6	1.7	1.9
566	Soybeans, dry, cooked, drained---	1 cup-----------	180	71	235	20	10	1.3	1.9	5.3
	Soy products:									
567	Miso-------------------------	1 cup-----------	276	53	470	29	13	1.8	2.6	7.3
568	Tofu, piece 2-1/2 by 2-3/4 by 1 in----------------------	1 piece---------	120	85	85	9	5	0.7	1.0	2.9
569	Sunflower seeds, dry, hulled-----	1 oz-----------	28	5	160	6	14	1.5	2.7	9.3
570	Tahini--------------------------	1 tbsp---------	15	3	90	3	8	1.1	3.0	3.5

[41] Cashews without salt contain 21 mg sodium per cup or 4 mg per oz.
[42] Cashews without salt contain 22 mg sodium per cup or 5 mg per oz.
[43] Macadamia nuts without salt contain 9 mg sodium per cup or 2 mg per oz.

Nutrients in Indicated Quantity

Cho-les-terol	Carbo-hydrate	Calcium	Phos-phorus	Iron	Potas-sium	Sodium	Vitamin A value (IU)	(RE)	Thiamin	Ribo-flavin	Niacin	Ascorbic acid	Item No.
Milli-grams	Grams	Milli-grams	Milli-grams	Milli-grams	Milli-grams	Milli-grams	Inter-national units	Retinol equiva-lents	Milli-grams	Milli-grams	Milli-grams	Milli-grams	
0	28	359	702	4.9	988	15	0	0	0.28	1.05	4.5	1	525
0	6	75	147	1.0	208	3	0	0	0.06	0.22	1.0	Tr	526
0	41	47	239	2.9	608	1	Tr	Tr	0.43	0.05	0.9	0	527
0	38	90	266	4.9	749	13	0	0	0.25	0.13	1.3	0	528
0	49	55	293	5.9	1,163	4	0	0	0.25	0.11	1.3	0	529
0	40	95	281	5.1	790	13	0	0	0.27	0.13	1.3	0	530
0	49	86	296	5.4	882	3	Tr	Tr	0.33	0.16	0.7	0	531
30	32	94	303	4.8	668	1,374	330	33	0.18	0.15	3.3	Tr	532
10	48	138	235	4.6	536	1,181	330	33	0.20	0.08	1.5	5	533
10	54	161	291	5.9	536	969	330	33	0.15	0.10	1.3	5	534
0	42	74	278	4.6	673	968	10	1	0.13	0.10	1.5	0	535
0	35	43	238	3.3	573	20	30	3	0.40	0.10	1.0	0	536
0	4	50	170	1.0	170	1	Tr	Tr	0.28	0.03	0.5	Tr	537
0	126	390	102	5.7	1,275	24	Tr	Tr	0.07	0.07	2.2	Tr	538
0	45	62	671	8.2	774	[41]877	0	0	0.27	0.27	1.9	0	539
0	9	13	139	1.7	160	[41]181	0	0	0.06	0.06	0.4	0	540
0	37	53	554	5.3	689	[42]814	0	0	0.55	0.23	2.3	0	541
0	8	12	121	1.2	150	[42]177	0	0	0.12	0.05	0.5	0	542
0	76	41	153	1.3	847	3	30	3	0.35	0.25	1.9	37	543
0	45	80	273	4.9	475	11	Tr	Tr	0.18	0.09	0.9	0	544
0	7	6	51	1.1	160	9	0	0	0.03	0.01	0.2	1	545
0	12	11	90	1.9	285	16	0	0	0.05	0.02	0.4	3	546
0	44	14	99	1.8	313	244	0	0	0.03	0.02	0.4	1	547
0	18	216	359	3.8	512	3	80	8	0.58	0.13	1.3	1	548
0	4	53	88	0.9	126	1	20	2	0.14	0.03	0.3	Tr	549
0	38	50	238	4.2	498	26	40	4	0.14	0.12	1.2	0	550
0	17	60	268	2.4	441	[43]348	10	1	0.29	0.15	2.7	0	551
0	4	13	57	0.5	93	[43]74	Tr	Tr	0.06	0.03	0.6	0	552
0	7	20	123	1.0	169	[44]190	Tr	Tr	0.06	0.06	1.3	0	553
0	6	31	131	0.9	165	[44]185	10	1	0.14	0.06	1.4	Tr	554
0	27	125	734	2.8	1,019	[45]626	0	0	0.42	0.15	21.5	0	555
0	5	24	143	0.5	199	[45]122	0	0	0.08	0.03	4.2	0	556
0	3	5	60	0.3	110	75	0	0	0.02	0.02	2.2	0	557
0	42	22	178	3.4	592	26	80	8	0.30	0.18	1.8	0	558
0	20	39	314	2.3	423	1	140	14	0.92	0.14	1.0	2	559
0	5	10	83	0.6	111	Tr	40	4	0.24	0.04	0.3	1	560
0	5	2	10	0.9	178	20	10	1	0.35	0.06	1.2	1	561
0	7	38	143	1.9	310	2	70	7	0.23	0.05	0.3	Tr	562
0	5	12	333	4.2	229	5	110	11	0.06	0.09	0.5	Tr	563
0	51	141	245	5.1	1,141	1,228	0	0	0.14	0.16	1.4	17	564
0	1	11	62	0.6	33	3	10	1	0.06	0.01	0.4	0	565
0	19	131	322	4.9	972	4	50	5	0.38	0.16	1.1	0	566
0	65	188	853	4.7	922	8,142	110	11	0.17	0.28	0.8	0	567
0	3	108	151	2.3	50	8	0	0	0.07	0.04	0.1	0	568
0	5	33	200	1.9	195	1	10	1	0.65	0.07	1.3	Tr	569
0	3	21	119	0.7	69	5	10	1	0.24	0.02	0.8	1	570

[Mixed nuts without salt contain 3 mg sodium per oz.
[Peanuts without salt contain 22 mg sodium per cup or 4 mg per oz.

Item No.	Foods, approximate measures, units, and weight (weight of edible portion only)		Grams	Water	Food energy	Pro-tein	Fat	Fatty acids		
								Satu-rated	Mono-unsatu-rated	Poly-unsatu-rated
			Grams	Per-cent	Cal-ories	Grams	Grams	Grams	Grams	Grams
	Legumes, Nuts, and Seeds—Con.									
	Walnuts:									
571	Black, chopped-----------------	1 cup----------	125	4	760	30	71	4.5	15.9	46.9
572		1 oz-----------	28	4	170	7	16	1.0	3.6	10.6
573	English or Persian, pieces or chips---------------------	1 cup----------	120	4	770	17	74	6.7	17.0	47.0
574		1 oz-----------	28	4	180	4	18	1.6	4.0	11.1
	Meat and Meat Products									
	Beef, cooked:[46]									
	Cuts braised, simmered, or pot roasted:									
	Relatively fat such as chuck blade:									
575	Lean and fat, piece, 2-1/2 by 2-1/2 by 3/4 in-------	3 oz-----------	85	43	325	22	26	10.8	11.7	0.9
576	Lean only from item 575----	2.2 oz---------	62	53	170	19	9	3.9	4.2	0.3
	Relatively lean, such as bottom round:									
577	Lean and fat, piece, 4-1/8 by 2-1/4 by 1/2 in-------	3 oz-----------	85	54	220	25	13	4.8	5.7	0.5
578	Lean only from item 577----	2.8 oz---------	78	57	175	25	8	2.7	3.4	0.3
	Ground beef, broiled, patty, 3 by 5/8 in:									
579	Lean------------------------	3 oz-----------	85	56	230	21	16	6.2	6.9	0.6
580	Regular---------------------	3 oz-----------	85	54	245	20	18	6.9	7.7	0.7
581	Heart, lean, braised-----------	3 oz-----------	85	65	150	24	5	1.2	0.8	1.6
582	Liver, fried, slice, 6-1/2 by 2-3/8 by 3/8 in[47]-----------	3 oz-----------	85	56	185	23	7	2.5	3.6	1.3
	Roast, oven cooked, no liquid added:									
	Relatively fat, such as rib:									
583	Lean and fat, 2 pieces, 4-1/8 by 2-1/4 by 1/4 in	3 oz-----------	85	46	315	19	26	10.8	11.4	0.9
584	Lean only from item 583----	2.2 oz---------	61	57	150	17	9	3.6	3.7	0.3
	Relatively lean, such as eye of round:									
585	Lean and fat, 2 pieces, 2-1/2 by 2-1/2 by 3/8 in	3 oz-----------	85	57	205	23	12	4.9	5.4	0.5
586	Lean only from item 585----	2.6 oz---------	75	63	135	22	5	1.9	2.1	0.2
	Steak:									
	Sirloin, broiled:									
587	Lean and fat, piece, 2-1/2 by 2-1/2 by 3/4 in-------	3 oz-----------	85	53	240	23	15	6.4	6.9	0.6
588	Lean only from item 587----	2.5 oz---------	72	59	150	22	6	2.6	2.8	0.3
589	Beef, canned, corned------------	3 oz-----------	85	59	185	22	10	4.2	4.9	0.4
590	Beef, dried, chipped------------	2.5 oz---------	72	48	145	24	4	1.8	2.0	0.2
	Lamb, cooked:									
	Chops, (3 per lb with bone):									
	Arm, braised:									
591	Lean and fat--------------	2.2 oz---------	63	44	220	20	15	6.9	6.0	0.9
592	Lean only from item 591----	1.7 oz---------	48	49	135	17	7	2.9	2.6	0.4
	Loin, broiled:									
593	Lean and fat--------------	2.8 oz---------	80	54	235	22	16	7.3	6.4	1.0
594	Lean only from item 593----	2.3 oz---------	64	61	140	19	6	2.6	2.4	0.4
	Leg, roasted:									
595	Lean and fat, 2 pieces, 4-1/8 by 2-1/4 by 1/4 in-------	3 oz-----------	85	59	205	22	13	5.6	4.9	0.8
596	Lean only from item 595------	2.6 oz---------	73	64	140	20	6	2.4	2.2	0.4
	Rib, roasted:									
597	Lean and fat, 3 pieces, 2-1/2 by 2-1/2 by 1/4 in-------	3 oz-----------	85	47	315	18	26	12.1	10.6	1.5
598	Lean only from item 597------	2 oz-----------	57	60	130	15	7	3.2	3.0	0.5

[46] Outer layer of fat was removed to within approximately 1/2 inch of the lean. Deposits of fat within the cut were not removed.

[47] Fried in vegetable shortening.

Nutrients in Indicated Quantity

Cho-les-terol	Carbo-hydrate	Calcium	Phos-phorus	Iron	Potas-sium	Sodium	Vitamin A value (IU)	(RE)	Thiamin	Ribo-flavin	Niacin	Ascorbic acid	Item No.
Milli-grams	Grams	Milli-grams	Milli-grams	Milli-grams	Milli-grams	Milli-grams	Inter-national units	Retinol equiva-lents	Milli-grams	Milli-grams	Milli-grams	Milli-grams	
0	15	73	580	3.8	655	1	370	37	0.27	0.14	0.9	Tr	571
0	3	16	132	0.9	149	Tr	80	8	0.06	0.03	0.2	Tr	572
0	22	113	380	2.9	602	12	150	15	0.46	0.18	1.3	4	573
0	5	27	90	0.7	142	3	40	4	0.11	0.04	0.3	1	574
87	0	11	163	2.5	163	53	Tr	Tr	0.06	0.19	2.0	0	575
66	0	8	146	2.3	163	44	Tr	Tr	0.05	0.17	1.7	0	576
81	0	5	217	2.8	248	43	Tr	Tr	0.06	0.21	3.3	0	577
75	0	4	212	2.7	240	40	Tr	Tr	0.06	0.20	3.0	0	578
74	0	9	134	1.8	256	65	Tr	Tr	0.04	0.18	4.4	0	579
76	0	9	144	2.1	248	70	Tr	Tr	0.03	0.16	4.9	0	580
164	0	5	213	6.4	198	54	Tr	Tr	0.12	1.31	3.4	5	581
410	7	9	392	5.3	309	90	[48]30,690	[48]9,120	0.18	3.52	12.3	23	582
72	0	8	145	2.0	246	54	Tr	Tr	0.06	0.16	3.1	0	583
49	0	5	127	1.7	218	45	Tr	Tr	0.05	0.13	2.7	0	584
62	0	5	177	1.6	308	50	Tr	Tr	0.07	0.14	3.0	0	585
52	0	3	170	1.5	297	46	Tr	Tr	0.07	0.13	2.8	0	586
77	0	9	186	2.6	306	53	Tr	Tr	0.10	0.23	3.3	0	587
64	0	8	176	2.4	290	48	Tr	Tr	0.09	0.22	3.1	0	588
80	0	17	90	3.7	51	802	Tr	Tr	0.02	0.20	2.9	0	589
46	0	14	287	2.3	142	3,053	Tr	Tr	0.05	0.23	2.7	0	590
77	0	16	132	1.5	195	46	Tr	Tr	0.04	0.16	4.4	0	591
59	0	12	111	1.3	162	36	Tr	Tr	0.03	0.13	3.0	0	592
78	0	16	162	1.4	272	62	Tr	Tr	0.09	0.21	5.5	0	593
60	0	12	145	1.3	241	54	Tr	Tr	0.08	0.18	4.4	0	594
78	0	8	162	1.7	273	57	Tr	Tr	0.09	0.24	5.5	0	595
65	0	6	150	1.5	247	50	Tr	Tr	0.08	0.20	4.6	0	596
77	0	19	139	1.4	224	60	Tr	Tr	0.08	0.18	5.5	0	597
50	0	12	111	1.0	179	46	Tr	Tr	0.05	0.13	3.5	0	598

[48] Value varies widely.

Item No.	Foods, approximate measures, units, and weight (weight of edible portion only)		Grams	Water Percent	Food energy Calories	Protein Grams	Fat Grams	Saturated Grams	Monounsaturated Grams	Polyunsaturated Grams
								Fatty acids		

Meat and Meat Products—Con.

Item No.	Foods, approximate measures, units, and weight (weight of edible portion only)		Grams	Water Percent	Food energy Calories	Protein Grams	Fat Grams	Saturated Grams	Monounsaturated Grams	Polyunsaturated Grams
	Pork, cured, cooked:									
	Bacon:									
599	Regular----------------------	3 medium slices	19	13	110	6	9	3.3	4.5	1.1
600	Canadian-style---------------	2 slices--------	46	62	85	11	4	1.3	1.9	0.4
	Ham, light cure, roasted:									
601	Lean and fat, 2 pieces, 4-1/8 by 2-1/4 by 1/4 in---------	3 oz------------	85	58	205	18	14	5.1	6.7	1.5
602	Lean only from item 601------	2.4 oz----------	68	66	105	17	4	1.3	1.7	0.4
603	Ham, canned, roasted, 2 pieces, 4-1/8 by 2-1/4 by 1/4 in-----	3 oz------------	85	67	140	18	7	2.4	3.5	0.8
	Luncheon meat:									
604	Canned, spiced or unspiced, slice, 3 by 2 by 1/2 in----	2 slices--------	42	52	140	5	13	4.5	6.0	1.5
605	Chopped ham (8 slices per 6 oz pkg)---------------------	2 slices--------	42	64	95	7	7	2.4	3.4	0.9
	Cooked ham (8 slices per 8-oz pkg):									
606	Regular-----------------	2 slices--------	57	65	105	10	6	1.9	2.8	0.7
607	Extra lean--------------	2 slices--------	57	71	75	11	3	0.9	1.3	0.3
	Pork, fresh, cooked:									
	Chop, loin (cut 3 per lb with bone):									
	Broiled:									
608	Lean and fat---------------	3.1 oz----------	87	50	275	24	19	7.0	8.8	2.2
609	Lean only from item 608----	2.5 oz----------	72	57	165	23	8	2.6	3.4	0.9
	Pan fried:									
610	Lean and fat---------------	3.1 oz----------	89	45	335	21	27	9.8	12.5	3.1
611	Lean only from item 610----	2.4 oz----------	67	54	180	19	11	3.7	4.8	1.3
	Ham (leg), roasted:									
612	Lean and fat, piece, 2-1/2 by 2-1/2 by 3/4 in------------	3 oz------------	85	53	250	21	18	6.4	8.1	2.0
613	Lean only from item 612------	2.5 oz----------	72	60	160	20	8	2.7	3.6	1.0
	Rib, roasted:									
614	Lean and fat, piece, 2-1/2 by 3/4 in--------------------	3 oz------------	85	51	270	21	20	7.2	9.2	2.3
615	Lean only from item 614------	2.5 oz----------	71	57	175	20	10	3.4	4.4	1.2
	Shoulder cut, braised:									
616	Lean and fat, 3 pieces, 2-1/2 by 2-1/2 by 1/4 in------------	3 oz------------	85	47	295	23	22	7.9	10.0	2.4
617	Lean only from item 616------	2.4 oz----------	67	54	165	22	8	2.8	3.7	1.0
	Sausages (See also Luncheon meats, items 604-607):									
618	Bologna, slice (8 per 8-oz pkg)	2 slices--------	57	54	180	7	16	6.1	7.6	1.4
619	Braunschweiger, slice (6 per 6-oz pkg)---------------------	2 slices--------	57	48	205	8	18	6.2	8.5	2.1
620	Brown and serve (10-11 per 8-oz pkg), browned-----------	1 link----------	13	45	50	2	5	1.7	2.2	0.5
621	Frankfurter (10 per 1-lb pkg), cooked (reheated)------------	1 frankfurter---	45	54	145	5	13	4.8	6.2	1.2
622	Pork link (16 per 1-lb pkg), cooked[50] ---------------------	1 link----------	13	45	50	3	4	1.4	1.8	0.5
	Salami:									
623	Cooked type, slice (8 per 8-oz pkg)-------------------	2 slices--------	57	60	145	8	11	4.6	5.2	1.2
624	Dry type, slice (12 per 4-oz pkg)---------------------	2 slices--------	20	35	85	5	7	2.4	3.4	0.6
625	Sandwich spread (pork, beef)---	1 tbsp----------	15	60	35	1	3	0.9	1.1	0.4
626	Vienna sausage (7 per 4-oz can)	1 sausage-------	16	60	45	2	4	1.5	2.0	0.3
	Veal, medium fat, cooked, bone removed:									
627	Cutlet, 4-1/8 by 2-1/4 by 1/2 in, braised or broiled-------	3 oz------------	85	60	185	23	9	4.1	4.1	0.6
628	Rib, 2 pieces, 4-1/8 by 2-1/4 by 1/4 in, roasted----------	3 oz------------	85	55	230	23	14	6.0	6.0	1.0

[49]Contains added sodium ascorbate. If sodium ascorbate is not added, ascorbic acid content is negligible.

Nutrients in Indicated Quantity

Cho-les-terol	Carbo-hydrate	Calcium	Phos-phorus	Iron	Potas-sium	Sodium	Vitamin A value		Thiamin	Ribo-flavin	Niacin	Ascorbic acid	Item No.
							(IU)	(RE)					
Milli-grams	Grams	Milli-grams	Milli-grams	Milli-grams	Milli-grams	Milli-grams	Inter-national units	Retinol equiva-lents	Milli-grams	Milli-grams	Milli-grams	Milli-grams	
16	Tr	2	64	0.3	92	303	0	0	0.13	0.05	1.4	6	599
27	1	5	136	0.4	179	711	0	0	0.38	0.09	3.2	10	600
53	0	6	182	0.7	243	1,009	0	0	0.51	0.19	3.8	0	601
37	0	5	154	0.6	215	902	0	0	0.46	0.17	3.4	0	602
35	Tr	6	188	0.9	298	908	0	0	0.82	0.21	4.3	[49]19	603
26	1	3	34	0.3	90	541	0	0	0.15	0.08	1.3	Tr	604
21	0	3	65	0.3	134	576	0	0	0.27	0.09	1.6	[49]8	605
32	2	4	141	0.6	189	751	0	0	0.49	0.14	3.0	[49]16	606
27	1	4	124	0.4	200	815	0	0	0.53	0.13	2.8	[49]15	607
84	0	3	184	0.7	312	61	10	3	0.87	0.24	4.3	Tr	608
71	0	4	176	0.7	302	56	10	1	0.83	0.22	4.0	Tr	609
92	0	4	190	0.7	323	64	10	3	0.91	0.24	4.6	Tr	610
72	0	3	178	0.7	305	57	10	1	0.84	0.22	4.0	Tr	611
79	0	5	210	0.9	280	50	10	2	0.54	0.27	3.9	Tr	612
68	0	5	202	0.8	269	46	10	1	0.50	0.25	3.6	Tr	613
69	0	9	190	0.8	313	37	10	3	0.50	0.24	4.2	Tr	614
56	0	8	182	0.7	300	33	10	2	0.45	0.22	3.8	Tr	615
93	0	6	162	1.4	286	75	10	3	0.46	0.26	4.4	Tr	616
76	0	5	151	1.3	271	68	10	1	0.40	0.24	4.0	Tr	617
31	2	7	52	0.9	103	581	0	0	0.10	0.08	1.5	[49]12	618
89	2	5	96	5.3	113	652	8,010	2,405	0.14	0.87	4.8	[49]6	619
9	Tr	1	14	0.1	25	105	0	0	0.05	0.02	0.4	0	620
23	1	5	39	0.5	75	504	0	0	0.09	0.05	1.2	[49]12	621
11	Tr	4	24	0.2	47	168	0	0	0.10	0.03	0.6	Tr	622
37	1	7	66	1.5	113	607	0	0	0.14	0.21	2.0	[49]7	623
16	1	2	28	0.3	76	372	0	0	0.12	0.06	1.0	[49]5	624
6	2	2	9	0.1	17	152	10	1	0.03	0.02	0.3	0	625
8	Tr	2	8	0.1	16	152	0	0	0.01	0.02	0.3	0	626
109	0	9	196	0.8	258	56	Tr	Tr	0.06	0.21	4.6	0	627
109	0	10	211	0.7	259	57	Tr	Tr	0.11	0.26	6.6	0	628

[49] One patty (8 per pound) of bulk sausage is equivalent to 2 links.

Item No.	Foods, approximate measures, units, and weight (weight of edible portion only)		Grams	Water Per-cent	Food energy Cal-ories	Pro-tein Grams	Fat Grams	Fatty acids		
								Saturated Grams	Mono-unsatu-rated Grams	Poly-unsatu-rated Grams
	Mixed Dishes and Fast Foods									
	Mixed dishes:									
629	Beef and vegetable stew, from home recipe-----------------	1 cup----------	245	82	220	16	11	4.4	4.5	0.5
630	Beef potpie, from home recipe, baked, piece, 1/3 of 9-in diam. pie[51] -----------------	1 piece---------	210	55	515	21	30	7.9	12.9	7.4
631	Chicken a la king, cooked, from home recipe------------	1 cup----------	245	68	470	27	34	12.9	13.4	6.2
632	Chicken and noodles, cooked, from home recipe------------	1 cup----------	240	71	365	22	18	5.1	7.1	3.9
	Chicken chow mein:									
633	Canned----------------------	1 cup----------	250	89	95	7	Tr	0.1	0.1	0.8
634	From home recipe-----------	1 cup----------	250	78	255	31	10	4.1	4.9	3.5
635	Chicken potpie, from home recipe, baked, piece, 1/3 of 9-in diam. pie[51] -------------	1 piece---------	232	57	545	23	31	10.3	15.5	6.6
636	Chili con carne with beans, canned----------------------	1 cup----------	255	72	340	19	16	5.8	7.2	1.0
637	Chop suey with beef and pork, from home recipe-------------	1 cup----------	250	75	300	26	17	4.3	7.4	4.2
	Macaroni (enriched) and cheese:									
638	Canned[52] ---------------------	1 cup----------	240	80	230	9	10	4.7	2.9	1.3
639	From home recipe[38] -----------	1 cup----------	200	58	430	17	22	9.8	7.4	3.6
640	Quiche Lorraine, 1/8 of 8-in diam. quiche[51] ---------------	1 slice---------	176	47	600	13	48	23.2	17.8	4.1
	Spaghetti (enriched) in tomato sauce with cheese:									
641	Canned----------------------	1 cup----------	250	80	190	6	2	0.4	0.4	0.5
642	From home recipe-------------	1 cup----------	250	77	260	9	9	3.0	3.6	1.2
	Spaghetti (enriched) with meat-balls and tomato sauce:									
643	Canned----------------------	1 cup----------	250	78	260	12	10	2.4	3.9	3.1
644	From home recipe-------------	1 cup----------	248	70	330	19	12	3.9	4.4	2.2
	Fast food entrees:									
	Cheeseburger:									
645	Regular---------------------	1 sandwich------	112	46	300	15	15	7.3	5.6	1.0
646	4 oz patty------------------	1 sandwich------	194	46	525	30	31	15.1	12.2	1.4
	Chicken, fried. See Poultry and Poultry Products (items 656-659).									
647	Enchilada-------------------	1 enchilada-----	230	72	235	20	16	7.7	6.7	0.6
648	English muffin, egg, cheese, and bacon-------------------	1 sandwich------	138	49	360	18	18	8.0	8.0	0.7
	Fish sandwich:									
649	Regular, with cheese---------	1 sandwich------	140	43	420	16	23	6.3	6.9	7.7
650	Large, without cheese--------	1 sandwich------	170	48	470	18	27	6.3	8.7	9.5
	Hamburger:									
651	Regular---------------------	1 sandwich------	98	46	245	12	11	4.4	5.3	0.5
652	4 oz patty------------------	1 sandwich------	174	50	445	25	21	7.1	11.7	0.6
653	Pizza, cheese, 1/8 of 15-in diam. pizza[51] ----------------	1 slice---------	120	46	290	15	9	4.1	2.6	1.3
654	Roast beef sandwich-----------	1 sandwich------	150	52	345	22	13	3.5	6.9	1.8
655	Taco-------------------------	1 taco---------	81	55	195	9	11	4.1	5.5	0.8

[38] Made with margarine.
[51] Crust made with vegetable shortening and enriched flour.

Nutrients in Indicated Quantity

Cholesterol	Carbohydrate	Calcium	Phosphorus	Iron	Potassium	Sodium	Vitamin A value		Thiamin	Riboflavin	Niacin	Ascorbic acid	Item No.
							(IU)	(RE)					
Milligrams	Grams	Milligrams	Milligrams	Milligrams	Milligrams	Milligrams	International units	Retinol equivalents	Milligrams	Milligrams	Milligrams	Milligrams	
71	15	29	184	2.9	613	292	5,690	568	0.15	0.17	4.7	17	629
42	39	29	149	3.8	334	596	4,220	517	0.29	0.29	4.8	6	630
221	12	127	358	2.5	404	760	1,130	272	0.10	0.42	5.4	12	631
103	26	26	247	2.2	149	600	430	130	0.05	0.17	4.3	Tr	632
8	18	45	85	1.3	418	725	150	28	0.05	0.10	1.0	13	633
75	10	58	293	2.5	473	718	280	50	0.08	0.23	4.3	10	634
56	42	70	232	3.0	343	594	7,220	735	0.32	0.32	4.9	5	635
28	31	82	321	4.3	594	1,354	150	15	0.08	0.18	3.3	8	636
68	13	60	248	4.8	425	1,053	600	60	0.28	0.38	5.0	33	637
24	26	199	182	1.0	139	730	260	72	0.12	0.24	1.0	Tr	638
44	40	362	322	1.8	240	1,086	860	232	0.20	0.40	1.8	1	639
285	29	211	276	1.0	283	653	1,640	454	0.11	0.32	Tr	Tr	640
3	39	40	88	2.8	303	955	930	120	0.35	0.28	4.5	10	641
8	37	80	135	2.3	408	955	1,080	140	0.25	0.18	2.3	13	642
23	29	53	113	3.3	245	1,220	1,000	100	0.15	0.18	2.3	5	643
89	39	124	236	3.7	665	1,009	1,590	159	0.25	0.30	4.0	22	644
44	28	135	174	2.3	219	672	340	65	0.26	0.24	3.7	1	645
104	40	236	320	4.5	407	1,224	670	128	0.33	0.48	7.4	3	646
19	24	97	198	3.3	653	1,332	2,720	352	0.18	0.26	Tr	Tr	647
213	31	197	290	3.1	201	832	650	160	0.46	0.50	3.7	1	648
56	39	132	223	1.8	274	667	160	25	0.32	0.26	3.3	2	649
91	41	61	246	2.2	375	621	110	15	0.35	0.23	3.5	1	650
32	28	56	107	2.2	202	463	80	14	0.23	0.24	3.8	1	651
71	38	75	225	4.8	404	763	160	28	0.38	0.38	7.8	1	652
56	39	220	216	1.6	230	699	750	106	0.34	0.29	4.2	2	653
55	34	60	222	4.0	338	757	240	32	0.40	0.33	6.0	2	654
21	15	109	134	1.2	263	456	420	57	0.09	0.07	1.4	1	655

[52]Made with corn oil.

Item No.	Foods, approximate measures, units, and weight (weight of edible portion only)		Water	Food energy	Pro-tein	Fat	Fatty acids		
							Satu-rated	Mono-unsatu-rated	Poly-unsatu-rated
	Poultry and Poultry Products	Grams	Per-cent	Cal-ories	Grams	Grams	Grams	Grams	Grams
	Chicken:								
	Fried, flesh, with skin:[53]								
	Batter dipped:								
656	Breast, 1/2 breast (5.6 oz with bones)-------------- 4.9 oz----------	140	52	365	35	18	4.9	7.6	4.3
657	Drumstick (3.4 oz with bones)------------------- 2.5 oz----------	72	53	195	16	11	3.0	4.6	2.7
	Flour coated:								
658	Breast, 1/2 breast (4.2 oz with bones)-------------- 3.5 oz----------	98	57	220	31	9	2.4	3.4	1.9
659	Drumstick (2.6 oz with bones)------------------- 1.7 oz----------	49	57	120	13	7	1.8	2.7	1.6
	Roasted, flesh only:								
660	Breast, 1/2 breast (4.2 oz with bones and skin)------- 3.0 oz----------	86	65	140	27	3	0.9	1.1	0.7
661	Drumstick, (2.9 oz with bones and skin)----------------- 1.6 oz----------	44	67	75	12	2	0.7	0.8	0.6
662	Stewed, flesh only, light and dark meat, chopped or diced-- 1 cup----------	140	67	250	38	9	2.6	3.3	2.2
663	Chicken liver, cooked------------ 1 liver--------	20	68	30	5	1	0.4	0.3	0.2
664	Duck, roasted, flesh only-------- 1/2 duck--------	221	64	445	52	25	9.2	8.2	3.2
	Turkey, roasted, flesh only:								
665	Dark meat, piece, 2-1/2 by 1-5/8 by 1/4 in-------------- 4 pieces--------	85	63	160	24	6	2.1	1.4	1.8
666	Light meat, piece, 4 by 2 by 1/4 in---------------------- 2 pieces--------	85	66	135	25	3	0.9	0.5	0.7
	Light and dark meat:								
667	Chopped or diced------------- 1 cup----------	140	65	240	41	7	2.3	1.4	2.0
668	Pieces (1 slice white meat, 4 by 2 by 1/4 in and 2 slices dark meat, 2-1/2 by 1-5/8 by 1/4 in)------- 3 pieces--------	85	65	145	25	4	1.4	0.9	1.2
	Poultry food products:								
	Chicken:								
669	Canned, boneless------------- 5 oz------------	142	69	235	31	11	3.1	4.5	2.5
670	Frankfurter (10 per 1-lb pkg) 1 frankfurter---	45	58	115	6	9	2.5	3.8	1.8
671	Roll, light (6 slices per 6 oz pkg)-------------------- 2 slices--------	57	69	90	11	4	1.1	1.7	0.9
	Turkey:								
672	Gravy and turkey, frozen----- 5-oz package----	142	85	95	8	4	1.2	1.4	0.7
673	Ham, cured turkey thigh meat (8 slices per 8-oz pkg)---- 2 slices--------	57	71	75	11	3	1.0	0.7	0.9
674	Loaf, breast meat (8 slices per 6-oz pkg)-------------- 2 slices--------	42	72	45	10	1	0.2	0.2	0.1
675	Patties, breaded, battered, fried (2.25 oz)------------ 1 patty---------	64	50	180	9	12	3.0	4.8	3.0
676	Roast, boneless, frozen, sea-soned, light and dark meat, cooked-------------------- 3 oz------------	85	68	130	18	5	1.6	1.0	1.4
	Soups, Sauces, and Gravies								
	Soups:								
	Canned, condensed:								
	Prepared with equal volume of milk:								
677	Clam chowder, New England-- 1 cup----------	248	85	165	9	7	3.0	2.3	1.1
678	Cream of chicken---------- 1 cup----------	248	85	190	7	11	4.6	4.5	1.6
679	Cream of mushroom--------- 1 cup----------	248	85	205	6	14	5.1	3.0	4.6
680	Tomato-------------------- 1 cup----------	248	85	160	6	6	2.9	1.6	1.1

[53] Fried in vegetable shortening.

Nutrients in Indicated Quantity

Cholesterol	Carbohydrate	Calcium	Phosphorus	Iron	Potassium	Sodium	Vitamin A value		Thiamin	Riboflavin	Niacin	Ascorbic acid	Item No.
							(IU)	(RE)					
Milligrams	Grams	Milligrams	Milligrams	Milligrams	Milligrams	Milligrams	International units	Retinol equivalents	Milligrams	Milligrams	Milligrams	Milligrams	
119	13	28	259	1.8	281	385	90	28	0.16	0.20	14.7	0	656
62	6	12	106	1.0	134	194	60	19	0.08	0.15	3.7	0	657
87	2	16	228	1.2	254	74	50	15	0.08	0.13	13.5	0	658
44	1	6	86	0.7	112	44	40	12	0.04	0.11	3.0	0	659
73	0	13	196	0.9	220	64	20	5	0.06	0.10	11.8	0	660
41	0	5	81	0.6	108	42	30	8	0.03	0.10	2.7	0	661
116	0	20	210	1.6	252	98	70	21	0.07	0.23	8.6	0	662
126	Tr	3	62	1.7	28	10	3,270	983	0.03	0.35	0.9	3	663
197	0	27	449	6.0	557	144	170	51	0.57	1.04	11.3	0	664
72	0	27	173	2.0	246	67	0	0	0.05	0.21	3.1	0	665
59	0	16	186	1.1	259	54	0	0	0.05	0.11	5.8	0	666
106	0	35	298	2.5	417	98	0	0	0.09	0.25	7.6	0	667
65	0	21	181	1.5	253	60	0	0	0.05	0.15	4.6	0	668
88	0	20	158	2.2	196	714	170	48	0.02	0.18	9.0	3	669
45	3	43	48	0.9	38	616	60	17	0.03	0.05	1.4	0	670
28	1	24	89	0.6	129	331	50	14	0.04	0.07	3.0	0	671
26	7	20	115	1.3	87	787	60	18	0.03	0.18	2.6	0	672
32	Tr	6	108	1.6	184	565	0	0	0.03	0.14	2.0	0	673
17	0	3	97	0.2	118	608	0	0	0.02	0.05	3.5	[54]0	674
40	10	9	173	1.4	176	512	20	7	0.06	0.12	1.5	0	675
45	3	4	207	1.4	253	578	0	0	0.04	0.14	5.3	0	676
22	17	186	156	1.5	300	992	160	40	0.07	0.24	1.0	3	677
27	15	181	151	0.7	273	1,047	710	94	0.07	0.26	0.9	1	678
20	15	179	156	0.6	270	1,076	150	37	0.08	0.28	0.9	2	679
17	22	159	149	1.8	449	932	850	109	0.13	0.25	1.5	68	680

[54]If sodium ascorbate is added, product contains 11 mg ascorbic acid.

Item No.	Foods, approximate measures, units, and weight (weight of edible portion only)		Grams	Water	Food energy	Pro-tein	Fat	Fatty acids		
								Saturated	Mono-unsaturated	Poly-unsaturated
			Grams	Percent	Calories	Grams	Grams	Grams	Grams	Grams
	Soups, Sauces, and Gravies—Con.									
	Soups:									
	Canned, condensed:									
	Prepared with equal volume of water:									
681	Bean with bacon-----------	1 cup----------	253	84	170	8	6	1.5	2.2	1.8
682	Beef broth, bouillon, consomme-----------------	1 cup----------	240	98	15	3	1	0.3	0.2	Tr
683	Beef noodle---------------	1 cup----------	244	92	85	5	3	1.1	1.2	0.5
684	Chicken noodle------------	1 cup----------	241	92	75	4	2	0.7	1.1	0.6
685	Chicken rice--------------	1 cup----------	241	94	60	4	2	0.5	0.9	0.4
686	Clam chowder, Manhattan----	1 cup----------	244	90	80	4	2	0.4	0.4	1.3
687	Cream of chicken----------	1 cup----------	244	91	115	3	7	2.1	3.3	1.5
688	Cream of mushroom---------	1 cup----------	244	90	130	2	9	2.4	1.7	4.2
689	Minestrone----------------	1 cup----------	241	91	80	4	3	0.6	0.7	1.1
690	Pea, green----------------	1 cup----------	250	83	165	9	3	1.4	1.0	0.4
691	Tomato--------------------	1 cup----------	244	90	85	2	2	0.4	0.4	1.0
692	Vegetable beef------------	1 cup----------	244	92	80	6	2	0.9	0.8	0.1
693	Vegetarian----------------	1 cup----------	241	92	70	2	2	0.3	0.8	0.7
	Dehydrated:									
	Unprepared:									
694	Bouillon------------------	1 pkt----------	6	3	15	1	1	0.3	0.2	Tr
695	Onion---------------------	1 pkt----------	7	4	20	1	Tr	0.1	0.2	Tr
	Prepared with water:									
696	Chicken noodle------------	1 pkt (6-fl-oz)	188	94	40	2	1	0.2	0.4	0.3
697	Onion---------------------	1 pkt (6-fl-oz)	184	96	20	1	Tr	0.1	0.2	0.1
698	Tomato vegetable----------	1 pkt (6-fl-oz)	189	94	40	1	1	0.3	0.2	0.1
	Sauces:									
	From dry mix:									
699	Cheese, prepared with milk---	1 cup----------	279	77	305	16	17	9.3	5.3	1.6
700	Hollandaise, prepared with water--------------------	1 cup----------	259	84	240	5	20	11.6	5.9	0.9
701	White sauce, prepared with milk---------------------	1 cup----------	264	81	240	10	13	6.4	4.7	1.7
	From home recipe:									
702	White sauce, medium[55]--------	1 cup----------	250	73	395	10	30	9.1	11.9	7.2
	Ready to serve:									
703	Barbecue-------------------	1 tbsp---------	16	81	10	Tr	Tr	Tr	0.1	0.1
704	Soy------------------------	1 tbsp---------	18	68	10	2	0	0.0	0.0	0.0
	Gravies:									
	Canned:									
705	Beef----------------------	1 cup----------	233	87	125	9	5	2.7	2.3	0.2
706	Chicken-------------------	1 cup----------	238	85	190	5	14	3.4	6.1	3.6
707	Mushroom------------------	1 cup----------	238	89	120	3	6	1.0	2.8	2.4
	From dry mix:									
708	Brown---------------------	1 cup----------	261	91	80	3	2	0.9	0.8	0.1
709	Chicken-------------------	1 cup----------	260	91	85	3	2	0.5	0.9	0.4
	Sugars and Sweets									
	Candy:									
710	Caramels, plain or chocolate---	1 oz-----------	28	8	115	1	3	2.2	0.3	0.1
	Chocolate:									
711	Milk, plain------------------	1 oz-----------	28	1	145	2	9	5.4	3.0	0.3
712	Milk, with almonds-----------	1 oz-----------	28	2	150	3	10	4.8	4.1	0.7
713	Milk, with peanuts-----------	1 oz-----------	28	1	155	4	11	4.2	3.5	1.5
714	Milk, with rice cereal-------	1 oz-----------	28	2	140	2	7	4.4	2.5	0.2
715	Semisweet, small pieces (60 per oz)-------------------	1 cup or 6 oz---	170	1	860	7	61	36.2	19.9	1.9
716	Sweet (dark)-----------------	1 oz-----------	28	1	150	1	10	5.9	3.3	0.3
717	Fondant, uncoated (mints, candy corn, other)-------------	1 oz-----------	28	3	105	Tr	0	0.0	0.0	0.0
718	Fudge, chocolate, plain--------	1 oz-----------	28	8	115	1	3	2.1	1.0	0.1
719	Gum drops--------------------	1 oz-----------	28	12	100	Tr	Tr	Tr	Tr	0.1

[55] Made with enriched flour, margarine, and whole milk.

Nutrients in Indicated Quantity

Cho-les-terol	Carbo-hydrate	Calcium	Phos-phorus	Iron	Potas-sium	Sodium	Vitamin A value		Thiamin	Ribo-flavin	Niacin	Ascorbic acid	Item No.
							(IU)	(RE)					
Milli-grams	Grams	Milli-grams	Milli-grams	Milli-grams	Milli-grams	Milli-grams	Inter-national units	Retinol equiva-lents	Milli-grams	Milli-grams	Milli-grams	Milli-grams	
3	23	81	132	2.0	402	951	890	89	0.09	0.03	0.6	2	681
Tr	Tr	14	31	0.4	130	782	0	0	Tr	0.05	1.9	0	682
5	9	15	46	1.1	100	952	630	63	0.07	0.06	1.1	Tr	683
7	9	17	36	0.8	55	1,106	710	71	0.05	0.06	1.4	Tr	684
7	7	17	22	0.7	101	815	660	66	0.02	0.02	1.1	Tr	685
2	12	34	59	1.9	261	1,808	920	92	0.06	0.05	1.3	3	686
10	9	34	37	0.6	88	986	560	56	0.03	0.06	0.8	Tr	687
2	9	46	49	0.5	100	1,032	0	0	0.05	0.09	0.7	1	688
2	11	34	55	0.9	313	911	2,340	234	0.05	0.04	0.9	1	689
0	27	28	125	2.0	190	988	200	20	0.11	0.07	1.2	2	690
0	17	12	34	1.8	264	871	690	69	0.09	0.05	1.4	66	691
5	10	17	41	1.1	173	956	1,890	189	0.04	0.05	1.0	2	692
0	12	22	34	1.1	210	822	3,010	301	0.05	0.05	0.9	1	693
1	1	4	19	0.1	27	1,019	Tr	Tr	Tr	0.01	0.3	0	694
Tr	4	10	23	0.1	47	627	Tr	Tr	0.02	0.04	0.4	Tr	695
2	6	24	24	0.4	23	957	50	5	0.05	0.04	0.7	Tr	696
0	4	9	22	0.1	48	635	Tr	Tr	0.02	0.04	0.4	Tr	697
0	8	6	23	0.5	78	856	140	14	0.04	0.03	0.6	5	698
53	23	569	438	0.3	552	1,565	390	117	0.15	0.56	0.3	2	699
52	14	124	127	0.9	124	1,564	730	220	0.05	0.18	0.1	Tr	700
34	21	425	256	0.3	444	797	310	92	0.08	0.45	0.5	3	701
32	24	292	238	0.9	381	888	1,190	340	0.15	0.43	0.8	2	702
0	2	3	3	0.1	28	130	140	14	Tr	Tr	0.1	1	703
0	2	3	38	0.5	64	1,029	0	0	0.01	0.02	0.6	0	704
7	11	14	70	1.6	189	117	0	0	0.07	0.08	1.5	0	705
5	13	48	69	1.1	259	1,373	880	264	0.04	0.10	1.1	0	706
0	13	17	36	1.6	252	1,357	0	0	0.08	0.15	1.6	0	707
2	14	66	47	0.2	61	1,147	0	0	0.04	0.09	0.9	0	708
3	14	39	47	0.3	62	1,134	0	0	0.05	0.15	0.8	3	709
1	22	42	35	0.4	54	64	Tr	Tr	0.01	0.05	0.1	Tr	710
6	16	50	61	0.4	96	23	30	10	0.02	0.10	0.1	Tr	711
5	15	65	77	0.5	125	23	30	8	0.02	0.12	0.2	Tr	712
5	13	49	83	0.4	138	19	30	8	0.07	0.07	1.4	Tr	713
6	18	48	57	0.2	100	46	30	8	0.01	0.08	0.1	Tr	714
0	97	51	178	5.8	593	24	30	3	0.10	0.14	0.9	Tr	715
0	16	7	41	0.6	86	5	10	1	0.01	0.04	0.1	Tr	716
0	27	2	Tr	0.1	1	57	0	0	Tr	Tr	Tr	0	717
1	21	22	24	0.3	42	54	Tr	Tr	0.01	0.03	0.1	Tr	718
0	25	2	Tr	0.1	1	10	0	0	0.00	Tr	Tr	0	719

Item No.	Foods, approximate measures, units, and weight (weight of edible portion only)		Water	Food energy	Pro-tein	Fat	Fatty acids Satu-rated	Mono-unsatu-rated	Poly-unsatu-rated
		Grams	Per-cent	Cal-ories	Grams	Grams	Grams	Grams	Grams
	Sugars and Sweets—Con.								
	Candy:								
720	Hard----------------------------	1 oz------------	28	1	110	0	0	0.0	0.0	0.0
721	Jelly beans---------------------	1 oz------------	28	6	105	Tr	Tr	Tr	Tr	0.1
722	Marshmallows--------------------	1 oz------------	28	17	90	1	0	0.0	0.0	0.0
723	Custard, baked------------------	1 cup-----------	265	77	305	14	15	6.8	5.4	0.7
724	Gelatin dessert prepared with gelatin dessert powder and water------------------------	1/2 cup---------	120	84	70	2	0	0.0	0.0	0.0
725	Honey, strained or extracted-----	1 cup-----------	339	17	1,030	1	0	0.0	0.0	0.0
726		1 tbsp----------	21	17	65	Tr	0	0.0	0.0	0.0
727	Jams and preserves--------------	1 tbsp----------	20	29	55	Tr	Tr	0.0	Tr	Tr
728		1 packet-------	14	29	40	Tr	Tr	0.0	Tr	Tr
729	Jellies-------------------------	1 tbsp----------	18	28	50	Tr	Tr	Tr	Tr	Tr
730		1 packet-------	14	28	40	Tr	Tr	Tr	Tr	Tr
731	Popsicle, 3-fl-oz size----------	1 popsicle------	95	80	70	0	0	0.0	0.0	0.0
	Puddings:								
	Canned:								
732	Chocolate------------------	5-oz can--------	142	68	205	3	11	9.5	0.5	0.1
733	Tapioca--------------------	5-oz can--------	142	74	160	3	5	4.8	Tr	Tr
734	Vanilla--------------------	5-oz can--------	142	69	220	2	10	9.5	0.2	0.1
	Dry mix, prepared with whole milk:								
	Chocolate:								
735	Instant-------------------	1/2 cup---------	130	71	155	4	4	2.3	1.1	0.2
736	Regular (cooked)-----------	1/2 cup---------	130	73	150	4	4	2.4	1.1	0.1
737	Rice----------------------	1/2 cup---------	132	73	155	4	4	2.3	1.1	0.1
738	Tapioca-------------------	1/2 cup---------	130	75	145	4	4	2.3	1.1	0.1
	Vanilla:								
739	Instant-------------------	1/2 cup---------	130	73	150	4	4	2.2	1.1	0.2
740	Regular (cooked)-----------	1/2 cup---------	130	74	145	4	4	2.3	1.0	0.1
	Sugars:								
741	Brown, pressed down-----------	1 cup-----------	220	2	820	0	0	0.0	0.0	0.0
	White:								
742	Granulated-----------------	1 cup-----------	200	1	770	0	0	0.0	0.0	0.0
743		1 tbsp----------	12	1	45	0	0	0.0	0.0	0.0
744		1 packet-------	6	1	25	0	0	0.0	0.0	0.0
745	Powdered, sifted, spooned into cup------------------	1 cup-----------	100	1	385	0	0	0.0	0.0	0.0
	Syrups:								
	Chocolate-flavored syrup or topping:								
746	Thin type------------------	2 tbsp----------	38	37	85	1	Tr	0.2	0.1	0.1
747	Fudge type-----------------	2 tbsp----------	38	25	125	2	5	3.1	1.7	0.2
748	Molasses, cane, blackstrap-----	2 tbsp----------	40	24	85	0	0	0.0	0.0	0.0
749	Table syrup (corn and maple)---	2 tbsp----------	42	25	122	0	0	0.0	0.0	0.0
	Vegetables and Vegetable Products								
750	Alfalfa seeds, sprouted, raw-----	1 cup-----------	33	91	10	1	Tr	Tr	Tr	0.1
751	Artichokes, globe or French, cooked, drained---------------	1 artichoke-----	120	87	55	3	Tr	Tr	Tr	0.1
	Asparagus, green:								
	Cooked, drained:								
	From raw:								
752	Cuts and tips--------------	1 cup-----------	180	92	45	5	1	0.1	Tr	0.2
753	Spears, 1/2-in diam. at base---------------------	4 spears--------	60	92	15	2	Tr	Tr	Tr	0.1
	From frozen:								
754	Cuts and tips--------------	1 cup-----------	180	91	50	5	1	0.2	Tr	0.3
755	Spears, 1/2-in diam. at base---------------------	4 spears--------	60	91	15	2	Tr	0.1	Tr	0.1
756	Canned, spears, 1/2-in diam. at base-------------------	4 spears--------	80	95	10	1	Tr	Tr	Tr	0.1
757	Bamboo shoots, canned, drained---	1 cup-----------	131	94	25	2	1	0.1	Tr	0.2

[56] For regular pack; special dietary pack contains 3 mg sodium.

Cholesterol	Carbohydrate	Calcium	Phosphorus	Iron	Potassium	Sodium	Vitamin A value (IU)	(RE)	Thiamin	Riboflavin	Niacin	Ascorbic acid	Item No.
Milligrams	Grams	Milligrams	Milligrams	Milligrams	Milligrams	Milligrams	International units	Retinol equivalents	Milligrams	Milligrams	Milligrams	Milligrams	
0	28	Tr	2	0.1	1	7	0	0	0.10	0.00	0.0	0	720
0	26	1	1	0.3	11	7	0	0	0.00	Tr	Tr	0	721
0	23	1	2	0.5	2	25	0	0	0.00	Tr	Tr	0	722
278	29	297	310	1.1	387	209	530	146	0.11	0.50	0.3	1	723
0	17	2	23	Tr	Tr	55	0	0	0.00	0.00	0.0	0	724
0	279	17	20	1.7	173	17	0	0	0.02	0.14	1.0	3	725
0	17	1	1	0.1	11	1	0	0	Tr	0.01	0.1	Tr	726
0	14	4	2	0.2	18	2	Tr	Tr	Tr	0.01	Tr	Tr	727
0	10	3	1	0.1	12	2	Tr	Tr	Tr	Tr	Tr	Tr	728
0	13	2	Tr	0.1	16	5	Tr	Tr	Tr	0.01	Tr	1	729
0	10	1	Tr	Tr	13	4	Tr	Tr	Tr	Tr	Tr	1	730
0	18	0	0	Tr	4	11	0	0	0.00	0.00	0.0	0	731
1	30	74	117	1.2	254	285	100	31	0.04	0.17	0.6	Tr	732
Tr	28	119	113	0.3	212	252	Tr	Tr	0.03	0.14	0.4	Tr	733
1	33	79	94	0.2	155	305	Tr	Tr	0.03	0.12	0.6	Tr	734
14	27	130	329	0.3	176	440	130	33	0.04	0.18	0.1	1	735
15	25	146	120	0.2	190	167	140	34	0.05	0.20	0.1	1	736
15	27	133	110	0.5	165	140	140	33	0.10	0.18	0.6	1	737
15	25	131	103	0.1	167	152	140	34	0.04	0.18	0.1	1	738
15	27	129	273	0.1	164	375	140	33	0.04	0.17	0.1	1	739
15	25	132	102	0.1	166	178	140	34	0.04	0.18	0.1	1	740
0	212	187	56	4.8	757	97	0	0	0.02	0.07	0.2	0	741
0	199	3	Tr	0.1	7	5	0	0	0.00	0.00	0.0	0	742
0	12	Tr	Tr	Tr	Tr	Tr	0	0	0.00	0.00	0.0	0	743
0	6	Tr	Tr	Tr	Tr	Tr	0	0	0.00	0.00	0.0	0	744
0	100	1	Tr	Tr	4	2	0	0	0.00	0.00	0.0	0	745
0	22	6	49	0.8	85	36	Tr	Tr	Tr	0.02	0.1	0	746
0	21	38	60	0.5	82	42	40	13	0.02	0.08	0.1	0	747
0	22	274	34	10.1	1,171	38	0	0	0.04	0.08	0.8	0	748
0	32	1	4	Tr	7	19	0	0	0.00	0.00	0.0	0	749
0	1	11	23	0.3	26	2	50	5	0.03	0.04	0.2	3	750
0	12	47	72	1.6	316	79	170	17	0.07	0.06	0.7	9	751
0	8	43	110	1.2	558	7	1,490	149	0.18	0.22	1.9	49	752
0	3	14	37	0.4	186	2	500	50	0.06	0.07	0.6	16	753
0	9	41	99	1.2	392	7	1,470	147	0.12	0.19	1.9	44	754
0	3	14	33	0.4	131	2	490	49	0.04	0.06	0.6	15	755
0	2	11	30	0.5	122	[56]278	380	38	0.04	0.07	0.7	13	756
0	4	10	33	0.4	105	9	10	1	0.03	0.03	0.2	1	757

Item No.	Foods, approximate measures, units, and weight (weight of edible portion only)		Grams	Water	Food energy	Pro-tein	Fat	Fatty acids		
								Saturated	Mono-unsaturated	Poly-unsaturated
	Vegetables and Vegetable Products—Con.		Grams	Percent	Calories	Grams	Grams	Grams	Grams	Grams
	Beans:									
	Lima, immature seeds, frozen, cooked, drained:									
758	Thick-seeded types (Ford-hooks)---------------------	1 cup-----------	170	74	170	10	1	0.1	Tr	0.3
759	Thin-seeded types (baby limas)---------------------	1 cup-----------	180	72	190	12	1	0.1	Tr	0.3
	Snap:									
	Cooked, drained:									
760	From raw (cut and French style)------------------	1 cup-----------	125	89	45	2	Tr	0.1	Tr	0.2
761	From frozen (cut)----------	1 cup-----------	135	92	35	2	Tr	Tr	Tr	0.1
762	Canned, drained solids (cut)	1 cup-----------	135	93	25	2	Tr	Tr	Tr	0.1
	Beans, mature. See Beans, dry (items 527-535) and Black-eyed peas, dry (item 536).									
	Bean sprouts (mung):									
763	Raw-----------------------	1 cup-----------	104	90	30	3	Tr	Tr	Tr	0.1
764	Cooked, drained----------------	1 cup-----------	124	93	25	3	Tr	Tr	Tr	Tr
	Beets:									
	Cooked, drained:									
765	Diced or sliced--------------	1 cup-----------	170	91	55	2	Tr	Tr	Tr	Tr
766	Whole beets, 2-in diam.------	2 beets---------	100	91	30	1	Tr	Tr	Tr	Tr
767	Canned, drained solids, diced or sliced-------------------	1 cup-----------	170	91	55	2	Tr	Tr	Tr	0.1
768	Beet greens, leaves and stems, cooked, drained-------------	1 cup-----------	144	89	40	4	Tr	Tr	0.1	0.1
	Black-eyed peas, immature seeds, cooked and drained:									
769	From raw-----------------	1 cup-----------	165	72	180	13	1	0.3	0.1	0.6
770	From frozen-----------------	1 cup-----------	170	66	225	14	1	0.3	0.1	0.5
	Broccoli:									
771	Raw----------------------	1 spear---------	151	91	40	4	1	0.1	Tr	0.3
	Cooked, drained:									
	From raw:									
772	Spear, medium--------------	1 spear---------	180	90	50	5	1	0.1	Tr	0.2
773	Spears, cut into 1/2-in pieces------------------	1 cup-----------	155	90	45	5	Tr	0.1	Tr	0.2
	From frozen:									
774	Piece, 4-1/2 to 5 in long--	1 piece---------	30	91	10	1	Tr	Tr	Tr	Tr
775	Chopped--------------------	1 cup-----------	185	91	50	6	Tr	Tr	Tr	0.1
	Brussels sprouts, cooked, drained:									
776	From raw, 7-8 sprouts, 1-1/4 to 1-1/2-in diam.-----------	1 cup-----------	155	87	60	4	1	0.2	0.1	0.4
777	From frozen---------------	1 cup-----------	155	87	65	6	1	0.1	Tr	0.3
	Cabbage, common varieties:									
778	Raw, coarsely shredded or sliced----------------------	1 cup-----------	70	93	15	1	Tr	Tr	Tr	0.1
779	Cooked, drained---------------	1 cup-----------	150	94	30	1	Tr	Tr	Tr	0.2
	Cabbage, Chinese:									
780	Pak-choi, cooked, drained------	1 cup-----------	170	96	20	3	Tr	Tr	Tr	0.1
781	Pe-tsai, raw, 1-in pieces------	1 cup-----------	76	94	10	1	Tr	Tr	Tr	0.1
782	Cabbage, red, raw, coarsely shredded or sliced------------	1 cup-----------	70	92	20	1	Tr	Tr	Tr	0.1
783	Cabbage, savoy, raw, coarsely shredded or sliced------------	1 cup-----------	70	91	20	1	Tr	Tr	Tr	Tr

[57] For green varieties; yellow varieties contain 101 IU or 10 RE.
[58] For green varieties; yellow varieties contain 151 IU or 15 RE.
[59] For regular pack; special dietary pack contains 3 mg sodium.

Nutrients in Indicated Quantity

Cho-les-terol	Carbo-hydrate	Calcium	Phos-phorus	Iron	Potas-sium	Sodium	Vitamin A value (IU)	Vitamin A value (RE)	Thiamin	Ribo-flavin	Niacin	Ascorbic acid	Item No.
Milli-grams	Grams	Milli-grams	Milli-grams	Milli-grams	Milli-grams	Milli-grams	Inter-national units	Retinol equiva-lents	Milli-grams	Milli-grams	Milli-grams	Milli-grams	
0	32	37	107	2.3	694	90	320	32	0.13	0.10	1.8	22	758
0	35	50	202	3.5	740	52	300	30	0.13	0.10	1.4	10	759
0	10	58	49	1.6	374	4	[57]830	[57]83	0.09	0.12	0.8	12	760
0	8	61	32	1.1	151	18	[58]710	[58]71	0.06	0.10	0.6	11	761
0	6	35	26	1.2	147	[59]339	[60]470	[60]47	0.02	0.08	0.3	6	762
0	6	14	56	0.9	155	6	20	2	0.09	0.13	0.8	14	763
0	5	15	35	0.8	125	12	20	2	0.06	0.13	1.0	14	764
0	11	19	53	1.1	530	83	20	2	0.05	0.02	0.5	9	765
0	7	11	31	0.6	312	49	10	1	0.03	0.01	0.3	6	766
0	12	26	29	3.1	252	[61]466	20	2	0.02	0.07	0.3	7	767
0	8	164	59	2.7	1,309	347	7,340	734	0.17	0.42	0.7	36	768
0	30	46	196	2.4	693	7	1,050	105	0.11	0.18	1.8	3	769
0	40	39	207	3.6	638	9	130	13	0.44	0.11	1.2	4	770
0	8	72	100	1.3	491	41	2,330	233	0.10	0.18	1.0	141	771
0	10	205	86	2.1	293	20	2,540	254	0.15	0.37	1.4	113	772
0	9	177	74	1.8	253	17	2,180	218	0.13	0.32	1.2	97	773
0	2	15	17	0.2	54	7	570	57	0.02	0.02	0.1	12	774
0	10	94	102	1.1	333	44	3,500	350	0.10	0.15	0.8	74	775
0	13	56	87	1.9	491	33	1,110	111	0.17	0.12	0.9	96	776
0	13	37	84	1.1	504	36	910	91	0.16	0.18	0.8	71	777
0	4	33	16	0.4	172	13	90	9	0.04	0.02	0.2	33	778
0	7	50	38	0.6	308	29	130	13	0.09	0.08	0.3	36	779
0	3	158	49	1.8	631	58	4,370	437	0.05	0.11	0.7	44	780
0	2	59	22	0.2	181	7	910	91	0.03	0.04	0.3	21	781
0	4	36	29	0.3	144	8	30	3	0.04	0.02	0.2	40	782
0	4	25	29	0.3	161	20	700	70	0.05	0.02	0.2	22	783

[60] For green varieties; yellow varieties contain 142 IU or 14 RE.
[61] For regular pack; special dietary pack contains 78 mg sodium.

Item No.	Foods, approximate measures, units, and weight (weight of edible portion only)			Water	Food energy	Pro-tein	Fat	Fatty acids		
								Saturated	Mono-unsaturated	Poly-unsaturated
	Vegetables and Vegetable Products—Con.		Grams	Per-cent	Cal-ories	Grams	Grams	Grams	Grams	Grams
	Carrots:									
	Raw, without crowns and tips, scraped:									
784	Whole, 7-1/2 by 1-1/8 in, or strips, 2-1/2 to 3 in long	1 carrot or 18 strips--------	72	88	30	1	Tr	Tr	Tr	0.1
785	Grated----------------------	1 cup-----------	110	88	45	1	Tr	Tr	Tr	0.1
	Cooked, sliced, drained:									
786	From raw---------------------	1 cup-----------	156	87	70	2	Tr	0.1	Tr	0.1
787	From frozen-----------------	1 cup-----------	146	90	55	2	Tr	Tr	Tr	0.1
788	Canned, sliced, drained solids	1 cup-----------	146	93	35	1	Tr	0.1	Tr	0.1
	Cauliflower:									
789	Raw, (flowerets)---------------	1 cup-----------	100	92	25	2	Tr	Tr	Tr	0.1
	Cooked, drained:									
790	From raw (flowerets)---------	1 cup-----------	125	93	30	2	Tr	Tr	Tr	0.1
791	From frozen (flowerets)------	1 cup-----------	180	94	35	3	Tr	0.1	Tr	0.2
	Celery, pascal type, raw:									
792	Stalk, large outer, 8 by 1-1/2 in (at root end)-------------	1 stalk---------	40	95	5	Tr	Tr	Tr	Tr	Tr
793	Pieces, diced------------------	1 cup-----------	120	95	20	1	Tr	Tr	Tr	0.1
	Collards, cooked, drained:									
794	From raw (leaves without stems)	1 cup-----------	190	96	25	2	Tr	0.1	Tr	0.2
795	From frozen (chopped)----------	1 cup-----------	170	88	60	5	1	0.1	0.1	0.4
	Corn, sweet:									
	Cooked, drained:									
796	From raw, ear 5 by 1-3/4 in--	1 ear-----------	77	70	85	3	1	0.2	0.3	0.5
	From frozen:									
797	Ear, trimmed to about 3-1/2 in long------------------	1 ear-----------	63	73	60	2	Tr	0.1	0.1	0.2
798	Kernels-------------------	1 cup-----------	165	76	135	5	Tr	Tr	Tr	0.1
	Canned:									
799	Cream style------------------	1 cup-----------	256	79	185	4	1	0.2	0.3	0.5
800	Whole kernel, vacuum pack----	1 cup-----------	210	77	165	5	1	0.2	0.3	0.5
	Cowpeas. See Black-eyed peas, immature (items 769,770), mature (item 536).									
801	Cucumber, with peel, slices, 1/8 in thick (large, 2-1/8-in diam.; small, 1-3/4-in diam.)--	6 large or 8 small slices	28	96	5	Tr	Tr	Tr	Tr	Tr
802	Dandelion greens, cooked, drained	1 cup-----------	105	90	35	2	1	0.1	Tr	0.3
803	Eggplant, cooked, steamed--------	1 cup-----------	96	92	25	1	Tr	Tr	Tr	0.1
804	Endive, curly (including esca-role), raw, small pieces-------	1 cup-----------	50	94	10	1	Tr	Tr	Tr	Tr
805	Jerusalem-artichoke, raw, sliced	1 cup-----------	150	78	115	3	Tr	0.0	Tr	Tr
	Kale, cooked, drained:									
806	From raw, chopped-------------	1 cup-----------	130	91	40	2	1	0.1	Tr	0.3
807	From frozen, chopped----------	1 cup-----------	130	91	40	4	1	0.1	Tr	0.3
808	Kohlrabi, thickened bulb-like stems, cooked, drained, diced--	1 cup-----------	165	90	50	3	Tr	Tr	Tr	0.1
	Lettuce, raw:									
	Butterhead, as Boston types:									
809	Head, 5-in diam-------------	1 head----------	163	96	20	2	Tr	Tr	Tr	0.2
810	Leaves----------------------	1 outer or 2 inner leaves--	15	96	Tr	Tr	Tr	Tr	Tr	Tr
	Crisphead, as iceberg:									
811	Head, 6-in diam-------------	1 head----------	539	96	70	5	1	0.1	Tr	0.5
812	Wedge, 1/4 of head----------	1 wedge---------	135	96	20	1	Tr	Tr	Tr	0.1
813	Pieces, chopped or shredded--	1 cup-----------	55	96	5	1	Tr	Tr	Tr	0.1
814	Looseleaf (bunching varieties including romaine or cos), chopped or shredded pieces---	1 cup-----------	56	94	10	1	Tr	Tr	Tr	0.1

[62] For regular pack; special dietary pack contains 61 mg sodium.
[63] For yellow varieties; white varieties contain only a trace of vitamin A.

							Vitamin A value						
Cho-les-terol	Carbo-hydrate	Calcium	Phos-phorus	Iron	Potas-sium	Sodium	(IU)	(RE)	Thiamin	Ribo-flavin	Niacin	Ascorbic acid	Item No.
Milli-grams	Grams	Milli-grams	Milli-grams	Milli-grams	Milli-grams	Milli-grams	Inter-national units	Retinol equiva-lents	Milli-grams	Milli-grams	Milli-grams	Milli-grams	

Nutrients in Indicated Quantity

Cho-les-terol	Carbo-hydrate	Calcium	Phos-phorus	Iron	Potas-sium	Sodium	(IU)	(RE)	Thiamin	Ribo-flavin	Niacin	Ascorbic acid	Item No.
0	7	19	32	0.4	233	25	20,250	2,025	0.07	0.04	0.7	7	784
0	11	30	48	0.6	355	39	30,940	3,094	0.11	0.06	1.0	10	785
0	16	48	47	1.0	354	103	38,300	3,830	0.05	0.09	0.8	4	786
0	12	41	38	0.7	231	86	25,850	2,585	0.04	0.05	0.6	4	787
0	8	37	35	0.9	261	[62]352	20,110	2,011	0.03	0.04	0.8	4	788
0	5	29	46	0.6	355	15	20	2	0.08	0.06	0.6	72	789
0	6	34	44	0.5	404	8	20	2	0.08	0.07	0.7	69	790
0	7	31	43	0.7	250	32	40	4	0.07	0.10	0.6	56	791
0	1	14	10	0.2	114	35	50	5	0.01	0.01	0.1	3	792
0	4	43	31	0.6	341	106	150	15	0.04	0.04	0.4	8	793
0	5	148	19	0.8	177	36	4,220	422	0.03	0.08	0.4	19	794
0	12	357	46	1.9	427	85	10,170	1,017	0.08	0.20	1.1	45	795
0	19	2	79	0.5	192	13	[63]170	[63]17	0.17	0.06	1.2	5	796
0	14	2	47	0.4	158	3	[63]130	[63]13	0.11	0.04	1.0	3	797
0	34	3	78	0.5	229	8	[63]410	[63]41	0.11	0.12	2.1	4	798
0	46	8	131	1.0	343	[64]730	[63]250	[63]25	0.06	0.14	2.5	12	799
0	41	11	134	0.9	391	[65]571	[63]510	[63]51	0.09	0.15	2.5	17	800
0	1	4	5	0.1	42	1	10	1	0.01	0.01	0.1	1	801
0	7	147	44	1.9	244	46	12,290	1,229	0.14	0.18	0.5	19	802
0	6	6	21	0.3	238	3	60	6	0.07	0.02	0.6	1	803
0	2	26	14	0.4	157	11	1,030	103	0.04	0.04	0.2	3	804
0	26	21	117	5.1	644	6	30	3	0.30	0.09	2.0	6	805
0	7	94	36	1.2	296	30	9,620	962	0.07	0.09	0.7	53	806
0	7	179	36	1.2	417	20	8,260	826	0.06	0.15	0.9	33	807
0	11	41	74	0.7	561	35	60	6	0.07	0.03	0.6	89	808
0	4	52	38	0.5	419	8	1,580	158	0.10	0.10	0.5	13	809
0	Tr	5	3	Tr	39	1	150	15	0.01	0.01	Tr	1	810
0	11	102	108	2.7	852	49	1,780	178	0.25	0.16	1.0	21	811
0	3	26	27	0.7	213	12	450	45	0.06	0.04	0.3	5	812
0	1	10	11	0.3	87	5	180	18	0.03	0.02	0.1	2	813
0	2	38	14	0.8	148	5	1,060	106	0.03	0.04	0.2	10	814

[64] For regular pack; special dietary pack contains 8 mg sodium.
[65] For regular pack; special dietary pack contains 6 mg sodium.

Item No.	Foods, approximate measures, units, and weight (weight of edible portion only)		Grams	Water Per-cent	Food energy Cal-ories	Pro-tein Grams	Fat Grams	Fatty acids Satu-rated Grams	Mono-unsatu-rated Grams	Poly-unsatu-rated Grams
	Vegetables and Vegetable Products—Con.									
	Mushrooms:									
815	Raw, sliced or chopped---------	1 cup-----------	70	92	20	1	Tr	Tr	Tr	0.1
816	Cooked, drained----------------	1 cup-----------	156	91	40	3	1	0.1	Tr	0.3
817	Canned, drained solids---------	1 cup-----------	156	91	35	3	Tr	0.1	Tr	0.2
818	Mustard greens, without stems and midribs, cooked, drained-------	1 cup-----------	140	94	20	3	Tr	Tr	0.2	0.1
819	Okra pods, 3 by 5/8 in, cooked---	8 pods----------	85	90	25	2	Tr	Tr	Tr	Tr
	Onions:									
	Raw:									
820	Chopped---------------------	1 cup-----------	160	91	55	2	Tr	0.1	0.1	0.2
821	Sliced----------------------	1 cup-----------	115	91	40	1	Tr	0.1	Tr	0.1
822	Cooked (whole or sliced), drained---------------------	1 cup-----------	210	92	60	2	Tr	0.1	Tr	0.1
823	Onions, spring, raw, bulb (3/8-in diam.) and white portion of top	6 onions--------	30	92	10	1	Tr	Tr	Tr	Tr
824	Onion rings, breaded, par-fried, frozen, prepared--------------	2 rings---------	20	29	80	1	5	1.7	2.2	1.0
	Parsley:									
825	Raw-------------------------	10 sprigs-------	10	88	5	Tr	Tr	Tr	Tr	Tr
826	Freeze-dried----------------	1 tbsp----------	0.4	2	Tr	Tr	Tr	Tr	Tr	Tr
827	Parsnips, cooked (diced or 2 in lengths), drained-------------	1 cup-----------	156	78	125	2	Tr	0.1	0.2	0.1
828	Peas, edible pod, cooked, drained	1 cup-----------	160	89	65	5	Tr	0.1	Tr	0.2
	Peas, green:									
829	Canned, drained solids---------	1 cup-----------	170	82	115	8	1	0.1	0.1	0.3
830	Frozen, cooked, drained--------	1 cup-----------	160	80	125	8	Tr	0.1	Tr	0.2
	Peppers:									
831	Hot chili, raw-----------------	1 pepper--------	45	88	20	1	Tr	Tr	Tr	Tr
	Sweet (about 5 per lb, whole), stem and seeds removed:									
832	Raw-------------------------	1 pepper--------	74	93	20	1	Tr	Tr	Tr	0.2
833	Cooked, drained-------------	1 pepper--------	73	95	15	Tr	Tr	Tr	Tr	0.1
	Potatoes, cooked:									
	Baked (about 2 per lb, raw):									
834	With skin-------------------	1 potato--------	202	71	220	5	Tr	0.1	Tr	0.1
835	Flesh only------------------	1 potato--------	156	75	145	3	Tr	Tr	Tr	0.1
	Boiled (about 3 per lb, raw):									
836	Peeled after boiling--------	1 potato--------	136	77	120	3	Tr	Tr	Tr	0.1
837	Peeled before boiling-------	1 potato--------	135	77	115	2	Tr	Tr	Tr	0.1
	French fried, strip, 2 to 3-1/2 in long, frozen:									
838	Oven heated----------------	10 strips-------	50	53	110	2	4	2.1	1.8	0.3
839	Fried in vegetable oil------	10 strips-------	50	38	160	2	8	2.5	1.6	3.8
	Potato products, prepared:									
	Au gratin:									
840	From dry mix---------------	1 cup-----------	245	79	230	6	10	6.3	2.9	0.3
841	From home recipe-----------	1 cup-----------	245	74	325	12	19	11.6	5.3	0.7
842	Hashed brown, from frozen------	1 cup-----------	156	56	340	5	18	7.0	8.0	2.1
	Mashed:									
	From home recipe:									
843	Milk added-----------------	1 cup-----------	210	78	160	4	1	0.7	0.3	0.1
844	Milk and margarine added---	1 cup-----------	210	76	225	4	9	2.2	3.7	2.5
845	From dehydrated flakes (without milk), water, milk, butter, and salt added---------------------	1 cup-----------	210	76	235	4	12	7.2	3.3	0.5
846	Potato salad, made with mayonnaise-------------------	1 cup-----------	250	76	360	7	21	3.6	6.2	9.3
	Scalloped:									
847	From dry mix---------------	1 cup-----------	245	79	230	5	11	6.5	3.0	0.5
848	From home recipe-----------	1 cup-----------	245	81	210	7	9	5.5	2.5	0.4

[66] For regular pack; special dietary pack contains 3 mg sodium.
[67] For red peppers; green peppers contain 350 IU or 35 RE.
[68] For green peppers; red peppers contain 4,220 IU or 422 RE.

Nutrients in Indicated Quantity

Cholesterol	Carbohydrate	Calcium	Phosphorus	Iron	Potassium	Sodium	Vitamin A value (IU)	Vitamin A value (RE)	Thiamin	Riboflavin	Niacin	Ascorbic acid	Item No.
Milligrams	Grams	Milligrams	Milligrams	Milligrams	Milligrams	Milligrams	International units	Retinol equivalents	Milligrams	Milligrams	Milligrams	Milligrams	
0	3	4	73	0.9	259	3	0	0	0.07	0.31	2.9	2	815
0	8	9	136	2.7	555	3	0	0	0.11	0.47	7.0	6	816
0	8	17	103	1.2	201	663	0	0	0.13	0.03	2.5	0	817
0	3	104	57	1.0	283	22	4,240	424	0.06	0.09	0.6	35	818
0	6	54	48	0.4	274	4	490	49	0.11	0.05	0.7	14	819
0	12	40	46	0.6	248	3	0	0	0.10	0.02	0.2	13	820
0	8	29	33	0.4	178	2	0	0	0.07	0.01	0.1	10	821
0	13	57	48	0.4	319	17	0	0	0.09	0.02	0.2	12	822
0	2	18	10	0.6	77	1	1,500	150	0.02	0.04	0.1	14	823
0	8	6	16	0.3	26	75	50	5	0.06	0.03	0.7	Tr	824
0	1	13	4	0.6	54	4	520	52	0.01	0.01	0.1	9	825
0	Tr	1	2	0.2	25	2	250	25	Tr	0.01	Tr	1	826
0	30	58	108	0.9	573	16	0	0	0.13	0.08	1.1	20	827
0	11	67	88	3.2	384	6	210	21	0.20	0.12	0.9	77	828
0	21	34	114	1.6	294	[66]372	1,310	131	0.21	0.13	1.2	16	829
0	23	38	144	2.5	269	139	1,070	107	0.45	0.16	2.4	16	830
0	4	8	21	0.5	153	3	[67]4,840	[67]484	0.04	0.04	0.4	109	831
0	4	4	16	0.9	144	2	[68]390	[68]39	0.06	0.04	0.4	[69]95	832
0	3	3	11	0.6	94	1	[70]280	[70]28	0.04	0.03	0.3	[71]81	833
0	51	20	115	2.7	844	16	0	0	0.22	0.07	3.3	26	834
0	34	8	78	0.5	610	8	0	0	0.16	0.03	2.2	20	835
0	27	7	60	0.4	515	5	0	0	0.14	0.03	2.0	18	836
0	27	11	54	0.4	443	7	0	0	0.13	0.03	1.8	10	837
0	17	5	43	0.7	229	16	0	0	0.06	0.02	1.2	5	838
0	20	10	47	0.4	366	108	0	0	0.09	0.01	1.6	5	839
12	31	203	233	0.8	537	1,076	520	76	0.05	0.20	2.3	8	840
56	28	292	277	1.6	970	1,061	650	93	0.16	0.28	2.4	24	841
0	44	23	112	2.4	680	53	0	0	0.17	0.03	3.8	10	842
4	37	55	101	0.6	628	636	40	12	0.18	0.08	2.3	14	843
4	35	55	97	0.5	607	620	360	42	0.18	0.08	2.3	13	844
29	32	103	118	0.5	489	697	380	44	0.23	0.11	1.4	20	845
170	28	48	130	1.6	635	1,323	520	83	0.19	0.15	2.2	25	846
27	31	88	137	0.9	497	835	360	51	0.05	0.14	2.5	8	847
29	26	140	154	1.4	926	821	330	47	0.17	0.23	2.6	26	848

[69] For green peppers; red peppers contain 141 mg ascorbic acid.
[70] For green peppers; red peppers contain 2,740 IU or 274 RE.
[71] For green peppers; red peppers contain 121 mg ascorbic acid.

Item No.	Foods, approximate measures, units, and weight (weight of edible portion only)			Water	Food energy	Pro-tein	Fat	Fatty acids Satu-rated	Mono-unsatu-rated	Poly-unsatu-rated
	Vegetables and Vegetable Products—Con.		Grams	Per-cent	Cal-ories	Grams	Grams	Grams	Grams	Grams
849	Potato chips	10 chips	20	3	105	1	7	1.8	1.2	3.6
	Pumpkin:									
850	Cooked from raw, mashed	1 cup	245	94	50	2	Tr	0.1	Tr	Tr
851	Canned	1 cup	245	90	85	3	1	0.4	0.1	Tr
852	Radishes, raw, stem ends, rootlets cut off	4 radishes	18	95	5	Tr	Tr	Tr	Tr	Tr
853	Sauerkraut, canned, solids and liquid	1 cup	236	93	45	2	Tr	0.1	Tr	0.1
	Seaweed:									
854	Kelp, raw	1 oz	28	82	10	Tr	Tr	0.1	Tr	Tr
855	Spirulina, dried	1 oz	28	5	80	16	2	0.8	0.2	0.6
	Southern peas. See Black-eyed peas, immature (items 769,770), mature (item 536).									
	Spinach:									
856	Raw, chopped	1 cup	55	92	10	2	Tr	Tr	Tr	0.1
	Cooked, drained:									
857	From raw	1 cup	180	91	40	5	Tr	0.1	Tr	0.2
858	From frozen (leaf)	1 cup	190	90	55	6	Tr	0.1	Tr	0.2
859	Canned, drained solids	1 cup	214	92	50	6	1	0.2	Tr	0.4
860	Spinach souffle	1 cup	136	74	220	11	18	7.1	6.8	3.1
	Squash, cooked:									
861	Summer (all varieties), sliced, drained	1 cup	180	94	35	2	1	0.1	Tr	0.2
862	Winter (all varieties), baked, cubes	1 cup	205	89	80	2	1	0.3	0.1	0.5
	Sunchoke. See Jerusalem-arti-choke (item 805).									
	Sweetpotatoes: Cooked (raw, 5 by 2 in; about 2-1/2 per lb):									
863	Baked in skin, peeled	1 potato	114	73	115	2	Tr	Tr	Tr	0.1
864	Boiled, without skin	1 potato	151	73	160	2	Tr	0.1	Tr	0.2
865	Candied, 2-1/2 by 2-in piece	1 piece	105	67	145	1	3	1.4	0.7	0.2
	Canned:									
866	Solid pack (mashed)	1 cup	255	74	260	5	1	0.1	Tr	0.2
867	Vacuum pack, piece 2-3/4 by 1 in	1 piece	40	76	35	1	Tr	Tr	Tr	Tr
	Tomatoes:									
868	Raw, 2-3/5-in diam. (3 per 12 oz pkg.)	1 tomato	123	94	25	1	Tr	Tr	Tr	0.1
869	Canned, solids and liquid	1 cup	240	94	50	2	1	0.1	0.1	0.2
870	Tomato juice, canned	1 cup	244	94	40	2	Tr	Tr	Tr	0.1
	Tomato products, canned:									
871	Paste	1 cup	262	74	220	10	2	0.3	0.4	0.9
872	Puree	1 cup	250	87	105	4	Tr	Tr	Tr	0.1
873	Sauce	1 cup	245	89	75	3	Tr	0.1	0.1	0.2
874	Turnips, cooked, diced	1 cup	156	94	30	1	Tr	Tr	Tr	0.1
	Turnip greens, cooked, drained:									
875	From raw (leaves and stems)	1 cup	144	93	30	2	Tr	0.1	Tr	0.1
876	From frozen (chopped)	1 cup	164	90	50	5	1	0.2	Tr	0.3
877	Vegetable juice cocktail, canned	1 cup	242	94	45	2	Tr	Tr	Tr	0.1
	Vegetables, mixed:									
878	Canned, drained solids	1 cup	163	87	75	4	Tr	0.1	Tr	0.2
879	Frozen, cooked, drained	1 cup	182	83	105	5	Tr	0.1	Tr	0.1
880	Waterchestnuts, canned	1 cup	140	86	70	1	Tr	Tr	Tr	Tr

[1] Value not determined.
[72] With added salt; if none is added, sodium content is 58 mg.
[73] For regular pack; special dietary pack contains 31 mg sodium.
[74] With added salt; if none is added, sodium content is 24 mg.

Nutrients in Indicated Quantity

Cho-les-terol	Carbo-hydrate	Calcium	Phos-phorus	Iron	Potas-sium	Sodium	Vitamin A value (IU)	Vitamin A value (RE)	Thiamin	Ribo-flavin	Niacin	Ascorbic acid	Item No.
Milli-grams	Grams	Milli-grams	Milli-grams	Milli-grams	Milli-grams	Milli-grams	Inter-national units	Retinol equiva-lents	Milli-grams	Milli-grams	Milli-grams	Milli-grams	
0	10	5	31	0.2	260	94	0	0	0.03	Tr	0.8	8	849
0	12	37	74	1.4	564	2	2,650	265	0.08	0.19	1.0	12	850
0	20	64	86	3.4	505	12	54,040	5,404	0.06	0.13	0.9	10	851
0	1	4	3	0.1	42	4	Tr	Tr	Tr	0.01	0.1	4	852
0	10	71	47	3.5	401	1,560	40	4	0.05	0.05	0.3	35	853
0	3	48	12	0.8	25	66	30	3	0.01	0.04	0.1	(1)	854
0	7	34	33	8.1	386	297	160	16	0.67	1.04	3.6	3	855
0	2	54	27	1.5	307	43	3,690	369	0.04	0.10	0.4	15	856
0	7	245	101	6.4	839	126	14,740	1,474	0.17	0.42	0.9	18	857
0	10	277	91	2.9	566	163	14,790	1,479	0.11	0.32	0.8	23	858
0	7	272	94	4.9	740	[72] 683	18,780	1,878	0.03	0.30	0.8	31	859
184	3	230	231	1.3	201	763	3,460	675	0.09	0.30	0.5	3	860
0	8	49	70	0.6	346	2	520	52	0.08	0.07	0.9	10	861
0	18	29	41	0.7	896	2	7,290	729	0.17	0.05	1.4	20	862
0	28	32	63	0.5	397	11	24,880	2,488	0.08	0.14	0.7	28	863
0	37	32	41	0.8	278	20	25,750	2,575	0.08	0.21	1.0	26	864
8	29	27	27	1.2	198	74	4,400	440	0.02	0.04	0.4	7	865
0	59	77	133	3.4	536	191	38,570	3,857	0.07	0.23	2.4	13	866
0	8	9	20	0.4	125	21	3,190	319	0.01	0.02	0.3	11	867
0	5	9	28	0.6	255	10	1,390	139	0.07	0.06	0.7	22	868
0	10	62	46	1.5	530	[73] 391	1,450	145	0.11	0.07	1.8	36	869
0	10	22	46	1.4	537	[74] 881	1,360	136	0.11	0.08	1.6	45	870
0	49	92	207	7.8	2,442	[75] 170	6,470	647	0.41	0.50	8.4	111	871
0	25	38	100	2.3	1,050	[76] 50	3,400	340	0.18	0.14	4.3	88	872
0	18	34	78	1.9	909	[77] 1,482	2,400	240	0.16	0.14	2.8	32	873
0	8	34	30	0.3	211	78	0	0	0.04	0.04	0.5	18	874
0	6	197	42	1.2	292	42	7,920	792	0.06	0.10	0.6	39	875
0	8	249	56	3.2	367	25	13,080	1,308	0.09	0.12	0.8	36	876
0	11	27	41	1.0	467	883	2,830	283	0.10	0.07	1.8	67	877
0	15	44	68	1.7	474	243	18,990	1,899	0.08	0.08	0.9	8	878
0	24	46	93	1.5	308	64	7,780	778	0.13	0.22	1.5	6	879
0	17	6	27	1.2	165	11	10	1	0.02	0.03	0.5	2	880

[75] With no added salt; if salt is added, sodium content is 2,070 mg.
[76] With no added salt; if salt is added, sodium content is 998 mg.
[77] With salt added.

Item No.	Foods, approximate measures, units, and weight (weight of edible portion only)		Water	Food energy	Pro-tein	Fat	Fatty acids		
							Satu-rated	Mono-unsatu-rated	Poly-unsatu-rated
	Miscellaneous Items	Grams	Per-cent	Cal-ories	Grams	Grams	Grams	Grams	Grams
	Baking powders for home use:								
	Sodium aluminum sulfate:								
881	With monocalcium phosphate monohydrate	1 tsp	3	2	5	Tr	0	0.0	0.0	0.0
882	With monocalcium phosphate monohydrate, calcium sulfate	1 tsp	2.9	1	5	Tr	0	0.0	0.0	0.0
883	Straight phosphate	1 tsp	3.8	2	5	Tr	0	0.0	0.0	0.0
884	Low sodium	1 tsp	4.3	1	5	Tr	0	0.0	0.0	0.0
885	Catsup	1 cup	273	69	290	5	1	0.2	0.2	0.4
886		1 tbsp	15	69	15	Tr	Tr	Tr	Tr	Tr
887	Celery seed	1 tsp	2	6	10	Tr	1	Tr	0.3	0.1
888	Chili powder	1 tsp	2.6	8	10	Tr	Tr	0.1	0.1	0.2
	Chocolate:								
889	Bitter or baking	1 oz	28	2	145	3	15	9.0	4.9	0.5
	Semisweet, see Candy, (item 715).								
890	Cinnamon	1 tsp	2.3	10	5	Tr	Tr	Tr	Tr	Tr
891	Curry powder	1 tsp	2	10	5	Tr	Tr	(1)	(1)	(1)
892	Garlic powder	1 tsp	2.8	6	10	Tr	Tr	Tr	Tr	Tr
893	Gelatin, dry	1 envelope	7	13	25	6	Tr	Tr	Tr	Tr
894	Mustard, prepared, yellow	1 tsp or individual packet	5	80	5	Tr	Tr	Tr	0.2	Tr
	Olives, canned:								
895	Green	4 medium or 3 extra large	13	78	15	Tr	2	0.2	1.2	0.1
896	Ripe, Mission, pitted	3 small or 2 large	9	73	15	Tr	2	0.3	1.3	0.2
897	Onion powder	1 tsp	2.1	5	5	Tr	Tr	Tr	Tr	Tr
898	Oregano	1 tsp	1.5	7	5	Tr	Tr	Tr	Tr	0.1
899	Paprika	1 tsp	2.1	10	5	Tr	Tr	Tr	Tr	0.2
900	Pepper, black	1 tsp	2.1	11	5	Tr	Tr	Tr	Tr	Tr
	Pickles, cucumber:								
901	Dill, medium, whole, 3-3/4 in long, 1-1/4-in diam.	1 pickle	65	93	5	Tr	Tr	Tr	Tr	0.1
902	Fresh-pack, slices 1-1/2-in diam., 1/4 in thick	2 slices	15	79	10	Tr	Tr	Tr	Tr	Tr
903	Sweet, gherkin, small, whole, about 2-1/2 in long, 3/4-in diam.	1 pickle	15	61	20	Tr	Tr	Tr	Tr	Tr
	Popcorn. See Grain Products, (items 497-499).								
904	Relish, finely chopped, sweet	1 tbsp	15	63	20	Tr	Tr	Tr	Tr	Tr
905	Salt	1 tsp	5.5	0	0	0	0	0.0	0.0	0.0
906	Vinegar, cider	1 tbsp	15	94	Tr	Tr	0	0.0	0.0	0.0
	Yeast:								
907	Baker's, dry, active	1 pkg	7	5	20	3	Tr	Tr	0.1	Tr
908	Brewer's, dry	1 tbsp	8	5	25	3	Tr	Tr	Tr	0.0

[1] Value not determined.

Nutrients in Indicated Quantity

Cho-les-terol	Carbo-hydrate	Calcium	Phos-phorus	Iron	Potas-sium	Sodium	Vitamin A value (IU)	(RE)	Thiamin	Ribo-flavin	Niacin	Ascorbic acid	Item No.
Milli-grams	Grams	Milli-grams	Milli-grams	Milli-grams	Milli-grams	Milli-grams	Inter-national units	Retinol equiva-lents	Milli-grams	Milli-grams	Milli-grams	Milli-grams	
0	1	58	87	0.0	5	329	0	0	0.00	0.00	0.0	0	881
0	1	183	45	0.0	4	290	0	0	0.00	0.00	0.0	0	882
0	1	239	359	0.0	6	312	0	0	0.00	0.00	0.0	0	883
0	1	207	314	0.0	891	Tr	0	0	0.00	0.00	0.0	0	884
0	69	60	137	2.2	991	2,845	3,820	382	0.25	0.19	4.4	41	885
0	4	3	8	0.1	54	156	210	21	0.01	0.01	0.2	2	886
0	1	35	11	0.9	28	3	Tr	Tr	0.01	0.01	0.1	Tr	887
0	1	7	8	0.4	50	26	910	91	0.01	0.02	0.2	2	888
0	8	22	109	1.9	235	1	10	1	0.01	0.07	0.4	0	889
0	2	28	1	0.9	12	1	10	1	Tr	Tr	Tr	1	890
0	1	10	7	0.6	31	1	20	2	0.01	0.01	0.1	Tr	891
0	2	2	12	0.1	31	1	0	0	0.01	Tr	Tr	Tr	892
0	0	1	0	0.0	2	6	0	0	0.00	0.00	0.0	0	893
0	Tr	4	4	0.1	7	63	0	0	Tr	0.01	Tr	Tr	894
0	Tr	8	2	0.2	7	312	40	4	Tr	Tr	Tr	0	895
0	Tr	10	2	0.2	2	68	10	1	Tr	Tr	Tr	0	896
0	2	8	7	0.1	20	1	Tr	Tr	0.01	Tr	Tr	Tr	897
0	1	24	3	0.7	25	Tr	100	10	0.01	Tr	0.1	1	898
0	1	4	7	0.5	49	1	1,270	127	0.01	0.04	0.3	1	899
0	1	9	4	0.6	26	1	Tr	Tr	Tr	0.01	Tr	0	900
0	1	17	14	0.7	130	928	70	7	Tr	0.01	Tr	4	901
0	3	5	4	0.3	30	101	20	2	Tr	Tr	Tr	1	902
0	5	2	2	0.2	30	107	10	1	Tr	Tr	Tr	1	903
0	5	3	2	0.1	30	107	20	2	Tr	Tr	0.0	1	904
0	0	14	3	Tr	Tr	2,132	0	0	0.00	0.00	0.0	0	905
0	1	1	1	0.1	15	Tr	0	0	0.00	0.00	0.0	0	906
0	3	3	90	1.1	140	4	Tr	Tr	0.16	0.38	2.6	Tr	907
0	3	[78]17	140	1.4	152	10	Tr	Tr	1.25	0.34	3.0	Tr	908

[78] Value may vary from 6 to 60 mg.

Index